PROGRESS IN BRAIN RESEARCH

VOLUME 26

DEVELOPMENTAL NEUROLOGY

PROGRESS IN BRAIN RESEARCH

PROGRESS IN BRAIN RESEARCH

VOLUME 26

DEVELOPMENTAL NEUROLOGY

EDITED BY

C. G. BERNHARD

Department of Physiology, Nobel Institute, Stockholm (Sweden)

AND

J. P. SCHADÉ

Central Institute for Brain Research, Amsterdam (The Netherlands)

ELSEVIER PUBLISHING COMPANY

AMSTERDAM / LONDON / NEW YORK

1967

ELSEVIER PUBLISHING COMPANY
335 JAN VAN GALENSTRAAT, P.O. BOX 211, AMSTERDAM

AMERICAN ELSEVIER PUBLISHING COMPANY, INC.
52 VANDERBILT AVENUE, NEW YORK, N.Y. 10017

ELSEVIER PUBLISHING COMPANY LIMITED
RIPPLESIDE COMMERCIAL ESTATE, BARKING, ESSEX

LIBRARY OF CONGRESS CATALOG CARD NUMBER 67-12771

WITH 135 ILLUSTRATIONS

PRINTED IN THE NETHERLANDS

List of Contributors

K.-E. ÅSTRÖM, Department of Pathology, Sabbatsbergs Sjukhys, Stockholm (Sweden).

C. G. BERNHARD, Department of Physiology, Karolinska Institutet, Stockholm (Sweden).

A. P. C. BOT, Netherlands Central Institute for Brain Research, Amsterdam (The Netherlands).

M. A. CORNER, Netherlands Central Institute for Brain Research, Amsterdam (The Netherlands).

G. M. KOLMODIN, Department of Physiology, Karolinska Institutet, Stockholm (Sweden).

K. MELLER, Max-Planck-Institut für Hirnforschung, Abteilung für Allgemeine Neurologie, Köln-Merheim (Germany).

B. A. MEYERSON, Department of Physiology, Karolinska Institutet, Stockholm (Sweden).

M. E. MOLLIVER, The Johns Hopkins University, Baltimore, Md. (U.S.A.)

J. P. SCHADÉ, Netherlands Central Institute for Brain Research, Amsterdam, (The Netherlands).

J. SEDLÁČEK, Netherlands Central Institute for Brain Research, Amsterdam (The Netherlands).

R. STOECKART, Netherlands Central Institute for Brain Research, Amsterdam (The Netherlands).

H. H. VAN DER HELM, Netherlands Central Institute for Brain Research, Amsterdam (The Netherlands).

J. VOS, Netherlands Central Institute for Brain Research, Amsterdam (The Netherlands).

W. WECHSLER, Max-Planck-Institut für Hirnforschung, Abteilung für Allgemeine Neurologie, Köln-Merheim (Germany).

Other volumes in this series:

Volume 1: *Brain Mechanisms*
Specific and Unspecific Mechanisms of Sensory Motor Integration
Edited by G. Moruzzi, A. Fessard and H. H. Jasper

Volume 2: *Nerve, Brain and Memory Models*
Edited by Norbert Wiener† and J. P. Schadé

Volume 3: *The Rhinencephalon and Related Structures*
Edited by W. Bargmann and J. P. Schadé

Volume 4: *Growth and Maturation of the Brain*
Edited by D. P. Purpura and J. P. Schadé

Volume 5: *Lectures on the Diencephalon*
Edited by W. Bargmann and J. P. Schadé

Volume 6: *Topics in Basic Neurology*
Edited by W. Bargmann and J. P. Schadé

Volume 7: *Slow Electrical Processes in the Brain*
by N. A. Aladjalova

Volume 8: *Biogenic Amines*
Edited by Harold E. Himwich and Williamina A. Himwich

Volume 9: *The Developing Brain*
Edited by Williamina A. Himwich and Harold E. Himwich

Volume 10: *The Structure and Function of the Epiphysis Cerebri*
Edited by J. Ariëns Kappers and J. P. Schadé

Volume 11: *Organization of the Spinal Cord*
Edited by J. C. Eccles and J. P. Schadé

Volume 12: *Physiology of Spinal Neurons*
Edited by J. C. Eccles and J. P. Schadé

Volume 13: *Mechanisms of Neural Regeneration*
Edited by M. Singer and J. P. Schadé

Volume 14: *Degeneration Patterns in the Nervous System*
Edited by M. Singer and J. P. Schadé

Volume 15: *Biology of Neuroglia*
Edited by E. D. P. De Robertis and R. Carrea

Volume 16: *Horizons in Neuropsychopharmacology*
Edited by Williamina A. Himwich and J. P. Schadé

Volume 17: *Cybernetics of the Nervous System*
Edited by Norbert Wiener† and J. P. Schadé

Volume 18: *Sleep Mechanisms*
Edited by K. Akert, Ch. Bally and J. P. Schadé

Volume 19: *Experimental Epilepsy*
by A. Kreindler

Volume 20: *Pharmacology and Physiology of the Reticular Formation*
Edited by A. V. Valdman

Volume 21A: *Correlative Neurosciences. Part A: Fundamental Mechanisms*
Edited by T. Tokizane and J. P. Schadé

Volume 21B: *Correlative Neurosciences. Part B: Clinical Studies*
Edited by T. Tokizane and J. P. Schadé

Volume 22: *Brain Reflexes*
Edited by E. A. Asratyan

Volume 23: *Sensory Mechanisms*
Edited by Y. Zotterman

Volume 24: *Carbon Monoxide Poisoning*
Edited by H. Bour and I. McA. Ledingham

Volume 25: *The Cerebellum*
Edited by C. A. Fox and R. S. Snider

Volume 27: *Structure and Function of the Limbic System*
Edited by W. Ross Adey and T. Tokizane

Volume 28: *Anticholinergic Drugs*
Edited by P. B. Bradley and M. Fink

Volume 29: *Brain-Barrier System*
Edited by A. Lajtha and D. H. Ford

Volume 30: *Cerebral Circulation*
Edited by W. Luyendijk

Contents

On the Early Development of the Isocortex in Fetal Sheep

KARL-ERIK ÅSTRÖM

Departments of Pathology II and Physiology II, Karolinska Institutet, Stockholm (Sweden)

INTRODUCTION

This work, which has been carried out during the last 5 years, concerns early development in fetal lambs. Its original purpose was to provide anatomical data for the interpretation of physiological phenomena (Bernhard *et al.*, 1959, 1967; Meyerson, 1964; Eidelberg *et al.*, 1965; Kolmodin and Meyerson, 1966; Molliver, 1967). It is also hoped that this study may contribute to the understanding of cerebral morphogenesis in general, and to that of ungulates in particular. It was based mainly upon the Golgi method, and deals only with qualitative aspects of the minute neuroanatomy.

HISTORICAL SURVEY

The basic concepts of neurogenesis were developed during the latter half of the 19th century by Kölliker (1896), Cajal (1906, 1911, 1960), His (1904) and others. The early evolution of the forebrain is similar in all vertebrates. The isocortex develops from the dorsal, bulging part of the telencephalic vesicles, whereas the basal part will subsequently constitute the rhinencephalon, the allocortex and the striatum. The following is concerned only with the isocortex and the underlying parts of the telencephalic wall.

The basic structure of the telencephalic wall can be recognized when the three layers, the matrix, the mantle and the marginal, have been formed. The development of neuroblasts and spongioblasts in the innermost layer represents the primary differentiation of the neuroectodermal cells. The spongioblasts have been described, *inter alia*, by Cajal, who called them epithelial cells. Their cell bodies are situated in the matrix. The inner, thicker, and shorter processes extend to the internal limiting membrane. The outer, thinner processes are known as radiating fibers, owing to their orientation. Most of them proceed to the outer surface. These fibers are numerous in the early stages and dominate the picture in many Golgi sections (see *e.g.* Fig. 8). Cajal suggested that they serve as a temporary supporting framework in the brain vesicles until the nerve and glial elements have become sufficiently mature. Later, they atrophy, and disappear. Some spongioblasts remain close to the ventricle,

* Present Address: Department of Pathology, Sabbatsbergs Sjukhus, Stockholm, Va. (Sweden).

References p. 57–59

where they will form the ependyma and the subependymal glial zone; but the majority migrate outwards to become glial cells. Lorente de Nó has pointed out that the glial cells invade the outer zones later than do the neuroblasts; and he called their movement 'the second migration' (1933).

In the early phase, the mantle zone contains neuroblasts, and the marginal zone is more or less without cells. In the course of the ensuing outward migration, cells accumulate in the outer part of the mantle zone to form a primordial pyramidal layer, and proceed into the marginal zone. These two layers constitute the cortical plate of the prospective isocortex. All the neuroblasts will eventually reach this plate (holocortex according to M. Rose, 1926), and there will be no subcortical nuclei.

The cortical plate — especially the pyramidal layer — grows by addition of new cells. Migration of these cells occurs during a certain phase of embryological development, the length of which is not known for sheep. Angevine and Sidman (1961) have shown that cells, which were formed at the same time mostly occupy the same stratum in the pyramidal zone; and that newly formed cells migrate beyond those already present in the zone. Consequently, cells in the deeper strata of the pyramidal zone were formed earlier, and appeared in the layer before the more superficial cells.

A prospective 'white' matter zone is formed concomitantly with the cortical plate. Both descending axons from cortical cells, and ascending fibers from cells at lower levels of the neuraxis, penetrate into the mantle zone and form a heavy system of fibers, which contributes in separating the cortex from the matrix.

The morphological differentiation of nerve cells within the isocortical plate has been studied mainly along two lines.

The first line of investigation has been concerned with the aggregation of cells in concentric layers, which is such a striking feature of the adult mammalian cortex; it has been studied especially in material stained according to Nissl's method. Up to a certain embryological stage the pyramidal layer is made up of cells situated closely to one another, with small dark nuclei and containing little cytoplasm, as seen in the Nissl pictures. Therefore, the layer appears as a dark homogeneous band when seen under low magnification (see *e.g.* Fig. 2, La py). Stratification then occurs through the formation of lighter zones alternating with the dark regions, and eventually a 6-layered cortex can be recognized. Brodman (1909) attached considerable importance to this original type, which he called 'the tectogenetic fundamental type of 6 layers'. He claimed that the regional differences in cytoarchitectonics can be interpreted as modifications of the original elementary pattern. He also asserted that the fundamental type is similar in all mammals, and therefore that structural differences between homologous regions in mammals can be looked upon as species-determined modifications of the basic plan. Lorente de Nó (1933, 1938) has challenged the validity of these concepts.

The second line of investigation on cortical development deals with the detailed structure of nerve cells and their connections. It has been based mainly upon the Golgi method. Such studies were conducted by other research workers including Vignal (1888), Retzius (1891, 1893), Kölliker (1896) and especially by Cajal (1906, 1911, 1960) and Lorente de Nó (1933). Conel (1939–1959) has made a comprehensive study of the postnatal development of the cortex in man, and Rabinowicz (1964) has extended these investigations to cover the 8th month of the prenatal period. In recent years the Golgi method has been used especially for quantitative determinations and in connection with neurophysiological studies in embryos and young animals (Eayrs and Goodhead, 1959; Purpura *et al.*, 1960; Noback and Purpura, 1961; Purpura *et al.*, 1964; Marty, 1962; Marty and Scherrer, 1964; Scheibel, 1962; Scheibel and Scheibel, 1964; Kobayashi *et al.*, 1964; Schadé and Van Groenigen, 1961; Schadé *et al.*, 1964).

Cajal described the two main types of nerve cells in the marginal zone: polygonal or stellate cells, with short axons and elongated cells, with enormous processes, that proceed horizontally, *i.e.* parallel with the hemispherical surface. These types of cells can be recognized also in embryos and young animals (see Cajal, 1960; Retzius, 1891, 1893). The elongated cells, which are frequently called Cajal–Retzius cells, become atrophied: the adult forms lack ascending branches from the horizontal dendrites which are numerous during fetal life.

In the adult stage the cells and fibers in the marginal layer have a mainly horizontal orientation, whereas in the pyramidal zone these elements are largely directed towards the hemispherical surface. This pattern is also seen early in embryonic life; in fact, it seems to be present immediately after the two layers have been formed within the cortical plate. The primitive pyramidal cells have a bipolar shape. The apical, thicker process is directed towards the surface, where it either ends in a thickening or is branched. The other end of the cell body tapers and continues inward as a thin thread (the prospective axis cylinder).

The further differentiation of the primitive bipolar cells has been particularly well described by Cajal (see *e.g.*, 1906) who mainly examined brains from mice and rabbits. This differentiation comprises development of descending and basal dendrites, branching of basal and apical dendrites, outgrowth of axon collaterals, and formation of spines on the apical dendrites. The terminal branches of the apical dendrites are the first to appear. Then come descending and basal dendrites and side-branches on the apical shafts, beginning from below. At first, the axon collaterals appear proximally on the axons of the large pyramidal cells as tiny processes. Subsequently, they grow and divide; more collaterals appear further away from the cell body, and processes will be seen also on the axons of the smaller pyramidal cells. The appearance of spines on the apical shafts signifies the functional maturation of the neurons. The development of cells with short axons is less well known, since they are rarely stained in the fetal and newborn animals.

The differentiation of the pyramidal cells starts in the deeper part of the layer, especially in the large cells in the middle stratum.

The formation of neurofibrils and Nissl bodies within the cortical neurons has been described by several authors, including Cajal (see *e.g.*, 1911). Flexner (1951) and collaborators studied the development and growth of nuclei, nucleoli and Nissl bodies, as well as the biochemical differentiation in the fetal cortex, and correlated these parameters to functions.

The prenatal formation of cerebral gyri in sheep was described by Anthony and

References p. 57–59

Grzybowski (1937), and an account of the pattern of sulci in adult animals was given by Landacre (1930). J. Rose studied the cytoarchitectonic structure of the sheep cortex as seen mainly in sections stained according to the Nissl method (1942). Romanes (1947) has described the prenatal medullation of the sheep's nervous system.

NOMENCLATURE

The neopallial wall, *i.e.* the suprastriatal portion of the telencephalic vesicle, appears to be made up of zones, which are concentric during the lissencephalic stage (see *e.g.* Figs. 10 and 11).

(I) *The germinal layer* or *matrix* surrounds the lateral ventricle. Here, most cells will leave the zone and migrate outwards to become nerve and glial cells after maturation. However, the internal limiting membrane, the ependyma and the subependymal glial zone will remain.

(II) *The intermediate layer* or *zone* represents the prospective white matter of the cerebral hemispheres. It is transversed by migrating neuroblasts and spongioblasts and by the radiating fibers of the epithelial cells, the general orientation of which is seen in Fig. 11. An inner subzone will contain the callosal, and projection fibers in addition to the numerous migrating cells. The outer part is less rich in fibers and cells; it will become the convolutional white matter.

(III) *The cortical plate*, the prospective isocortex, consists of two layers.

(a) The cell-dense *pyramidal layer* or zone will become strata II–VI of the 6-layered isocortex.

(b) The *marginal layer* or zone, which will become the first stratum of the isocortex, is also called the plexiform or molecular layer, the lamina or stratum zonalis, the velum marginalis, etc.

The following nomenclature, the names being mostly descriptive of cortical nerve cells, has been adopted especially from Kölliker (1896), Cajal (1911) and Lorente de Nó (1938). In the marginal layer, there are fusiform, triangular and polygonal cells, and the elongated Cajal–Retzius cells; and in the remaining strata, pyramidal cells, star or stellate cells and spindle cells. According to the appearance of their axons there are: cells with short (Golgi II) and long axons; cells with ascending (Martinotti cells) and descending axons; cells with horizontal axons, long and short (in the marginal zone); cells with intracortical distribution only; and cells with axons of association and projection.

The descriptive terms outer–inner, superficial–deep, superior–inferior, outwards –inwards, will be used to refer to the position of structures within the wall of the telencephalon in relation to its surface. Horizontal usually means parallel with the hemispherical surface.

The definition of epithelial cells and radiating fibers was given in the introduction.

MATERIALS AND METHODS

All fetuses were used for neurophysiological studies (for technique see Bernhard *et al.*

TABLE I

Weight of specimen (g)	*Estimated fetal age in days*	*Histological method*
1.1	20–25	Cresyl violet
5.7	42	,,
6.5	43	,,
12	48	Golgi
14.5	49	,,
16	51	,,
19	52	,,
20	52	,,
25	53	,,
25	53	,,
27	54	,,
28	54	,,
29	54	,,
35	56	Palmgren
37	57	Golgi
39	57	Cresyl violet
42	58	Golgi
47	59	,,
49	59	,,
50	59	,,
50	59	,,
50	59	Cresyl violet
55	60	Golgi
56	60	,,
60	60	Cresyl violet
60	60	Palmgren
61	60	Golgi
66	60	,,
69	61	,,
75	61	,,
75	61	,,
92	62	,,
94	62	,,
95	63	Cresyl violet
128	65	Golgi
147	66	,,
175	70	,,
180	71	Cresyl violet
187	71	Golgi
265	79	,,
275	80	Cresyl violet
360	82	Golgi
450	89	Cresyl violet
468	90	Golgi

References p. 57–59

1959; Eidelberg *et al.*, 1965a,b). They were in good condition throughout the experiments; and the histological material was obtained immediately after the animals were killed. The smallest specimen (weight 1.1 g) was fixed *in toto*. From the remaining specimens the brain was removed and fixed either intact or in pieces.

Unless otherwise stated, the descriptions refer to the middle part of the convex aspect of the telencephalic vesicle, *i.e.* the part that eventually develops into the parietal area.

Cox's modification of Golgi's method was used in a few cases, but was found to be less satisfactory, since it does not show the axons and their collaterals very clearly. Consequently, the study was based upon the original, rapid Golgi method. (For technical details see *e.g.* Cajal, 1894, and Von Lenhossék, 1895.) The fixed and stained blocks were embedded in celloidin and serially sectioned at 100 μ. To clarify the fine details of individual cells in such sections, *e.g.* the course of an axon and its collaterals, it is usually necessary to study the thick sections under high magnification and by focusing up and down. Thus, individual elements may be followed over distances of several hundred microns. Microphotographs can never adequately illustrate the results of such studies and, therefore, drawings have to be made, despite the time that this technique requires. The disadvantages of a microphotograph, compared with a drawing, are evident from Figs. 20A and C. The technique of preparing the drawings was described in a previous publication (Åström, 1953).

Great care has been taken to accurately depict the relative size and length of the different components of a cell, as well as the situation of these components in relation to each other and to the surface of the brain and the borders of the pyramidal cell zone. However, the reciprocal position of the cells side-ways is not necessarily the same as that in the sections. Occasionally, the cells have seen 'spread out' somewhat in order to make the drawings clearer. Cells, as well as blood vessels, radiating fibers, glia cells etc., have been omitted for the same reason.

Sections from paraffin-embedded material were stained with cresyl violet, and according to Palmgren's method for axis cylinders.

Material was obtained from about 70 specimens, 44 of which were used in this study (see the Table). Exact gestational age is not known, since the ewes had been settled in the field. Hence fetal age was estimated, from the weight of the fetus, according to Barcroft's curves (1946).

RESULTS

1.1-g fetus

The study was based upon a series of horizontal sections, stained with cresyl violet. Figs. 1A and B illustrate two of these sections (not consecutive). The large lateral ventricles (Ve l) are enclosed posteriorly by the striatal (Str) and rhinencephalic structures (Lo py), and anteriorly and laterally by the thin evaginated walls of the telencephalic vesicles. The most primitive parts of the neopallium, which is in the process of further development, are within the limbic zones along the choroid fissure

(Fig. 1B); the telencephalic wall consists here mainly of a homogeneous cell-rich lamina, *i.e.* the matrix. Differentiation, as well as the thickness of the hemispherical wall, increases towards the anterior, superior and posterior edges and then further along the lateral convex wall. A primordial isocortex (Co is) is visible only within the most highly differentiated area, *i.e.* the middle part of the bulging convex wall of the hemispherical vesicles at the level of, and anterior to, the striate body. Consequently, this area contains all the elementary layers of the primitive neopallium. These layers are as follows (Figs. 1C and D).

(1) The matrix (Mx), the innermost layer, is densely populated. It forms a dark layer along the inner aspect of the telencephalic vesicles, and constitutes a third or more of the ventricle wall (Fig. 1C). The nuclei are mostly elongated, and have a radial orientation. The chromatin is finely stippled, and usually there is at least one nucleolus. A faintly stained, amorphous, basophilic cytoplasmic material is occasionally seen at one or both ends of the nucleus. The cells frequently form columns with 20 cells or more in a row. The inner apical processes insert on the internal limiting membrane. Close to this membrane, many germinal cells are in mitotic division.

(2) The mantle layer (Mn) is less densely populated and the nuclei are lighter (Fig. 1D). They are about as large as those in the matrix, and many of them also have the same oblong shape, whereas others are more spherical. Pale, thin bipolar processes are sometimes noted. A network of thin filaments can be seen between the cells. The cells lack the regular orientation of those in the matrix but, in general, the long axes of the cells in the inner part tend to be directed anteroposteriorly, whereas the cells in the outer part become oriented more perpendicularly to the surface. The inner region is more densely populated than the outer region and is well demarcated from the matrix.

(3) The pyramidal cell layer (La py), although thin, is densely populated, averaging 3–5 cells in depth (Fig. 1D). The name is inappropriate, since the perikarya have not, as yet, a pyramidal shape, but it is retained for convenience. Most of the nuclei are comparatively large, with finely stippled chromatin and one or more nucleoli; they appear to be better developed than those in the mantle zone. The nuclei usually have a pear-like shape, the enlarged end being directed outwards. Faintly stained clumps of cytoplasm at both ends of the nucleus give the cell a bipolar appearance. Presumably the thicker, outer processes represent apical dendrites which seem to extend into the marginal layer. The inner processes taper rapidly. The cells are less densely situated in the deeper part of the pyramidal layer where a fine, loose reticulum is seen between them. The zone also contains some smaller, darker and more spherically shaped nuclei.

(4) The marginal layer (La ma) contains sparse cells in a reticulum of fine filaments, which is loose in the outer, and somewhat denser in the inner, part (Fig. 1D). The cells are scattered throughout the layer, but are more numerous near the surface. The larger nuclei are frequently elongated, the long axes being parallel to the surface; they contain fine chromatin particles and mostly 1–2 nucleoli. These nuclei evidently belong to nerve cells, which are bipolar and emit dendrites parallel to the surface. The proximal parts of such processes are, in fact, occasionally visible even in these cresyl

References p. 57–59

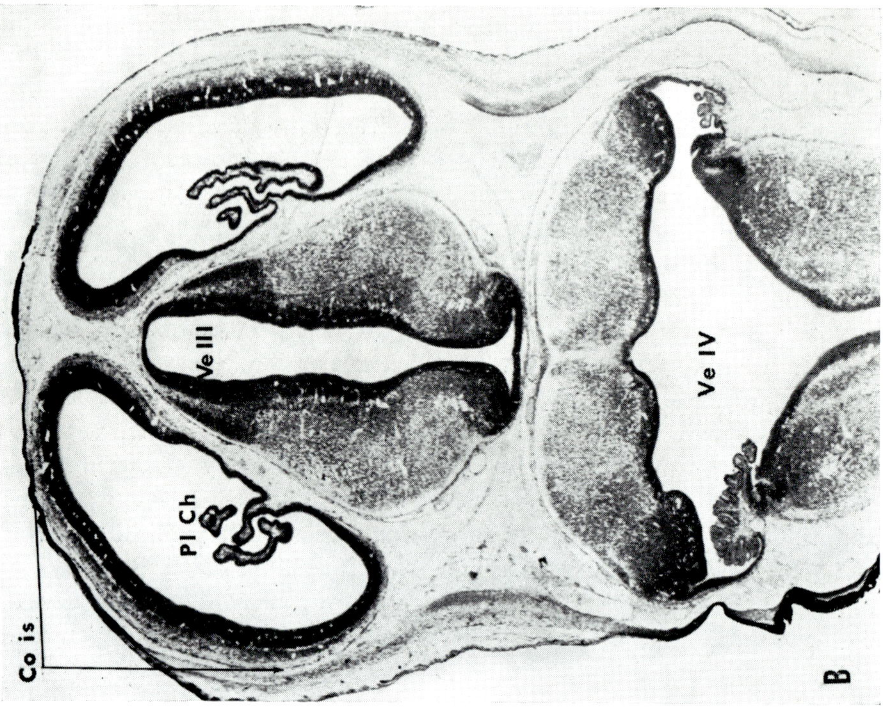
Co is
Pl Ch
Ve III
Ve IV
B

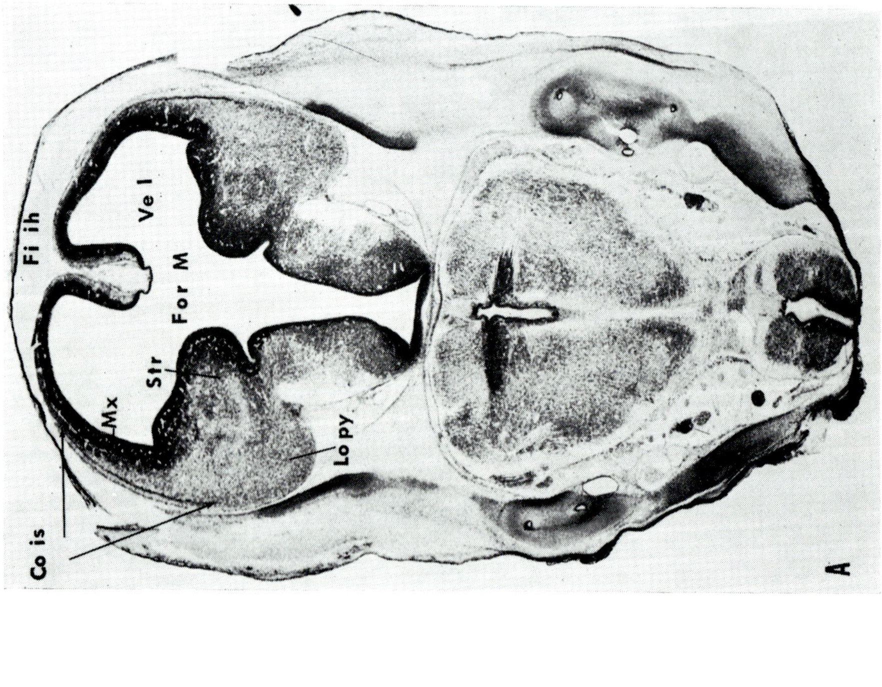
Co is
Mx
Str
For M
Ve I
Fi ih
Lo py
A

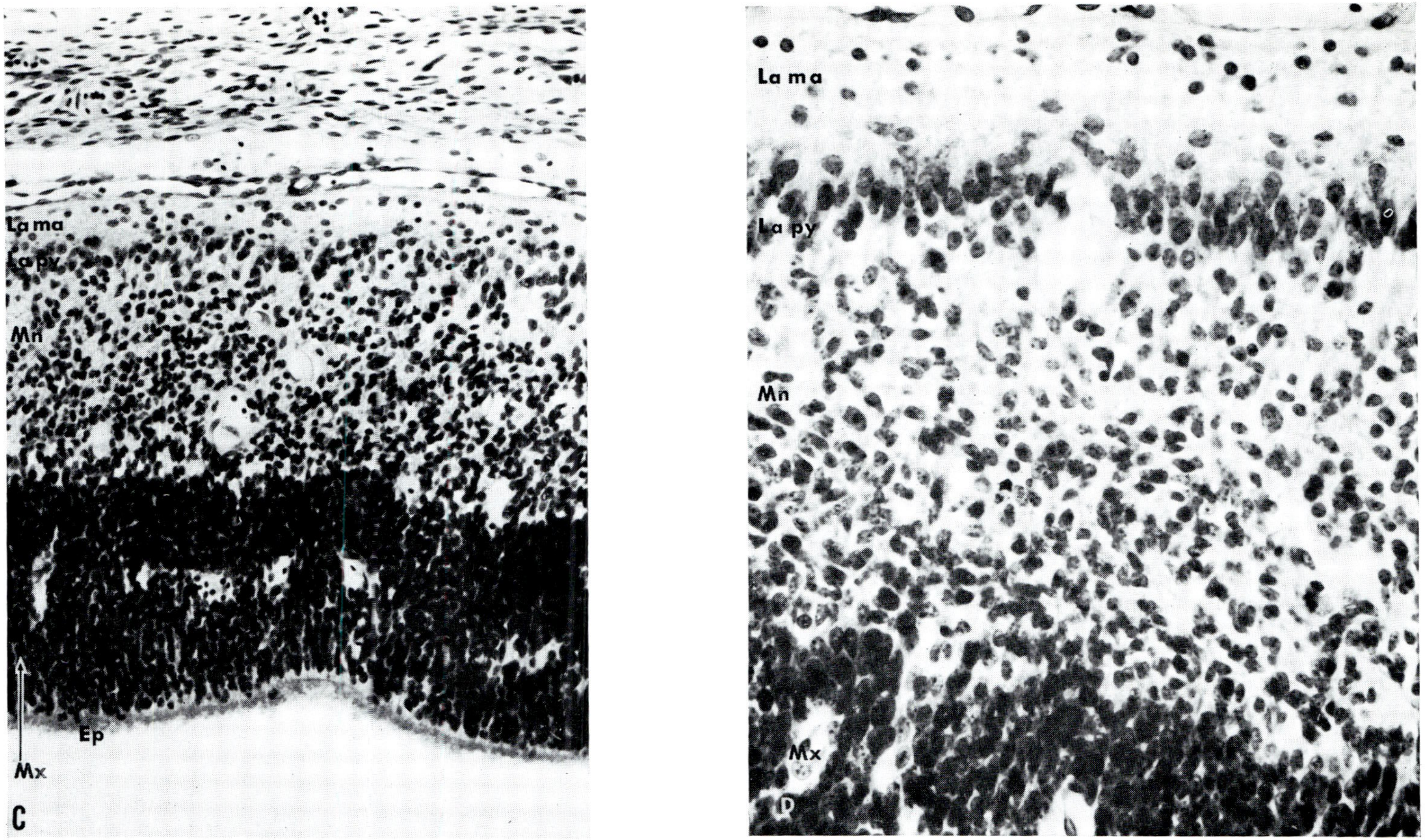

Fig. 1. 1.1-gram fetus, estimated age 20–25 days. Horizontal sections. Cresyl violet. (A and B) Upper part of figure, forebrain with telencephalic vesicles and diencephalon; lower part of figure, rhombencephalon with 4th ventricle, × 18 and 25. Co is = isocortical plate; Fi ih = interhemispherical fissure; For M = foramen Monroi; Lo py = pyriform lobe; Mx = matrix; Pl ch = choroid plexus, invaginated at choroid fissure; Str = striatum; Ve 1 = lateral ventricle; Ve III = third ventricle; Ve IV = 4th ventricle. (C) Telencephalic wall with incipient formation of isocortical plate (La ma + La py) and broad matrix (Mx). Hemispherical surface upwards and lateral ventricle downwards, × 240. Mn = mantle layer or zone; Ep = ependyma. (D) Telencephalic wall in higher magnification. Columns of germinal cells in matrix (Mx). Migrating neuroblasts in mantle zone (Mn). Differentiated cells in pyramidal (La py) and marginal (La ma) layers, × 500.

References p. 57–59

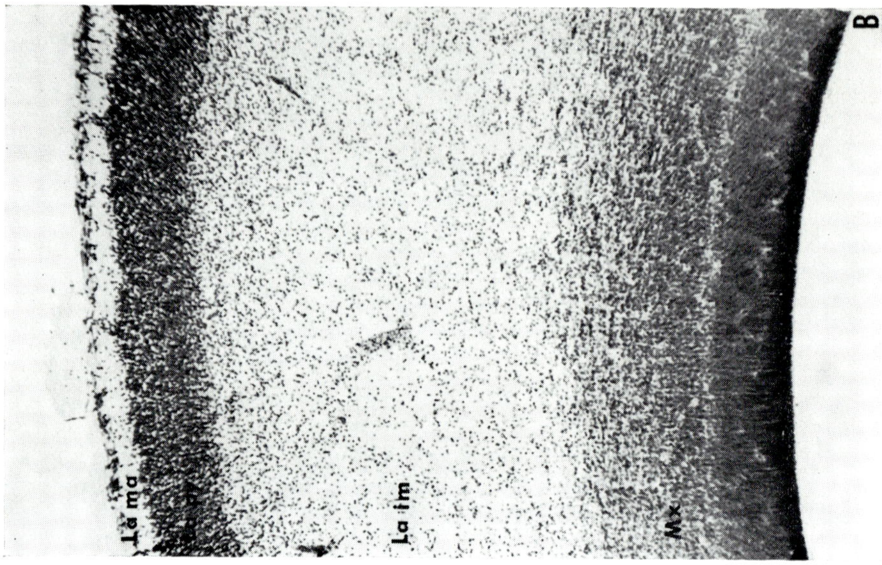
La ma
La im
Mx
B

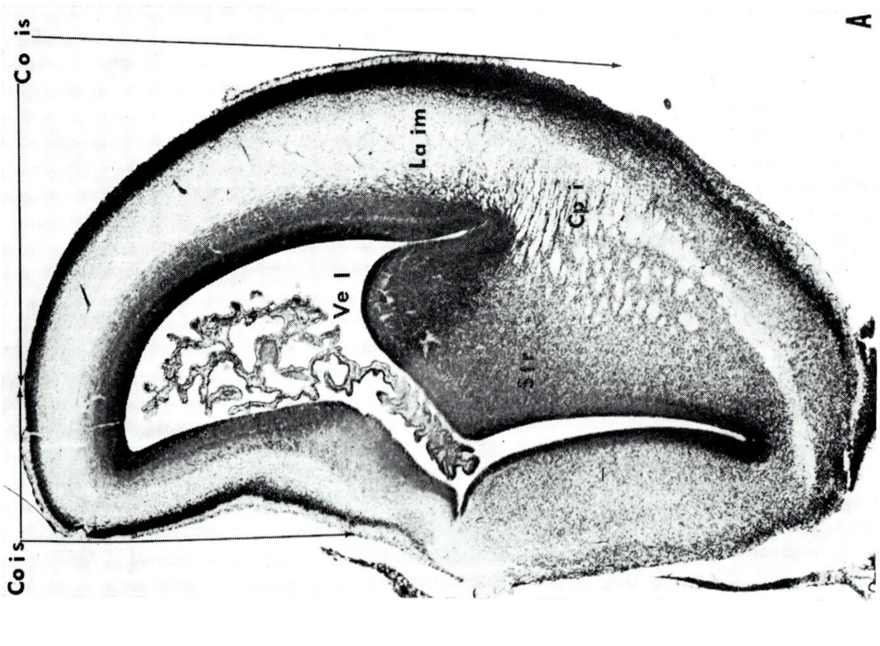
Co is
Co is
La im
Cp i
Ve l
Str
A

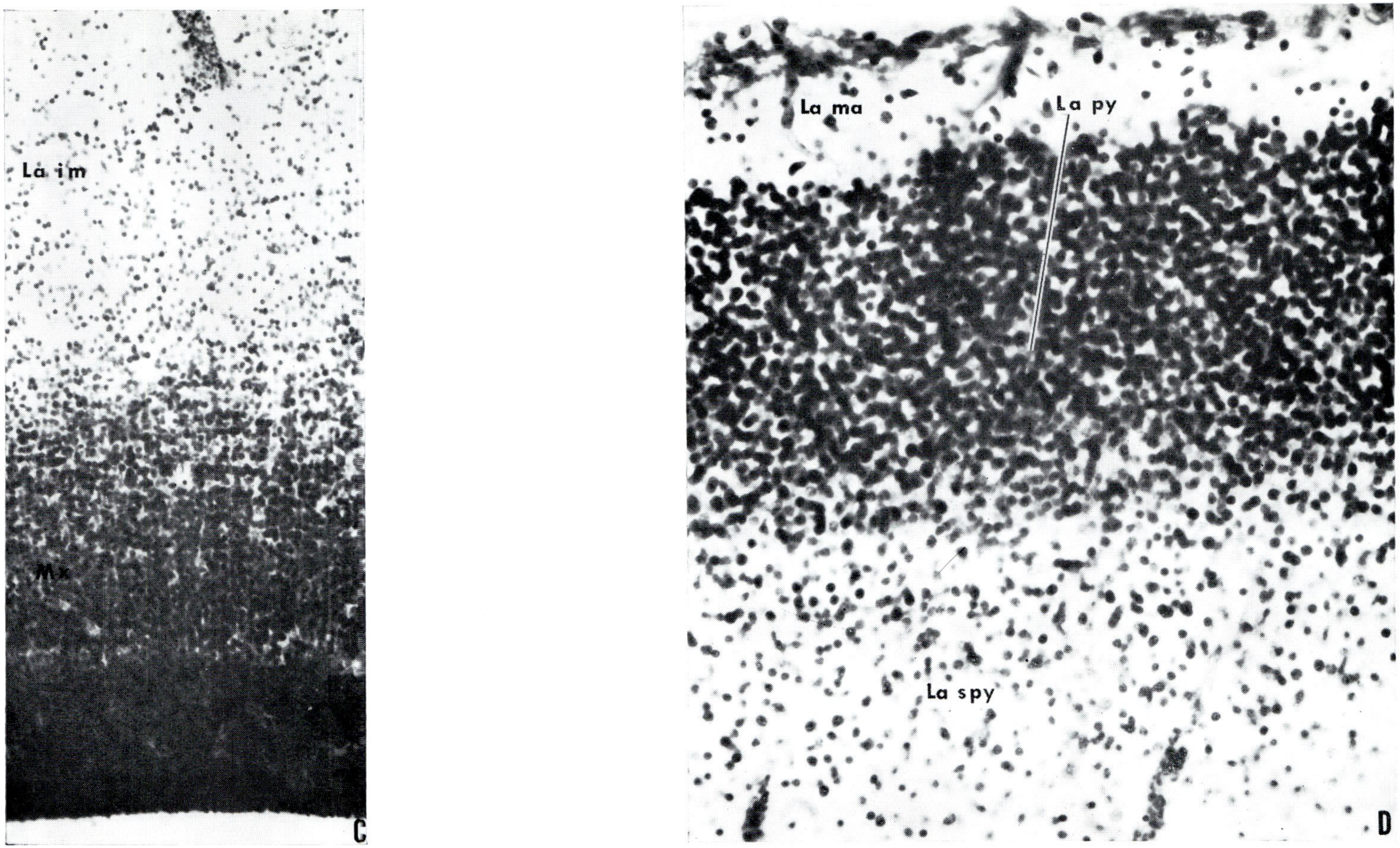

Fig. 2. 6.5-gram fetus, estimated age 43 days. Cresyl violet. (A) Coronal section through one hemisphere. Isocortical plate (Co is) is completely developed in neopallial wall. Incipient formation of 'white matter' (La im) and of internal capsule (Cp i)? × 28. Ve l = lateral ventricle; Str = striatum. (B) Detail of (A). Lateral telencephalic wall with 4 layers: Mx, matrix; La im, intermediate layer; La py, pyramidal layer; La ma, marginal layer. Hemispherical surface is upwards, lateral ventricle downwards, × 120. (C) Detail of (B). Matrix (Mx) is divided by thin light line. Migrating neuroblasts in intermediate zone (La im), × 225. (D) Detail of (B). Differentiated horizontal cells in marginal layer (La ma). Considerable increase of pyramidal layer (La py) with homogeneous cells as seen in Nissl sections. Some rather well differentiated cells, presumably stellate cells, in subpyramidal zone(La spy), × 500.

violet stained sections. There are also darker, spherical or somewhat irregularly shaped nuclei at different depths of the marginal layer.

A thin zone (measuring about the breadth of a nucleus) is observed immediately beneath the external limiting membrane, which does not contain any cells, only thin, sparse filaments radiating towards the surface (ascending branches from Cajal–Retzius cells?).

6.5-g fetus

The study was based upon coronal sections stained with cresyl violet. Considerable changes have occurred (*cf.* Fig. 2A with Figs. 1A and B). The ventricle wall is thicker and the neopallium better developed; all the 4 layers above-mentioned are now visible along the superior circumference of the brain vesicles; the intermediate zone contains numerous fibers; many more neuroblasts have migrated into the pyramidal layer.

The *matrix* (Mx) comprises about a third of the neopallial wall (Figs. 2B and C). It is divided into two parts by a thin light line, which runs parallel with the internal limiting membrane (best seen under low magnification as in Fig. 2B).

The inner part is densely populated. The cells are similar to those in the matrix of the 1.1-g fetus but there are more mitoses, which reflect the intense development of the telencephalon. The cells lie less close outside the thin line previously referred to and many are becoming spherical or have assumed more irregular shapes. Their orientation is more irregular, and here they do not form columns. The chromatin of the nuclei is usually similar to that of the cells in the inner zone, but small dark rounded nuclei are occasionally observed. Here too, there are many mitoses.

The cells in the outermost part of the matrix seem to be separated by bundles of fibers, presumably from the corpus callosum, which encircle the upper part of the lateral ventricle. The outer border of the matrix is, therefore, indistinct.

The *intermediate layer* (La im) forms a contrast to the surrounding zones, since it is less rich in cells and, therefore, appears lighter (Fig. 2B). Its height is about half that of the neopallial wall. Between the cells are numerous fibers, most of which seem to run either parallel with, or radiate towards, the hemispherical surface. Most of the nuclei are smaller than those in the matrix; their chromatin is rather light, and they are spherical or slightly elongated towards the surface. All the cells here are probably neuroblasts.

The cells are more closely situated in the outermost part of the intermediate zone,

---

Fig. 3. 12-gram fetus, estimated age 48 days. Sagittal sections (not consecutive) through telencephalon with coverings. Golgi method, × 12. (A) Tangential section through the lateral hemispherical wall. Frontal end of brain to the right, occipital to the left. Occipital end of lateral ventricle (Ve 1) with choroid plexus seen on left side. Efferent and afferent fibers (Fb p) converge downwards and inwards. (B) Somewhat more medial section than A (same series). Convex pallial wall at top, striatum (Str) and internal capsule (Cp i) at bottom. Some projection fibers from internal capsule (Fb p) at right. (C) Same brain, other hemisphere. More medial section than (B). Frontal end of brain to the left, occipital to the right. Brain stem extends towards right and downwards. Decussation of corticofugal (Fb cf) and thalamocortical (R th) fibers at D. Pl ch = choroid plexus.

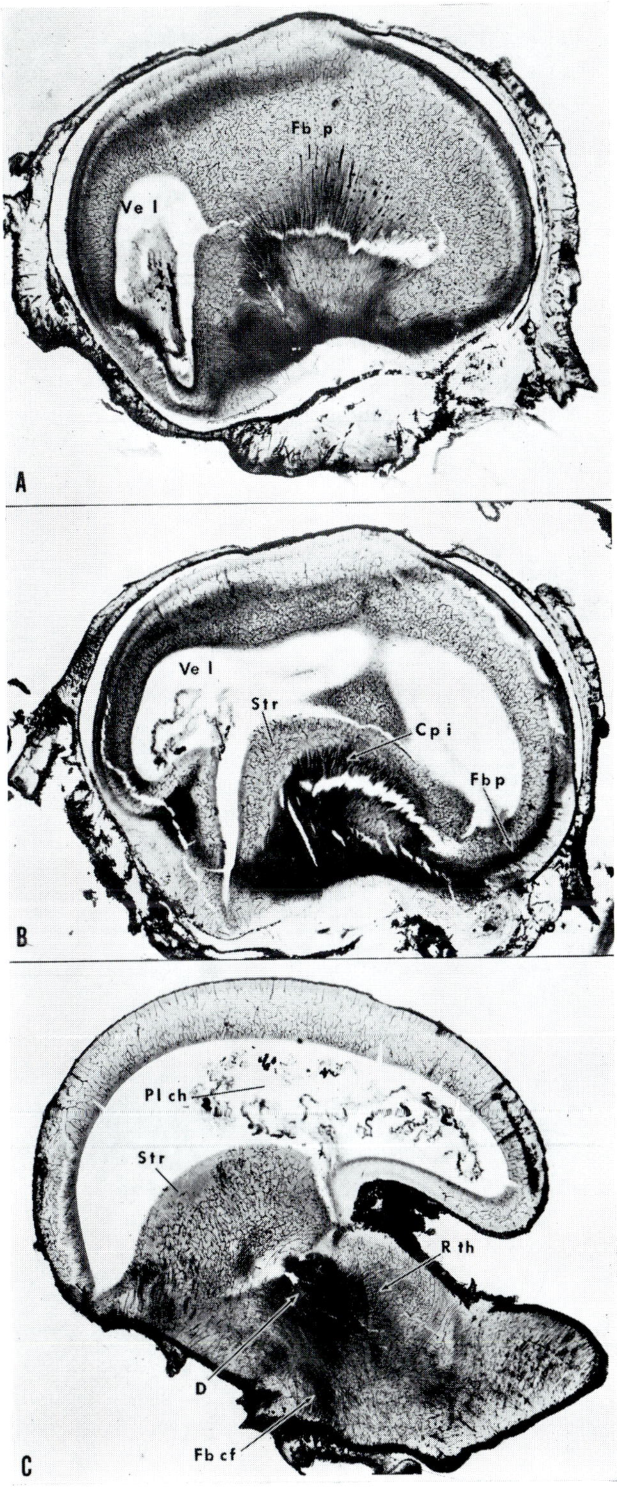

References p. 57–59

where a thin subcortical layer (La spy) can be recognized (Fig. 2D). Most cells here seem to be neuroblasts, but there are also more differentiated cells with larger, lighter nuclei and sparse cytoplasm. These cells may well be so-called stellate cells, which are seen in Golgi-stained sections from a 12-g fetus (*vide infra*).

The *pyramidal layer* (La py) is thickest in the lower part of the lateral wall where the depth averages 30–40 cells. The border with the marginal layer is better defined than that with the subcortical region. The cells are usually slightly separated from each other in all directions; they do not form any radiating columns. The nuclei are largely dark, spherical, comparatively small and occasionally surrounded by a thin rim of cytoplasm. The cells appear to be somewhat darker and more densely situated in the outermost stratum.

The large, well developed 'pyramidal' cells in the 1.1-g fetus seem to have become covered when more primitive cells migrated into the layer.

The *marginal layer* (La ma) has not changed much in comparison with the other

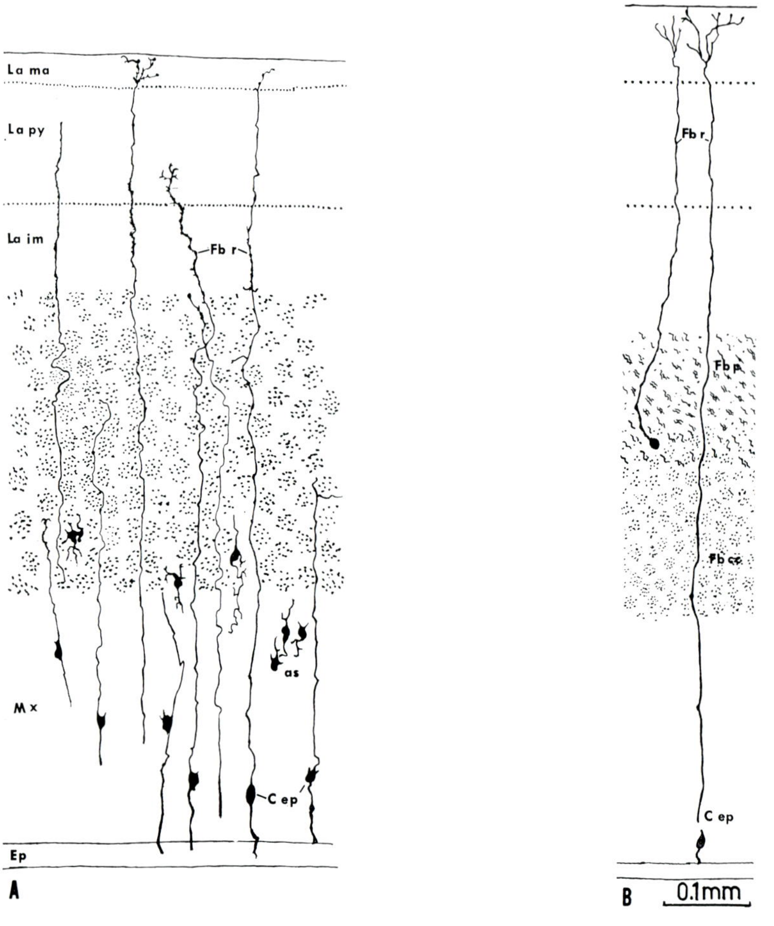

layers of the 6.5-g animal (Fig. 2D). The thickness of the layer is about the same as it is in the 1.1-g fetus. The well differentiated cells are somewhat larger and more clearly situated in the outer part of the layer, that is, subpially; the dominating orientation is still horizontal. The smaller, darker cells are seen at all depths.

Fig. 2A indicates that a primordial internal capsule (Cp i) has been formed. No fiber-stained preparations were available to confirm this.

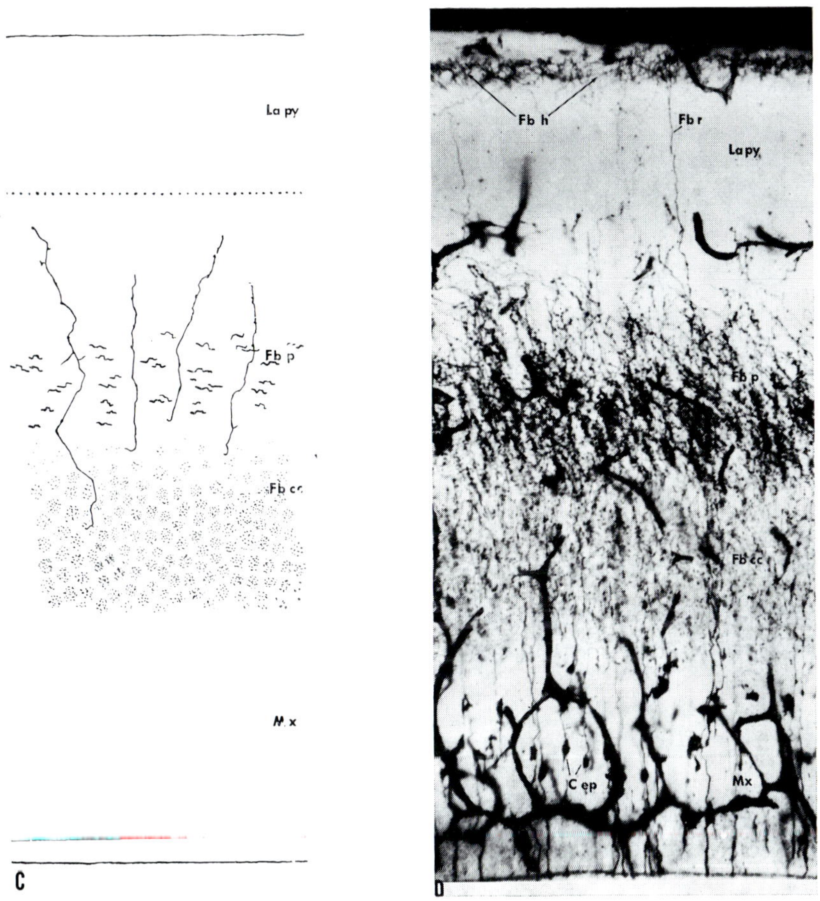

Fig. 4. 12-gram fetus (same as in Fig. 3). Cross sections through telencephalic wall. Surface is upwards and lateral ventricle with ependyma (Ep) is downwards. Wall is made up of concentric zones: matrix (Mx), intermediate (La im), pyramidal (La py), and marginal (La ma) layers. Golgi method. (A) Epithelial cells (C ep) in matrix (Mx) emit central extensions to ependyma. Their peripheral processes, the radiating fibers (Fb r), wind among bundles of fibers in intermediate layer, terminating mostly in the marginal zone. Small astrocytes (as) in matrix and inner part of intermediate layer. (B) Similar to (A). One epithelial cell body unusually far out in intermediate layer. (C) Callosal (Fb cc) and projection (Fb p) fibers in inner and outer parts of intermediate zone. Collaterals from the fibers terminate in the outermost part of layer. (D) Microphotograph. Precipitations on hemispherical surface. A few horizontal fibers (Fb h) in marginal zone, upper left. Other features as in A–C.

References p. 57–59

12-g fetus

The study was based upon a series of sagittal Golgi-stained sections (coronal sectioning was used in all of them). Figs. 3A, B, and C represent three of these sections (not consecutive). Fig. 3A is from a tangential section through the lateral hemispherical wall. The other two pictures show how the thin pallial wall bulges above the large lateral ventricle (Ve l) with its choroid plexus (Pl ch). The di- and mesencephalic structures are shown at the bottom of these pictures. The capillary network is clearly visible everywhere.

Attention was focused especially on the neopallial wall (Figs. 4–7).

The cell-dense *matrix* contains two types of cells.

(1) Primitive *astrocytes* (as). They are mostly small, with short, branching extensions; they are rather numerous in the matrix and the inner part of the intermediate layer (Fig. 4A). They either occur singly or form small groups. Some of the astrocytes are connected with blood vessels. No glial cells were seen nearer to the surface.

(2) The numerous *epithelial* cells (C ep) are bipolar and radially oriented. They have small cell bodies and thick inner extensions, which reach the internal limiting membrane (Figs. 4A and B). The cell bodies are scattered throughout the matrix. A few similar cells are seen in the intermediate zone (Fig. 4B, left).

The fundamental structure of the *intermediate layer* was rather distinct in this animal because of the simple structure of the brain, the successful impregnation of the material, and the instructive coronal sectioning. This zone contains numerous fibers. The following types can be recognized.

(1) The numerous radiating fibers (Fb r) from the epithelial cells, which penetrate the pallium everywhere (Figs. 4A and B), are approximately perpendicular to the ependymal and external surfaces of the cerebral vesicles, but the course of the individual fibers is tortuous, winding between the fasicles in the intermediate layer. They are thick, when compared for instance with the axons of the pyramidal cells. Some of them are rather uneven and covered with spines, whereas others are of uniform caliber and have a smooth surface. Most radiating fibers extend to the surface of the cerebral hemisphere; some of them emit short collateral branches, but a few elements terminate, at different depths in the intermediate layer, either in single knobs or in multiple short branches. The distal end is thicker and its surface less smooth than the other parts of each fiber.

(2) The fibers of the corpus callosum (Fb cc) are most prominent at about the anteroposterior levels of the striate body. The thin, cross-cut fibers form bundles in the deep part of the intermediate zone (Figs. 4C and D).

(3) Projection fibers (Fb p) are situated peripherally to the callosal elements (Figs. 4C and D). These fibers can be readily separated from the radiating fibers, since they are thinner, more tortuous and differently oriented. These thin, unmyelinated, efferent and afferent fibers radiate from the cortex towards the internal capsule and *vice versa* (Figs. 3A and B). The efferent fibers, which proceed from the cortical and subcortical cells (*vide infra*), descend through the midbrain to lower levels. The afferent fibers emanate from the thalamic radiation (Fig. 3C, R th).

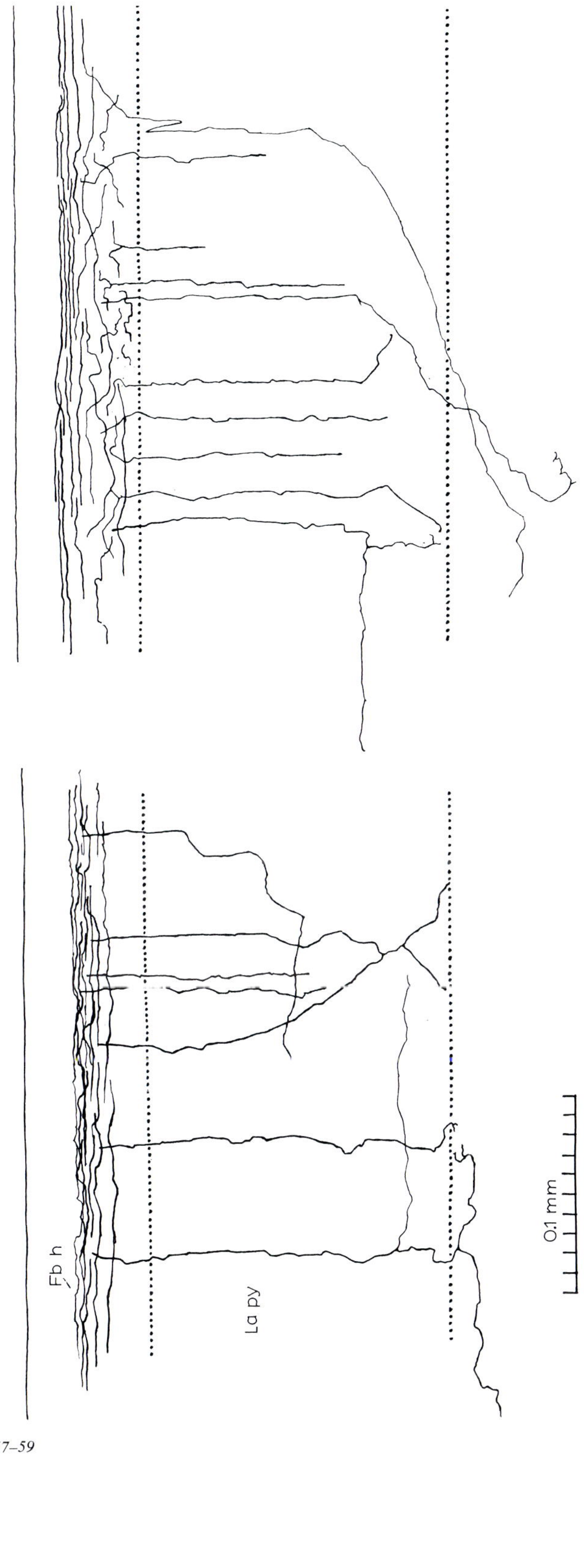

Fig. 5. 12-gram fetus (same animal as in Figs. 3 and 4). Descending collaterals from horizontal fibers (Fb h) in two different areas of marginal zone emit branches to lower part of pyramidal layer (La py) and subpyramidal areas. Hemispherical surface was covered by precipitates. Golgi method.

(4) Collaterals or endings in the more superficial part of the intermediate zone (Fig. 4C) seem to emanate exclusively from callosal fibers or from both callosal and thalamic elements. These thin filaments ascend and become slightly thicker distally; some of them have a few short branches. Descending collaterals from the marginal layer also reach the subcortical region (Fig. 5; *vide infra*).

Two types of cells were seen in the intermediate zone.

(1) The migrating *neuroblasts* are pear-shaped cells usually with short, peripheral processes.

(2) The larger *stellate cells* in the outer part of the intermediate zone are true nerve cells (Fig. 6). Their slender dendrites are frequently oriented in an antero-posterior direction, but rarely proceed towards the suiface. Some of them are long, and many exceed 250 μ. They mingle with the long, similarly oriented dendrites from the cortical nerve cells (Fig. 6, right), thereby forming a dense subcortical network.

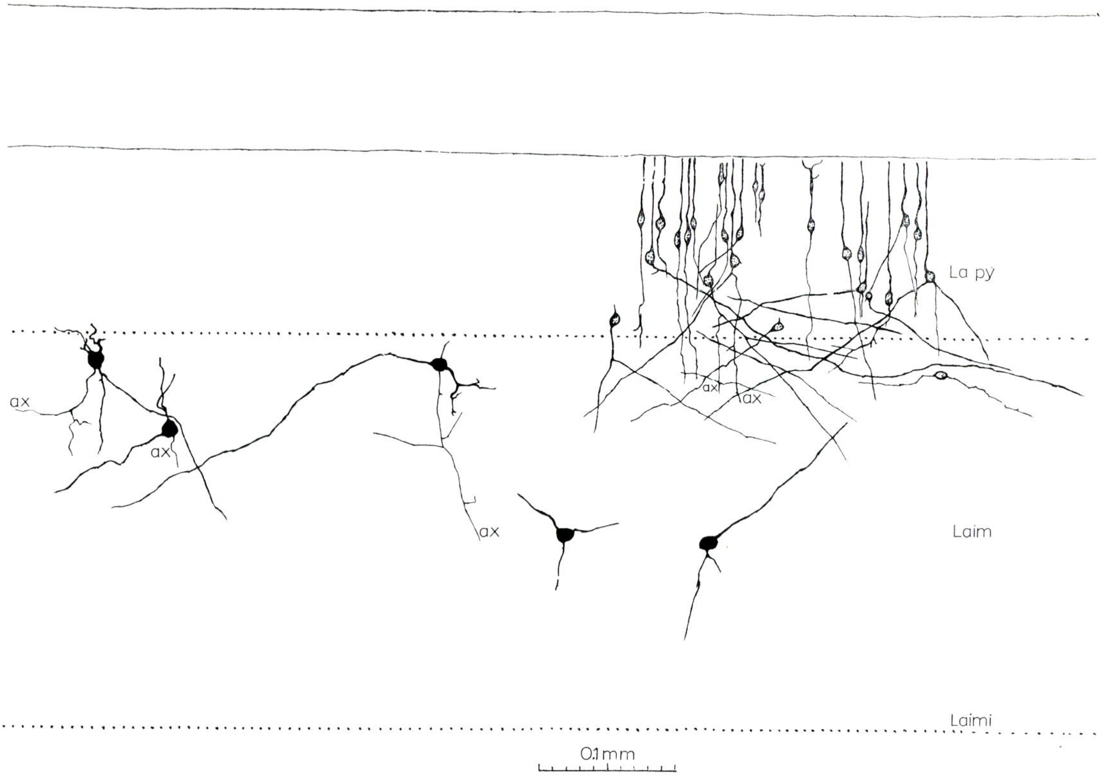

Fig. 6. 12-gram animal (same as in Figs. 3–5). Nerve cells in upper part of pyramidal layer (La py) have simple bipolar appearance. More highly developed cells in lower part of the layer have descending basal dendrites, some of them very long. Precipitations have covered terminal branches of apical dendrites. Stellate cells are situated in intermediate layer (La im), but should be considered as part of the primordial isocortex. Their long dendrites form a dense plexus together with those from the deep pyramidal cells. Stellate cell axons have collaterals. The Golgi sections reveal a differentiation of nerve cells and stratification in the primordial isocortex which is not seen in Nissl sections. Upper solid and upper dotted lines indicate borders of pyramidal layer. Lower dotted line, approximate border between outer and inner part (La imi) of intermediate zone.

Axons, some with collaterals, of stellate cells are also seen in Fig. 6. They will presumably form part of the system of projection fibers and descend to lower levels of the neuraxis.

The *pyramidal layer* is densely populated. The more superficial cells here have an

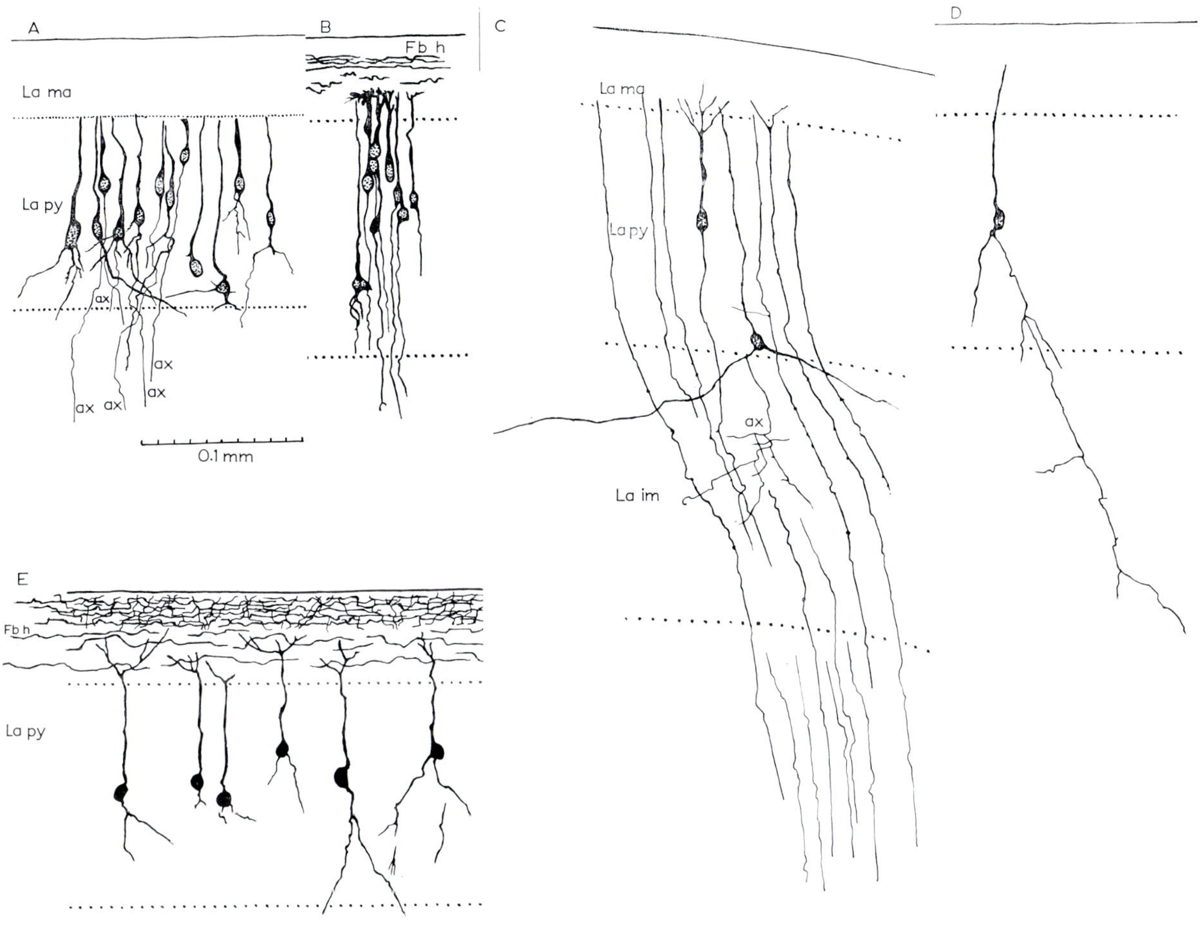

Fig. 7. 12-gram fetus (same as in Figs. 3–6). Pyramidal cells in various areas of the isocortex in the lateral wall of the telencephalon. Solid line, hemispherical surface. Dotted lines enclose pyramidal layer (La py). Golgi method. Magnification as in (E). (A and B) Immature bipolar cells in superficial part of pyramidal layer. Better development in deeper part of layer, where pyramidal cells have basal dendrites. Apical dendrites terminate in deep part of marginal layer (La ma), mostly forming a few short branches (B). Precipitations obscure marginal zone in (A). Thin axons (ax) descend towards intermediate zone. (C) Collaterals from axons (ax) of deep pyramidal cell terminate in outer part of intermediate zone (La im), where stellate cells were seen in Fig. 6. Apical dendrites of this cell terminate undivided in marginal zone. More superficial cell has no axon collaterals but more highly developed apical dendrite. Vertical lines represent radiating fibers. Inner dotted line: border between outer and inner part of intermediate layer. (D) Similar as (C). (E) Pyramidal cells with descending basal dendrites in inferior part of layer. Branches of apical dendrites in deeper part; numerous horizontal fibers in outer part of marginal zone.

References p. 57–59

immature bipolar appearance (Figs. 7A and B). The comparatively thick apical dendrites terminate in several branches within the deep part of the marginal layer beneath the horizontal fibers (Fig. 7B). The thinner basal processes at the opposite end of the perikaryon taper rapidly and proceed as very thin axons without collaterals, which can be followed to the intermediate zone.

The cells in the deeper part of the pyramidal layer are more highly developed (Figs. 6 and 7). Most of them have slender basal dendrites (usually 1 or 2 as seen on the sections). As a rule they are undivided, but occasionally they have one or two bifurcations. The dendrites descend more or less steeply in the direction of the frontal or occipital pole, as seen in the sagittal sections. Some basal dendrites terminate within the pyramidal layer itself (Figs. 7A–E). Others continue to the outer part of the intermediate zone (Figs. 6 and 7C) where, together with dendrites from stellate cells, they form a subcortical plexus (Fig. 6). The length of the basal dendrites varies from 10–20 μ up to about 300 μ (see *e.g.* the remarkable cells in Fig. 6).

The apical dendrites of the deep pyramidal cells ascend to the inner part of the marginal layer, where they terminate with or without ramifications (Figs. 7B–E). They are thicker than the basal dendrites of the same cells, but, on the whole, they are thinner than the apical dendrites of the more superficial cells.

The axons of the deep pyramidal cells descend into the intermediate zone, where they emit collaterals (see especially the complicated system of collaterals in Fig. 7C). They probably continue as projection fibers.

Thus, even at this early stage a differentiation can be observed: the pyramidal cells are more highly developed in the deeper part of the pyramidal zone.

Some fibers (Fb r) from the epithelial cells terminate within the pyramidal layer in flower-like formations or without branching (Fig. 4A).

The external part of the *marginal layer* contains numerous horizontal fibers (Fb h), which run parallel with the pial surface, chiefly in an anteroposterior direction (Figs. 4D, 5, 7B, and E). Furthermore, here the majority of the radiating fibers (Fb r) terminate in numerous branches (Fig. 4A). Thus, the interwoven horizontal and epithelial fibers form a complicated network in the outer part of the marginal zone.

The deep part of the marginal layer, which contains fewer horizontal fibers, receives the terminal ramifications of the apical dendrites (Figs. 7B–E). It should be emphasized that the apical dendrites of the pyramidal cells dissipate within the inner part of the marginal layer and do not extend — in contrast to the terminals of the epithelial fibers — to the hemispherical surface. This fact does not seem to have been fully appreciated previously.

The horizontal fibers emit thin *collaterals*, which descend to the deeper (more differentiated) stratum of the pyramidal layer and the subcortical area (Fig. 5). Most of them are undivided, but some have one or two branches. Several collaterals are seen running horizontally in the pyramidal layer, which means that they may be able to make contact with several cells in the same stratum. One collateral (Fig. 5, left part) is returning to the marginal layer.

Unfortunately, no cells were stained in the marginal layer of this preparation.

It should be repeated, that as yet no glial cells have migrated to the cortical layers.

14.5–20-g fetuses

The telencephalic wall is becoming thicker but, with regard to the Golgi-stained sections, there are no fundamentally new features compared with those of the 12-g fetus. Prominent elements are the epithelial fibers, which terminate at different depths of the wall. Neuroblasts migrate through the intermediate zone.

25–29-g fetuses

The pallial wall is much thicker; the intermediate zone especially has increased in volume. The epithelial fibers predominate in many Golgi-stained sections. Most of them originate in the pear-shaped small cells of the matrix and they terminate, as they did earlier, at different depths of the wall, mainly in the marginal layer. However,

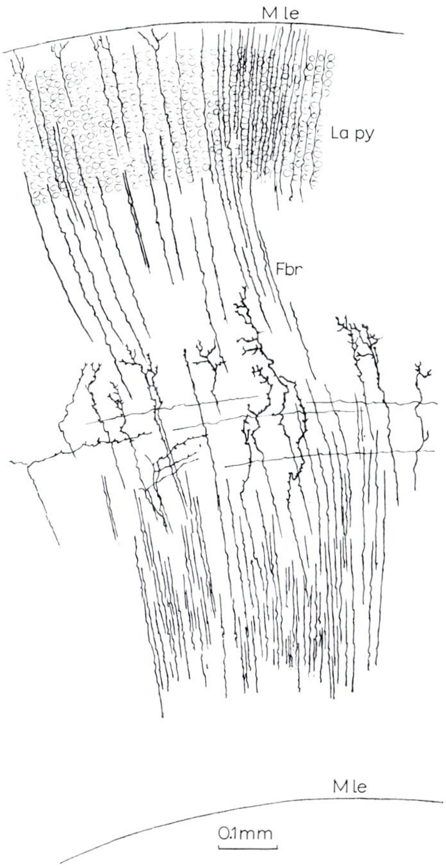

Fig. 8. 28-gram fetus, estimated age 54 days. Radiating fibers (Fbr) penetrate hemispherical wall. Most of them extend to marginal layer (top) but many terminate in forming branches in the intermediate zone. A few callosal fibers are seen. M le = external limiting membrane; M le = internal limiting membrane. Golgi method.

References p. 57–59

many thick, uneven terminal segments and multiple, sometimes flower-like, endings are prominent in the deep and in the middle parts of the intermediate zone, where they form a tangle (Fig. 8). A similar observation was made by Kölliker (1896) in a 4-month-old human fetus (*cf.* Fig. 8 with Fig. 814 in his work). The terminations in the marginal zone are somewhat more elaborate than earlier. The small astrocytes are numerous in the outer part of the matrix.

The inner part of the intermediate zone is filled with fibers, which run concentrically with the ependymal lining of the lateral ventricle as seen in the coronal sections. Most of the callosal fibers lie inferior to the projection and thalamic fibers.

There is a less dense network in the outer part of the intermediate zone which contains radiating fibers, projection fibers from the pyramidal cells, and collaterals from afferent and callosal fibers.

The small, dark, pear-shaped cell bodies of migrating neuroblasts are scattered over the whole intermediate layer, but are most numerous in its inner part, where they may form clusters between the bundles of circulating fibers.

Larger stellate cells are seen especially in the outer part of the intermediate zone and particularly in the subpyramidal region, where they form a stratum (Fig. 9B), which should be considered to be a stratum of the primitive cortex. The stellate cells are better differentiated than the primitive pyramidal cells as they were already at the 12-g stage (*cf.* Figs. 6 and 9). The perikaryon emits 2–4 dendrites; one of them is usually thicker than the others. Some of them bifurcate or emit short branches. The thick processes are as a rule directed inwards; the others run in all directions. Some of the dendrites penetrate into the pyramidal cell layer. There are also bipolar cells which are oriented parallel with the hemispherical surface. Many dendrites have been severed close to the cell body; consequently their possible further extension in an anterior or posterior direction cannot be observed in the coronal sections. No dendrite was seen, however, whose length was equal to that of the stellate cells in the 12-g fetus (Fig. 6). The axons of the stellate cells, some with collaterals, are directed inwards.

The cells in the *pyramidal layer* have small nuclei and are densely packed, especially in the most superficial stratum. They do not appear to be more highly differentiated than in the 12-g fetus, although the layer is about twice as thick. The neurons in the most superficial stratum have a primitive bipolar appearance (Fig. 9A). The branching of their apical dendrites in the deeper part of the marginal layer is somewhat more elaborate than it was earlier.

Fig. 9. (A and C) 28-gram fetus (same as in Fig. 8), estimated age 54 days. (B) 25-gram fetus, estimated age 53 days. Golgi method. (A and B) Composite picture of marginal and pyramidal (A) and subpyramidal (B) areas placed in correct relation to each other and to the surface. The selected areas have similar situation in lateral telencephalic wall. Stellate cells in (B) should be considered as deepest stratum of primordial isocortex although by definition they are situated in the intermediate zone (dotted line indicates upper border of zone). Most cells in superficial part of pyramidal layer are still of a primitive bipolar type. Deep pyramidal cells not stained in this area. Marginal zone contains 1 Cajal–Retzius cell (upper left). Dotted line: border between marginal and pyramidal layers. (C) Different types of horizontal cells in marginal layer. Three bipolar cells in pyramidal layer also shown at right.

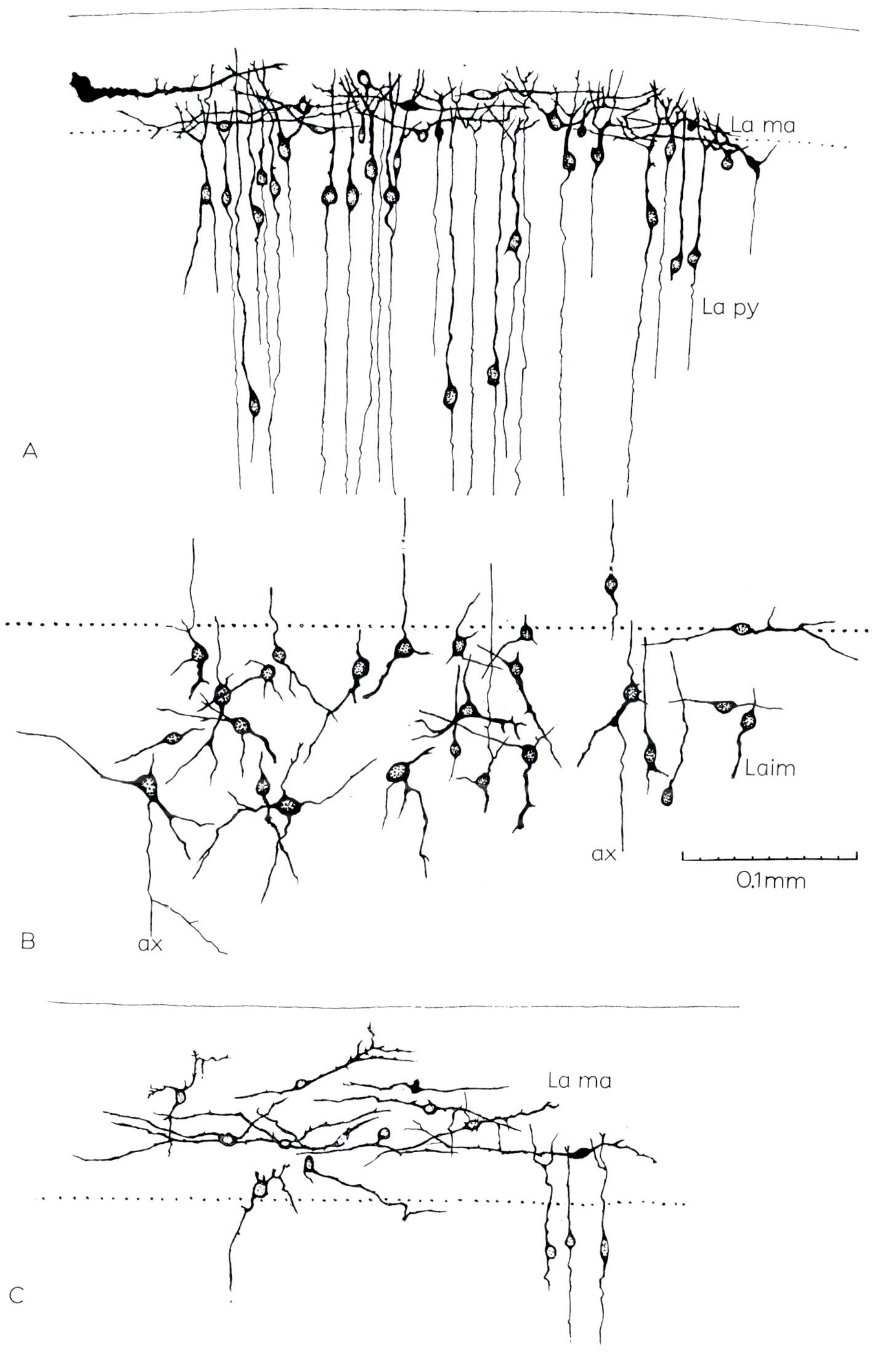

References p. 57–59

The nerve cells in the deep part of the pyramidal layer frequently emit 1–2 basal dendrites which run inwards vertically or obliquely (not seen in Fig. 9B). The long slender anteroposteriorly oriented dendrites of the 12-g fetus (Fig. 6) were never observed in these sections.

The *marginal layer* has about the same thickness as it had previously. The horizontal Cajal cells (Figs. 9A and C) are usually bipolar, but some cells emit 2 dendrites from either end of the cell body and unipolar, tripolar or neurons of other types are also visible. The nuclei are comparatively small, and the dendrites measure up to 100 μ. Fig. 9A (left) illustrates one large horizontal cell of the Cajal–Retzius type.

The horizontal cells mingle with the terminations of apical dendrites in the inferior part of the marginal layer. Furthermore, the region is transversed by horizontal and radiating fibers. The result is a dense plexus.

The superficial part of the marginal zone was difficult to study owing to precipitations; it is evident, however, that it contains numerous horizontal fibers and also some cells.

36–42-g fetuses

The hemispherical surface is still lissencephalic but a flattening of the dorsolateral aspect indicates the prospective formation of the suprasylvian gyrus (Figs. 10 and 11).

The fundamental structure of the pallial wall is not altered except for the migration of astrocytes, which will be described later. The study of a material, stained with cresyl violet and with silver according to Palmgren's method, has confirmed and extended the previous observations.

The portion of the *germinal layer*, which corresponds to the isocortex, surrounds the superior part of the ventricle at the level of the basal ganglia (Figs. 10 and 11). The thickness of the matrix (Mx) increases in a lateral direction (the pyramidal layer also becomes somewhat thicker laterally). Epithelial fibers extend from the germinal zone towards the surface. Their general direction has been outlined in Fig. 11.

The germinal zone can be divided into sublayers as it was in the 6.5-g fetus. The inner part is made up of densely packed cells which form columns outside the internal limiting membrane. Mitoses are rare in contrast to those seen in younger animals. The cells in the outer part are separated to some extent by a fine network of fibrils. The nuclei are usually smaller, darker and more pleomorphic than those in the inner sublayer, but some scattered, larger and lighter nuclei are also seen. Many cells, especially in the more peripheral part, are oriented parallel with the ependymal lining. Golgi sections show that the region contains many astrocytes with short branching processes. (These were already seen in the 12-g animal; see Fig. 4A.) The prospective subependymal glia zone might emanate from these cells.

The concentric parts of the *intermediate zone* are easy to recognize in the silver-stained section of Fig. 10 (*cf.* with Fig. 11). The *inner* part (La imi) contains the callosal and projection fibers, the callosal fibers running close to the germinal zone. The medial end of the subzone terminates at the corpus callosum (Co c), and the lateral end at the internal capsule (Cp i). Numerous pear-shaped, rather small and dark neuroblasts

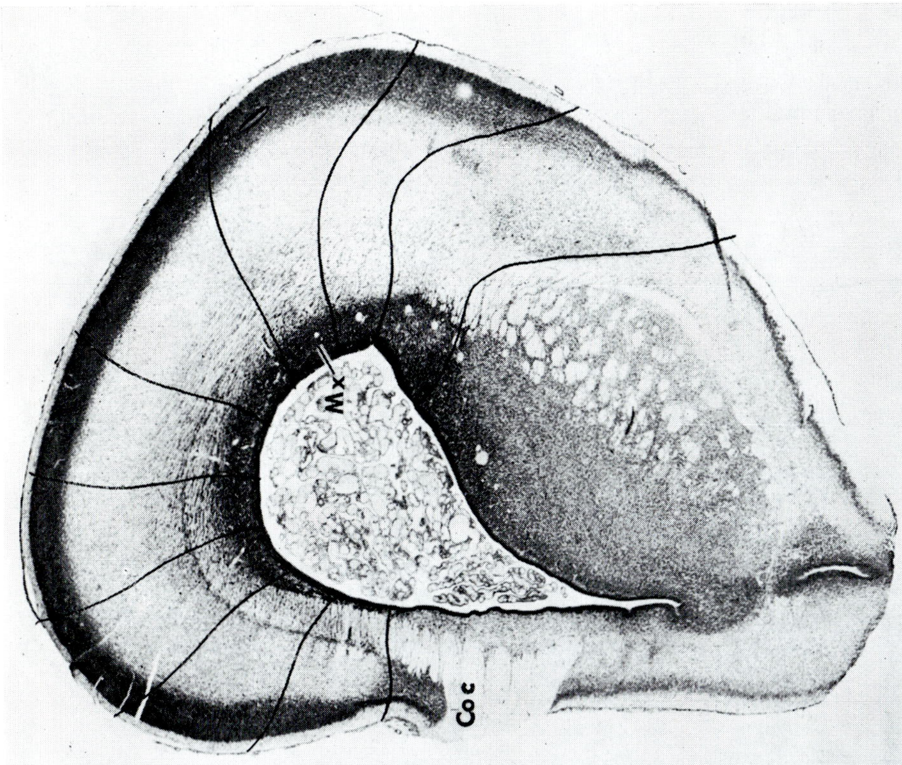

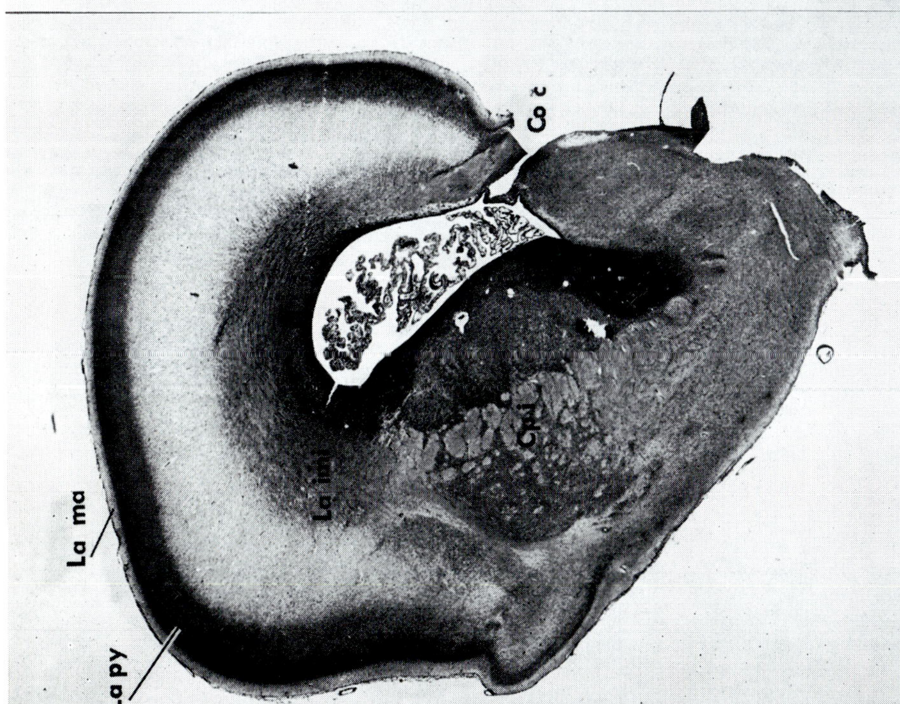

Fig. 10. 35-gram fetus, estimated age 56 days. Coronal section at level of anterior limb of internal capsule (Cp i). Concentric layering of neopallial wall which bulges lateral to and above lateral ventricle. Cell-rich matrix forms dark band along ventricle. Shading in innermost part of intermediate layer (La imi) is due to presence of numerous fibers and cells. Incipient stratification in pyramidal layer (La py). Palmgren's silver method, × 12. Co c = corpus callosum.

Fig. 11. 39-gram fetus, estimated age 57 days. Coronal section at level of genu of corpus callosum (Co c). Similar features as in Fig. 10. General direction of radiating fibers indicated by lines. Cresyl violet, × 15.

References p. 57–59

lie in clusters or rows between the circulating fibers. They have peripheral processes, and some also emit thin extensions in a central direction. Furthermore, there are some larger nuclei with light chromatin, and one or two nucleoli.

The *outer* part of the intermediate zone lacks the circulating fibers but there are numerous cells, many of which are more highly differentiated than those in the inner part. At least three types of cells can be recognized (Fig. 12). (1) The pear-shaped or round, small, dark cell bodies of the neuroblasts are less numerous than in the inner part. (2) The stellate cells increase in number towards the pyramidal layer. The nucleus is rounded; it has finely stippled chromatin, one or two nucleoli, and is larger than that in any other nerve cell of the neopallial wall at this stage. A thin rim of cytoplasm surrounds the nucleus or is visible along one of its sides. It is stained with silver, but true neurofibrils are not observed. The cell body emits several processes, one of which

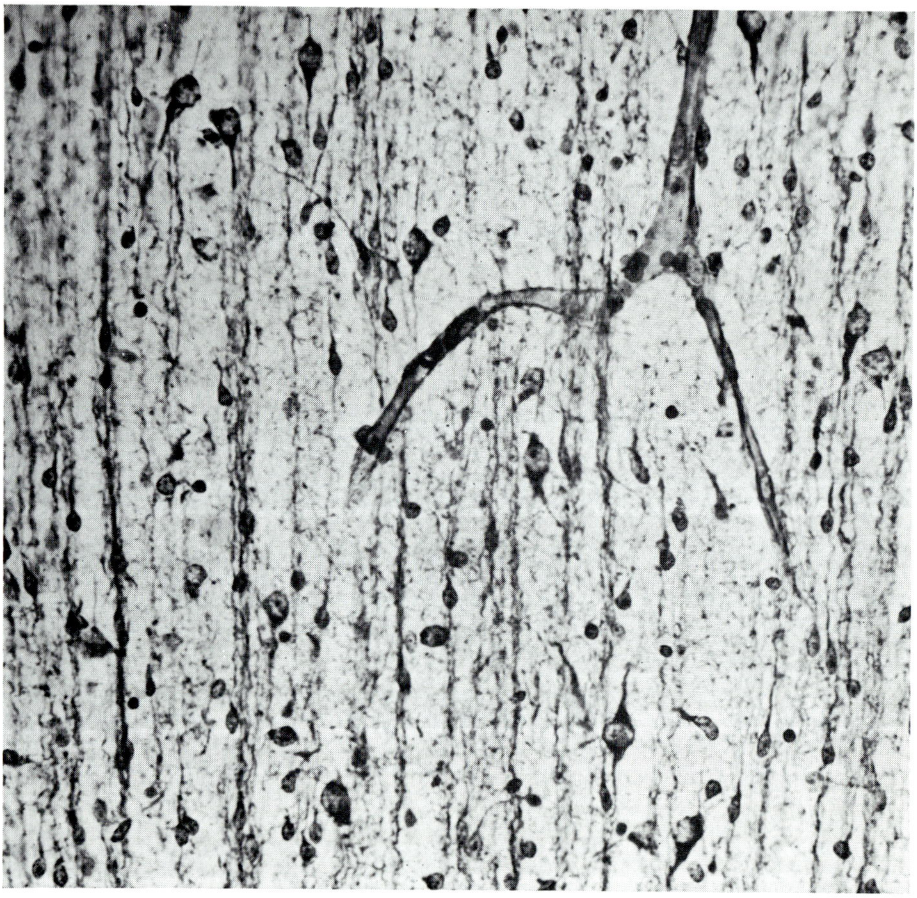

Fig. 12. 35-gram animal (same as in Fig. 10), estimated age 56 days. Outer part of intermediate zone. Bundles of radiating fibers run vertically towards surface (top). Tapering ends of pear-shaped neuroblasts are directed towards surface, *i.e.* upwards. Large stellate cells are well differentiated nerve cells. Tiny cells presumably belong to glial cells. Nuclei close to wall of capillary may belong to astrocytes. Large spaces between cells and radiating fibers. Palmgren's method, × 480.

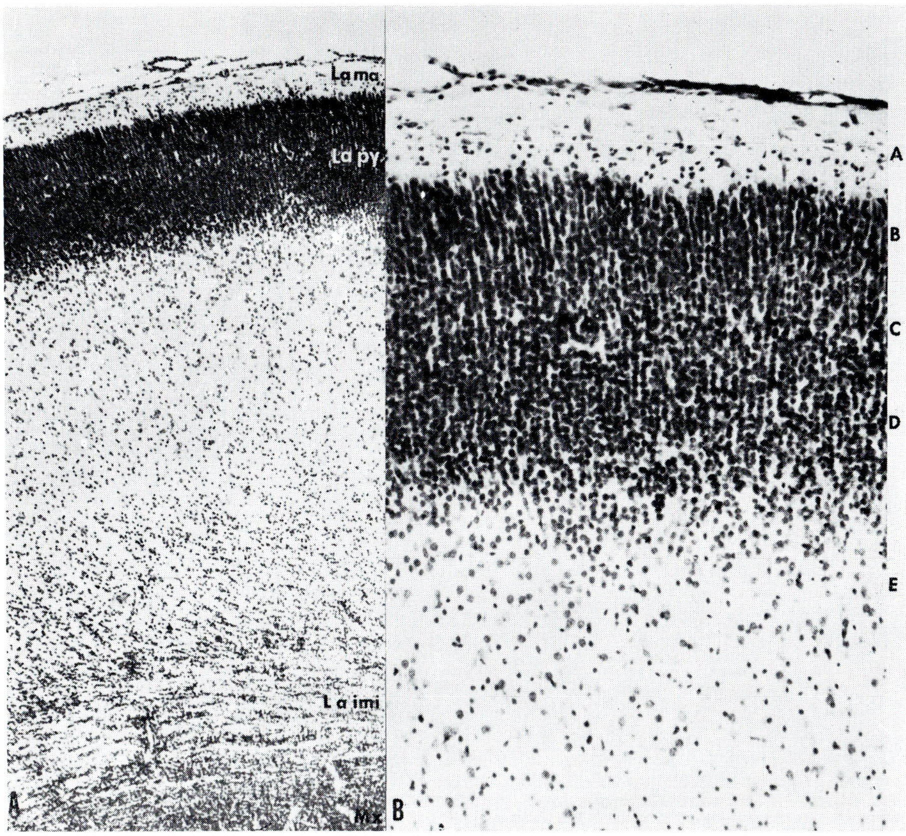

Fig. 13. 39-gram fetus, estimated age 57 days. Cresyl violet. (A) Detail of Fig. 11. Surface of hemispherical wall at top. Outer part of matrix (Mx) at bottom. Groups of cells separated by callosal and projection fibers in inner part of intermediate layer (La imi). Incipient stratification in pyramidal layer (La py) is due to formation of thin light band in middle part of layer, × 65. (B) Detail of (A). Five strata may be recognized in anlage of the isocortex. Marginal layer (A) is well developed, has largely same appearance as earlier. Pyramidal layer proper (B–D) still has a largely primitive appearance, but slight differences among nerve cells create an impression of stratification: cells in most superficial part (B) are least highly developed and most compactly situated; cells in middle part (C) are most highly developed and more widely separated than other cells. Transitional zone (E) between pyramidal layer proper and intermediate zone is less cell-rich, contains many highly developed stellate cells, and should be regarded as deepest layer in primordial isocortex. × 160.

is usually rather thick and directed inwards. These dendrites branch as has previously been described. (3) A few rather minute cells have small, dark, round or slightly irregular nuclei, no visible cytoplasm and no processes. Other cell bodies have the average size of the neuroblasts but do not emit any apical processes, and their long axes are frequently perpendicular to the radiating fibers. The nature of these elements is obscure. They do not have the appearance of nerve cells and probably belong to astrocytes (*vide infra*).

There are rather large spaces between the cells and bundles of radiating fibers in the outer part of the intermediate zone (Fig. 12). Microscopical examination under high magnification reveals a network of thin fibers (presumably axons, collaterals and astrogliotic fibrils). Furthermore, these spaces must contain dendrites (unstained) from the stellate and lower pyramidal nerve cells. The possibility that these spaces also contain a large amount of extracellular fluid has to be considered.

The *pyramidal layer* (La py) is considerably thicker than it was earlier; its depth corresponds to about 50–60 cells lying close to each other (Fig. 13). The nuclei of the most superficial pyramidal cells are smaller and darker than those of the other cortical cells, and usually have one nucleolus. They are elongated vertically, and form compact vertical columns, which are separated from each other by the radiating

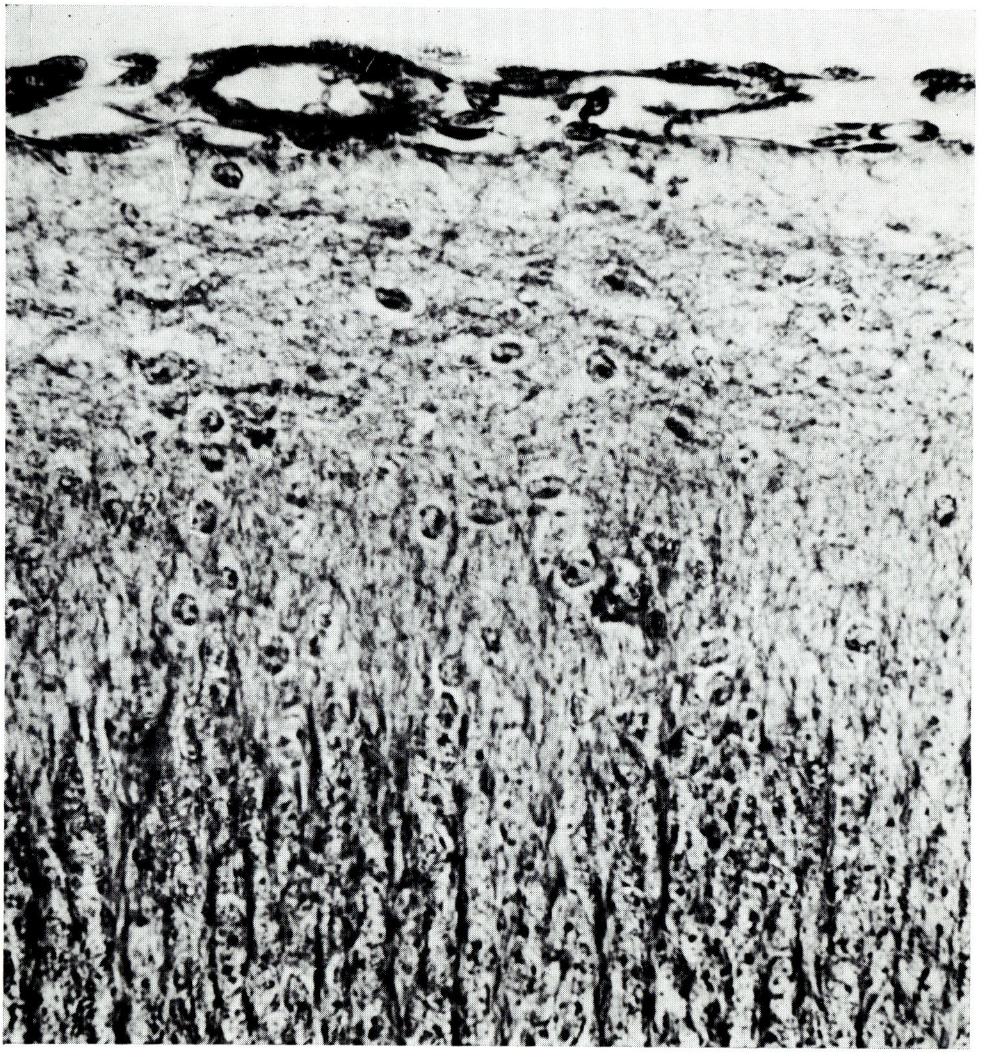

Fig. 14. 35-gram fetus (same as in Fig. 10), estimated age 56 days. Bundles of radiating fibers between columns of cells in superficial part of pyramidal layer proceed together with apical dendrites into lower part of marginal zone; their general orientation is perpendicular to the hemispherical surface. Horizontal fibers and cells in outer part of marginal zone have, in general, a course parallel with surface. Palmgren's method, × 760.

fibers, and apical dendrites (Figs. 13B and 14). Golgi-stained sections show that these cells have a simple, bipolar structure.

In the inferior part of the pyramidal layer the nuclei are larger, lighter, and more rounded; they are frequently surrounded by a thin rim of cytoplasm and have prominent nucleoli. The intercellular spaces are slightly wider and the columnar arrangement of the cells less evident. The widening of the intercellular spaces seems to be due to the more highly developed neuronal processes and the appearance of astrocytes.

When viewed under low magnification the middle stratum of the pyramidal layer stands out as a somewhat light band (Fig. 13); this is owing to the comparatively large size and light color of the nuclei and the widening of the intercellular spaces.

The deepest stratum of the pyramidal layer, which is characterized by a reduced cell density and an admixture of stellate neurons to the pyramidal cells, constitutes a transition to the intermediate zone.

To conclude, at this stage the primordial pyramidal layer displays 4 strata of alternative darker and lighter zones. Thus, including the marginal zone, a 5-layer cortex can be recognized (Fig. 13B, A–E).

The pyramidal layer also contains some dark, rather small nuclei which were not seen earlier. They probably belong to the astrocytes.

The *marginal layer* (La ma) is similar to that in the younger animals. The horizontal nerve cells have large oval nuclei with light chromatin and, usually, one nucleolus; the proximal parts of their dendrites contain clumps, which are stained with cresyl violet and silver. The region also contains cells with dark nuclei, usually without nucleoli (probably astrocytes).

The inner part of the marginal layer is denser, due, *inter alia*, to the terminal ramifications of the apical dendrites. The general direction of these elements and of the epithelial fibers, which extend to the outer area, is perpendicular to the surface (Fig. 14). The cells are more numerous than in the outer zone. Their nuclei are of different sizes and shapes; on the whole they are somewhat smaller and darker than those of the pyramidal cells, and usually have nucleoli.

Astrocytes have now appeared in the more superficial layers. In the pyramidal zone their cell bodies occupy especially the middle stratum and seem to contribute to the separation of the nerve cells referred to previously. Here, the astrocytes mimic the pyramidal neurons since they have cell bodies and apical dendrites (Fig. 15). As a rule, they can readily be distinguished, however, for the following reasons: an astrocyte lacks an axon; the cell body is more elongated; unlike the pyramidal cells, it is not triangular, and has a less smooth, more nodular surface, which is frequently covered by short thin processes; there are frequently two or more apical dendrites, which may follow a curved or an angular course instead of running vertically straight as do the dendrites in the pyramidal cells; the basal dendrites are shorter, thinner, more uneven; some astrocytic cell bodies or processes, or both, are attached to the capillaries (Fig. 15).

The astrocytes of the subpyramidal zone (Fig. 15, lower part) are different in shape. The cell bodies are plump, more rounded, and are usually covered by numerous short,

References p. 57–59

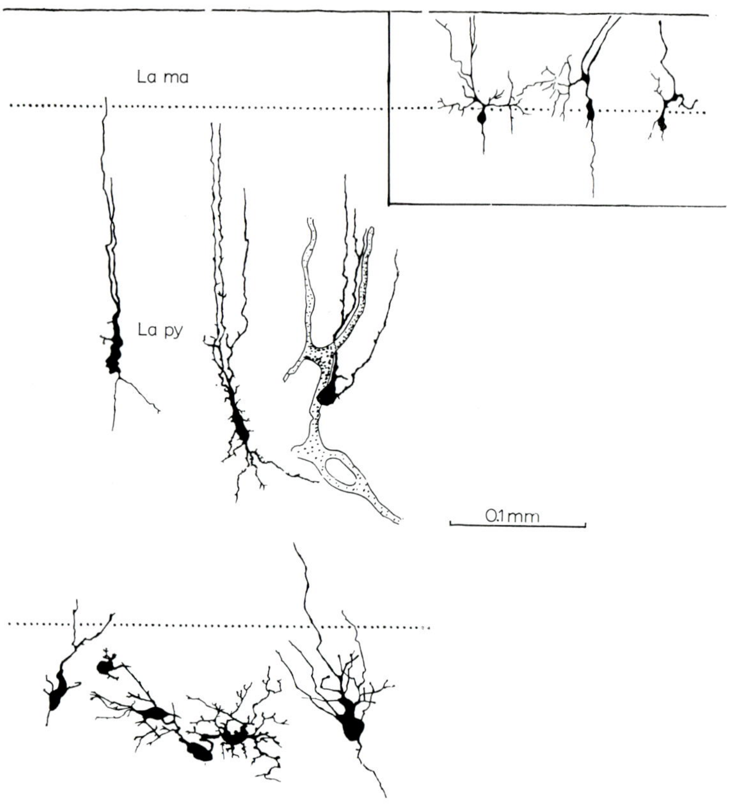

Fig. 15. 42-gram fetus, estimated age 58 days. Inset: 49-gram fetus, estimated age 59 days. Astrocytes in marginal (La ma), pyramidal (La py) and subpyramidal zones. One cell body is attached to capillary wall. Golgi method.

thin processes. Some longer dendrites penetrate into the pyramidal zone, but none extends as far as the surface.

It is a curious fact that the astrocytes in the pyramidal and subpyramidal layers resemble the neighboring nerve cells, *i.e.* the pyramidal neurons in the first place and the stellate cells in the second.

Heavy precipitations prevented the astrocytes from being investigated in the most superficial layers of any of the fetuses in this group (36–42 g). They were clearly seen in a specimen of 49 g, however (Fig. 15, inset). The small cell bodies are situated on the border between the pyramidal and the marginal zones, but most processes are directed outwards, and confined to the marginal layer. Usually one or two apical processes are comparatively thick, whereas the others are very delicate and extensively ramified. Occasionally, a thin dendrite is directed inwards, simulating an axon. Again, the similarity between these astrocytes and the neighboring nerve cells is striking. However, the astrocytes here are more irregularly shaped, their processes more ramified and frequently thinner than those of the neurons; many of them extend to the most superficial part of the marginal zone, whereas the apical dendrites of the nerve cells always terminate within the inner part of the zone.

47–50-g fetuses

The main change in this group is the appearance of corticopetal fibers throughout the neocortex (Fig. 16). They ascend from the intermediate zone, occasionally emit a few short collaterals when passing the pyramidal layer, and are dissolved in the marginal zone, where their terminal branches frequently run horizontally. In contrast to the radiating fibers, they are very delicate and tortuous, and — in most cases — cross the pyramidal layer obliquely. The exact origin of these afferent fibers is unknown, but it is conceivable, even likely, that they emanate from both callosal and thalamic elements. They were clearly seen for the first time in a fetus of 49 g. However, some observations, though admittedly incomplete, indicate that they already begin to penetrate the pyramidal cell layer in animals weighing 25 g.

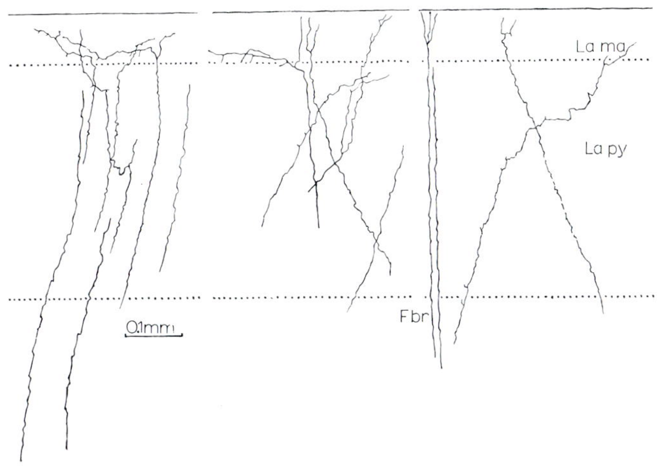

Fig. 16. 49-gram fetus, estimated age 59 days. Afferent 'oblique' fibers to pyramidal and marginal layers in three different areas of the isocortex in lateral hemispherical wall. Two radiating fibers (Fb r) in right picture. Golgi method.

61–75-g fetuses

The surface is still lissencephalic, and the general structure of the telencephalon remains largely unchanged. As before, the radiating fibers dominate in the *intermediate zone*, where many of them terminate. In one specimen, weighing 66 g, a series of neuroblasts (nb) were well impregnated in the outer part of the intermediate zone (Fig. 17B). Their pear-shaped cell bodies are bipolar. Thin axons run in a central direction, and the thicker, short, somewhat tortuous dendrites, which occasionally emit one or more thin branches, are directed towards the hemispherical surface. Some of the tips are enlarged, forming blunted ends. Astrocytes (as) and stellate cells (C st) are mingled with the neuroblasts.

The *pyramidal layer* still has a primitive character (Fig. 17A). However, the neurons

References p. 57–59

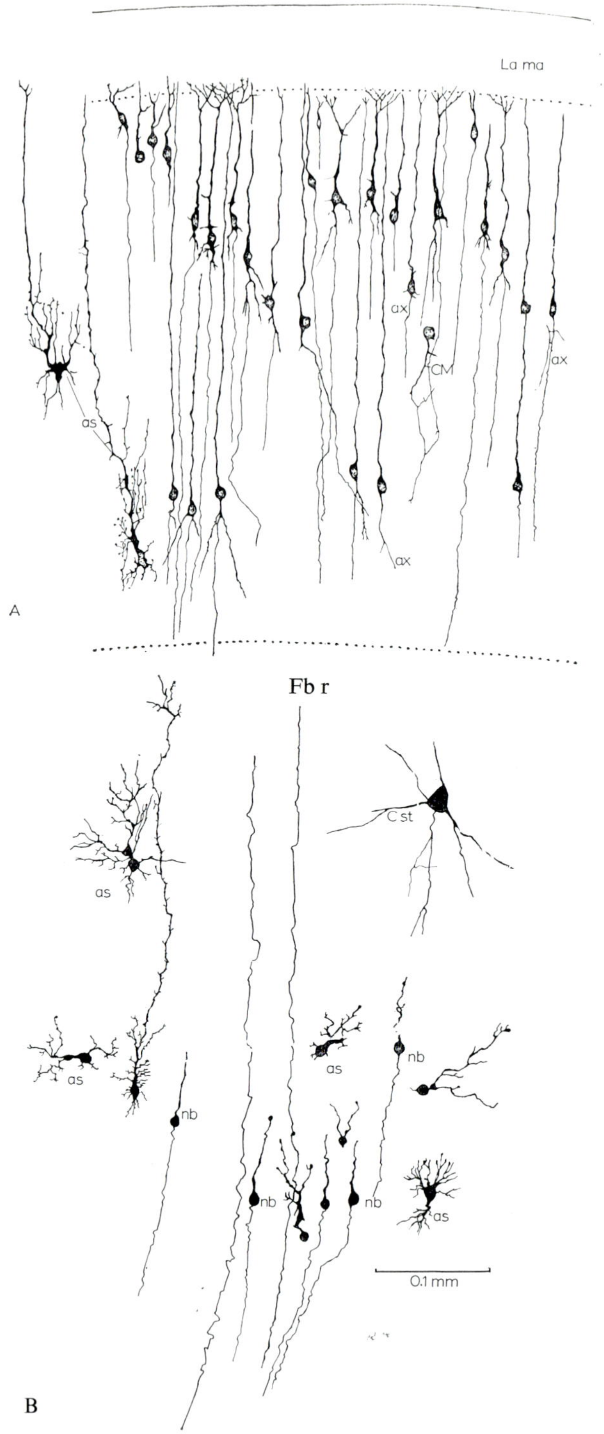

Fig. 17. 66-gram fetus, estimated age 60 days. Composite picture of pyramidal cells in one area (A) and of subpyramidal elements in an adjacent area (B) of same block, placed in correct relation to each other and to the surface. Golgi method. (A) Cells in superficial stratum of pyramidal layer have immature bipolar appearance. Cells in middle part are more highly developed than those in deeper stratum of layer; some of them have long descending basal dendrites. Martinotti cell with ascending axon (C M). Short axon collaterals (ax) on cell at right. Two astrocytes on left side of picture. (B) Neuroblasts (nb), astrocytes (as), stellate cell (C st) and radiating fibers (Fb r) in subpyramidal area.

in the middle stratum of the layer are more highly developed than those in the younger animals, and some of them have attained the typical pyramidal shape. Several dendrites emanate from the base of the cell bodies. Most of them are short but there are also some long, slender, basal dendrites, which descend to lower strata, but never to the subcortical areas. The apical dendrites bifurcate in the marginal zone as usual, ramification being somewhat more elaborate than in younger aminals. The shafts of many apical dendrites also have a few short branches.

The cells in the inferior part of the layer are less well developed than those in the middle. The cell bodies are rounded and somewhat smaller, lack basal dendrites or have one or two short descending processes; and, in the marginal zone, their apical dendrites either divide slightly or do not divide at all.

The neurons in the most superficial stratum of the pyramidal zone have the bipolar appearance of undifferentiated cells.

Most axons of the pyramidal cells are smooth and undivided, but the very first traces of the incipient development of collaterals can be observed in a small number of them (Fig. 17A, right). All axons descend to the intermediate zone.

Nearly all nerve cells in the pyramidal layer have apical dendrites, which extend to the marginal zone. However, one cell without an apical dendrite is seen in Fig. 17A (CM). In contrast to the pyramidal cells, the axon of this neuron proceeds to the surface and is therefore a true Martinotti cell. The appearance of this type of cell signals an important forthcoming change in the structure of the pyramidal layer.

The apical dendrites of the pyramidal cells branch more elaborately than earlier, and extend further into the superficial parts of the marginal zone (but never as far as the astrocytes and the epithelial fibers).

Afferent fibers descend, as they did previously, from the marginal to the pyramidal layer where they seem to terminate, especially in its middle part. The ascending fibers cross the pyramidal cell layer obliquely and end in the marginal zone; some collaterals proceed also to the middle part of the pyramidal cell layer.

The *astrocytes* are present at all levels of the cortex and dominate the picture in many Golgi-stained sections. They are more highly developed and many of them are connected to blood vessels (more of them than previously?), mostly via perivascular feet, but sometimes through the astrocytic cell body itself. Fig. 17A shows two representative cells (as), one in the middle and the other in the deep part of the pyramidal layer.

95-g fetus

A shallow impression on the dorsolateral aspect of the telencephalic surface represents the prospective suprasylvian gyrus.

Sections stained with cresyl violet show elements of a new type which have smaller and darker nuclei, lack visible nucleoli and seem to belong to astrocytes (Fig. 18A). A few similar cells were already visible in the 39-g fetus, but they have now increased in number and are almost as common as the pyramidal cells. They are present everywhere in the layer but are most abundant in its middle and its deep strata.

References p. 57–59

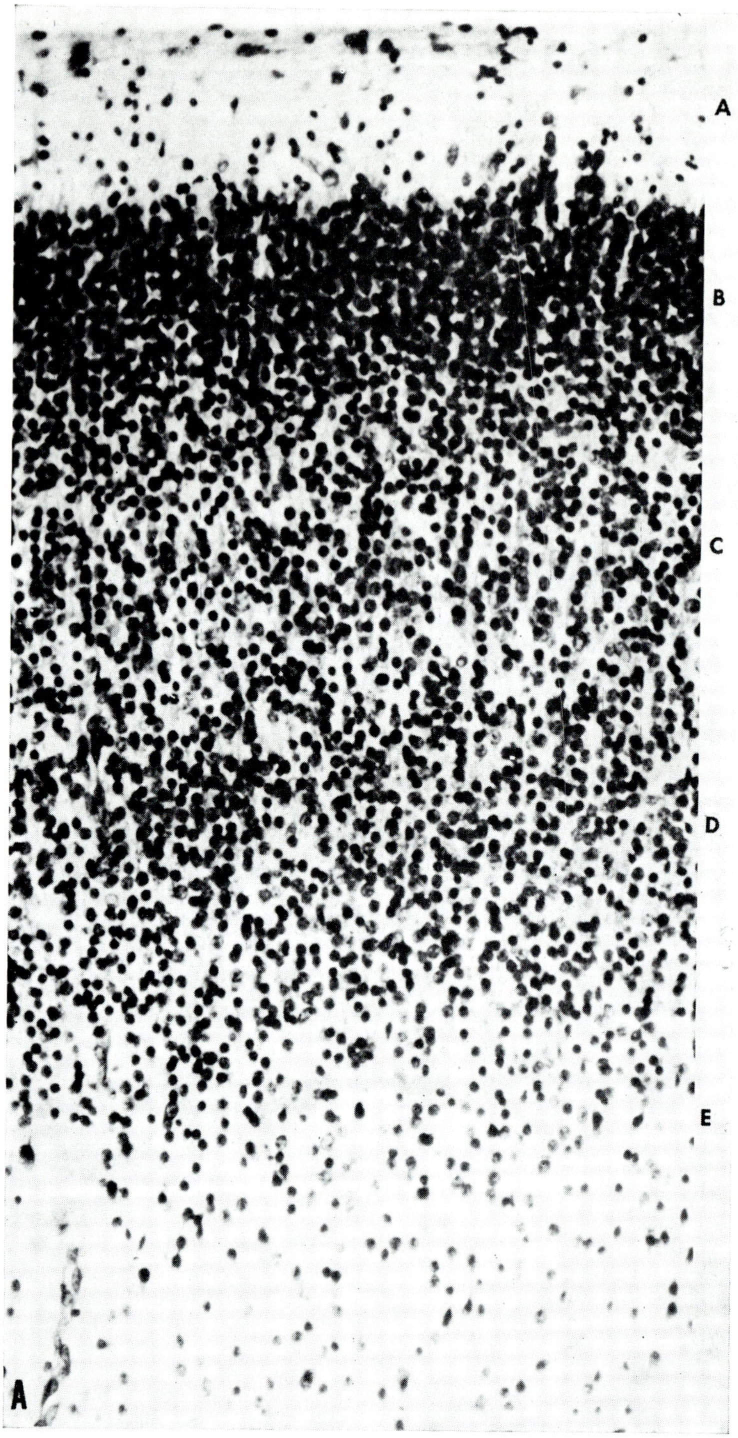

Fig. 18A. 95-gram fetus, estimated age 62 days. Stratification more evident than in younger animals (*cf.* 39-gram fetus in Fig. 13B). Cresyl violet, × 400.

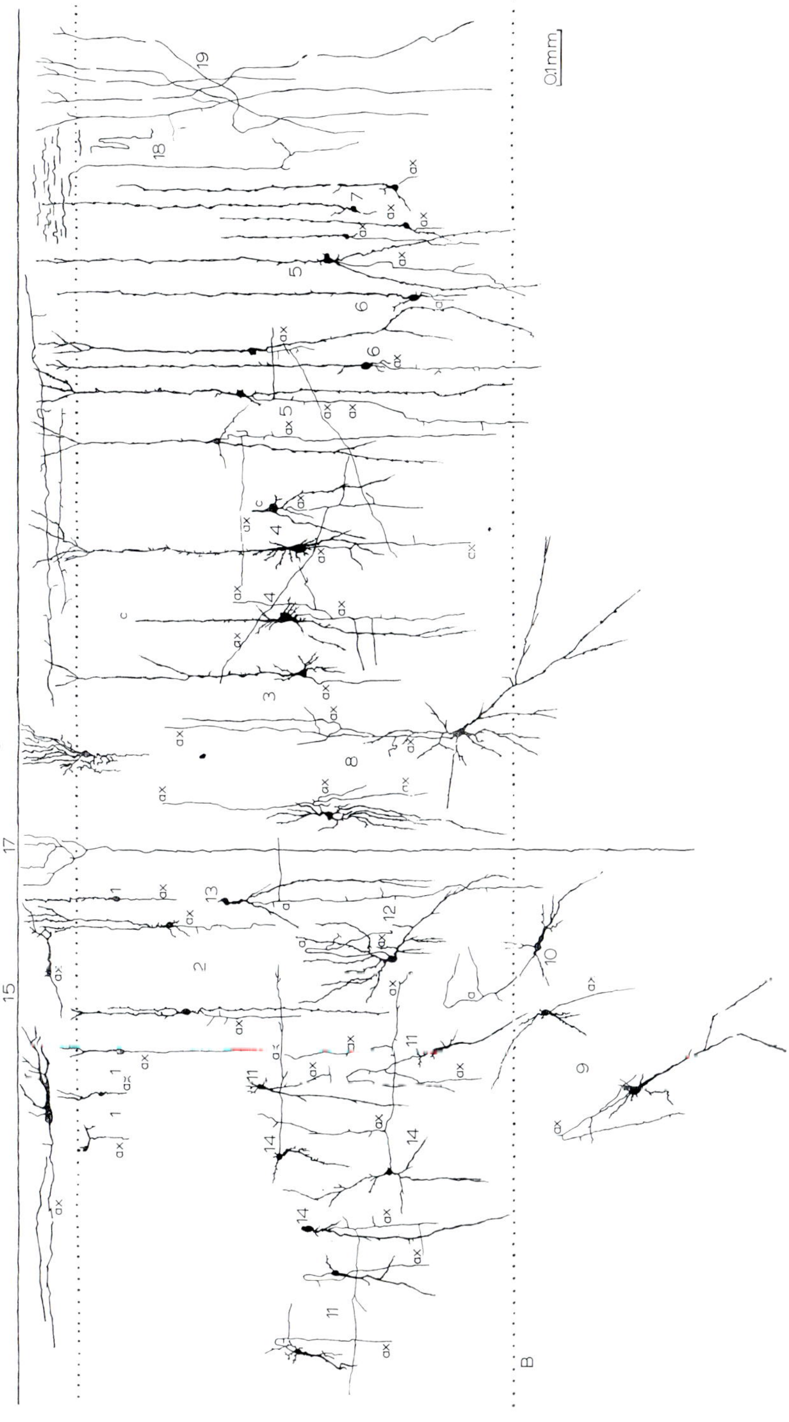

Fig. 18B. 94-gram fetus, estimated age 62 days. Golgi method. Much fuller information on cortical differentiation is obtained from Golgi sections than from corresponding Nissl picture in (A). 1 = simple bipolar cells in superficial part of pyramidal layer; 2 = somewhat deeper and more highly developed cell, whose axon has short collaterals; 3, 4, 5 = pyramidal cells in middle part of layer; some have long axon collaterals, basal and apical dendrites are more highly developed; 6, 7 = deep pyramidal cells are less well developed than those in middle stratum; 8 = Martinotti cells with ascending axons; 9, 10 = stellate cells in subpyramidal zone of the type seen in younger specimens; 11, 12, 13, 14 = stellate cells in pyramidal layer, not seen in younger specimens; 15 = horizontal cells in marginal layer; 16 = astrocyte; 17 = radiating fiber; 18 = descending afferent fibers to pyramidal layer; 19 = ascending 'oblique' afferent fibers.

The 4-layer stratification of the pyramidal zone is more evident than it was in the 39-g fetus (*cf.* Figs. 13B and 18A) owing to the further development and separation of the nerve cells in the middle part (C). Many cells here have comparatively large nuclei with light, scattered chromatin, a prominent nucleolus, and cytoplasm containing a fine dust-like material (Nissl-bodies?). The nerve cells in the lower part of the zone (D) are also somewhat more highly developed, whereas those in the most superficial stratum (B) are still crowded, and have the same shape as in younger animals.

Many small dark nuclei in the inner part of the marginal zone (A) indicate the presence of numerous astrocytes. There seem to be less neuroblasts and more astrocytes in the intermediate zone than earlier. The stellate cells are seen mainly in the subpyramidal zone (stratum E in Fig. 18A).

However, sections stained with cresyl violet give an incomplete picture of the cortical development at this stage. Examination of a series of successfully impregnated Golgi sections (Fig. 18B) showed that dramatic changes had occurred in the 95-g fetus, compared with that of 75 g. The fundamentally new changes are: (1) the development of collaterals on the axons from the pyramidal cells, and (2) the appearance of stellate cells in the pyramidal zone.

The details in Fig. 18B were drawn from impregnated cells in a series of sections of one block. All the cells illustrated were situated within the same very limited region of the anterior part of the parietal area.

Cells 3–7 in Fig. 18B are reminiscent of those in the middle and the inferior strata of the 66-g fetus (Fig. 17A). However, an important difference is the development of collaterals on many of their axons. The axons of the cells in the middle stratum (4, 5) may have as many as 4 collaterals which can be up to 300 μ long. Their course is largely horizontal, and they seem to constitute a primitive band of Baillarger. At least one recurrent, *i.e.* ascending collateral was also seen (No. 4, left). All axons seem to descend to subpyramidal areas (some have been cut off in the section).

The dendrites of the cells in the middle pyramidal stratum are also more highly developed than they were earlier. Cells 3–4 now have a true pyramidal shape; their basal dendrites are more numerous, the apical extensions are thicker and they have branches proximally and even indications of 'spines'. Other cells are smaller (5) but have long descending dendrites, some of which extend to the lower border of the pyramidal layer. This type of cell has been seen in all previous Golgi sections.

The cells in the lower part of the pyramidal layer (6, 7) are less well developed; the cell body is small and has few, if any, basal dendrites, the apical extension proceeds to, but does not ramify in the marginal zone, and the axon has either short collaterals or none at all.

The cells in the uppermost strata are also less well developed than those in the middle part of the pyramidal layer. The most superficial neurons (1) still have a simple bipolar appearance. Deeper cells (2) may have double apical dendrites, basal processes and short axon collaterals.

In contrast to the cells described, the stellate neurons in the left part of Fig. 18B (11–14) were not observed earlier in the pyramidal zone. They lack apical dendrites (by definition of normal stellate cells) and have various shapes. Frequently the perikaryon has several short, thin branches and one or two larger descending branches (11, 13, 14), but some cells have one (14) or more (12) ascending dendrites.

The axons of the stellate cells ramify within the pyramidal layer, horizontally and vertically (11, 14). Most of the axons seem to terminate within the pyramidal zone, but some do descend to lower levels (*e.g.* 13).

The stellate cells in the pyramidal zone have the same appearance as those in the subcortical area (9, 10) where this type of cell was already seen at the 12-g stage (Fig. 6).

Two neurons (8) differ from the other stellate cells, since their axons, which are extensively ramified, ascend (presumably to the marginal layer) but have been cut off. They are true Martinotti cells.

The afferent cortical fibers are of the type previously observed (Fig. 18B, right). Oblique fibers ascend from the 'white matter' (19), and collaterals descend from the horizontal fibers (18). The marginal layer and the middle part of the pyramidal zone are the receiving stations. The horizontal cells in the marginal layer (15) appear unchanged. The picture also shows one astrocyte (16) and the termination of one epithelial fiber in the marginal zone (17).

The cortical astrocytes have further developed (Fig. 19). Their endings form, together with the terminations of the radiating fibers (Fb r), a dense tangle in the marginal zone (La ma), in which neurons, nerve fibers and the ramifications of apical dendrites are embedded. The astrocytes have numerous connections with blood vessels, as is seen in the picture.

147-g fetus

The cells in the middle stratum of the pyramidal layer have somewhat more highly developed basal dendrites (Fig. 20), but their general appearance is the same as in the 95-g animal. Recurrent axon collaterals are now seen to extend to the marginal zone (Fig. 20A). Two cells with ascending axons (C M), and one cell with short branches (Golgi-II?) are seen on the right side of Fig. 20A.

180–187-g fetuses

An incipient gyration is now clearly visible (Fig. 21A). The prospective parietal gyrus is to the right of the suprasylvian fissure on the dorsolateral aspect of the hemisphere.

The cell-stained sections (Figs. 21A and B) reveal a higher degree of cortical development than was previously observed. There is a 4-layer stratification of alternating dark and light bands in the pyramidal layer (in the medial wall even a 5-layering is recognizable). The most superficial cells are still those least well developed. They are densely packed, and form a dark stratum. The remaining cells are further apart from each other, have large nuclei with light chromatin, and visible cytoplasm.

The Golgi section of the 187-g fetus in Fig. 22 shows that the superficial cells in the pyramidal layer have retained their primitive bipolar appearance, whereas the cells in the intermediate part of the layer have still more highly developed basal dendrites

References p. 57–59

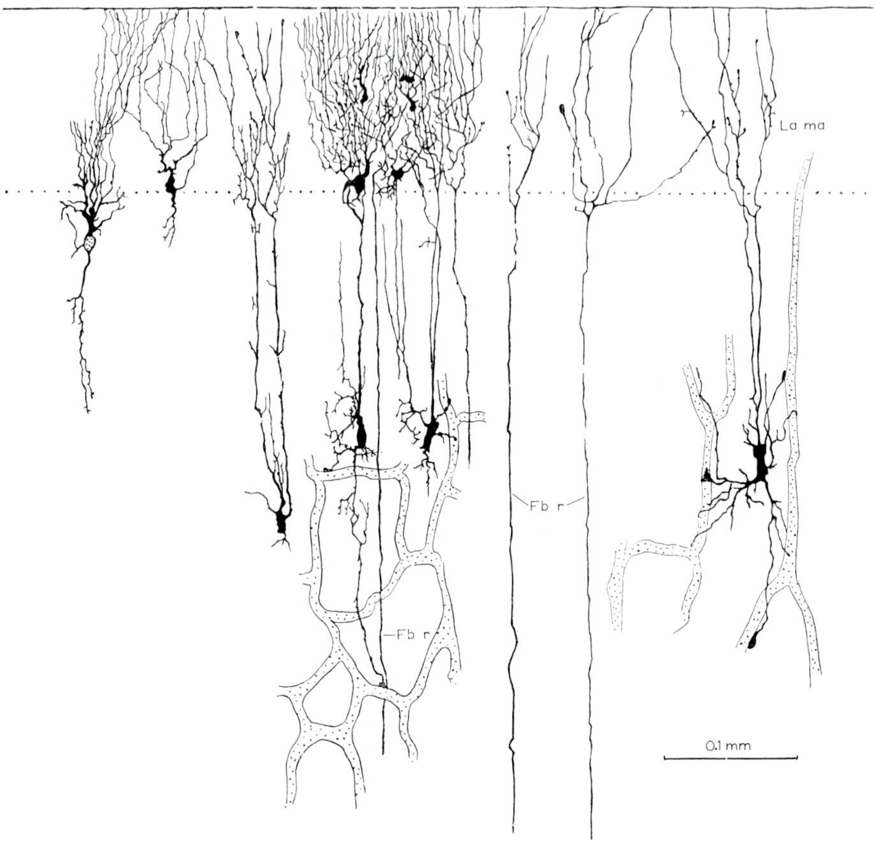

Fig. 19. 94-gram fetus (same animal and area as in Fig. 18B), estimated age 62 days. Well developed astrocytes in pyramidal and marginal layers. Some have connections with capillaries. Radiating fibers (Fb r). Golgi method.

than they had earlier. The cells in the deeper parts are not clearly visible in this preparation. However, the scrutiny of other sections indicates that, though more highly developed, they still do not have a true pyramidal shape.

265-g fetus

The superficial cells retain a simple primitive appearance, whereas there are many well developed pyramidal cells in the other layers.

450–460-g fetuses

The gyration of the cerebral hemispheres is rather advanced (Fig. 23A), and there is a clear 6-layer stratification of the cortex. Even in the most superficial stratum (Fig. 23B) the cells are much more fully developed and are situated further apart from each other than previously; the nuclei are large and light, and the cytoplasm contains

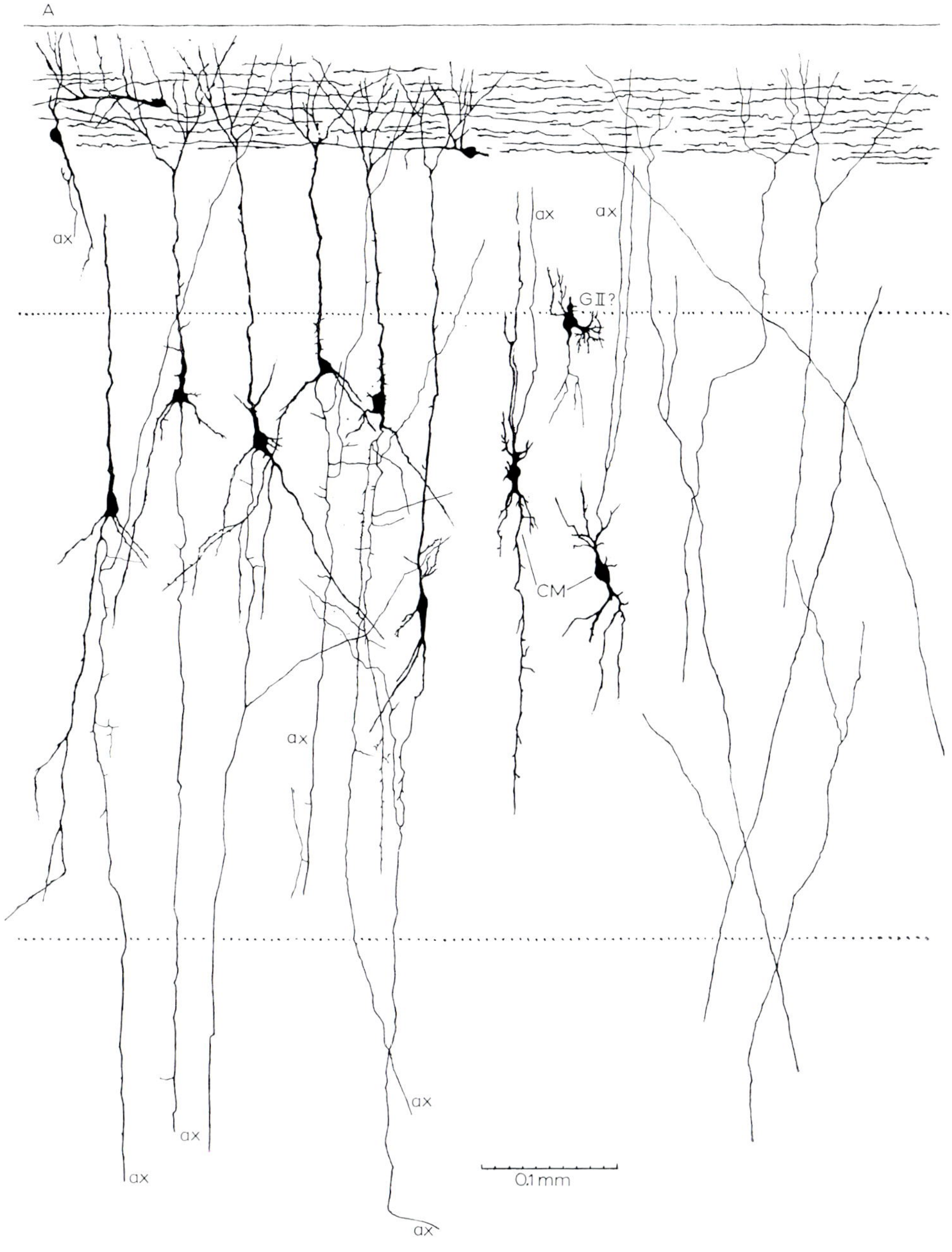

Fig. 20. 147-gram fetus, estimated age 66 days. Golgi method. (A) Still more highly developed cells in middle stratum of pyramidal layer. Recurrent collaterals extend to marginal zone. Two Martinotti cells (C M) and possibly one Golgi II type of cell (GII?). 'Oblique' afferent fibers to the right. Upper dotted line indicates approximate lower border of superficial stratum in pyramidal layer. Lower dotted line represents inferior border of pyramidal layer. (B) Adjacent area to (A). Cells in middle stratum have long descending dendrites. Deep cells are still less highly developed. Terminal branches of apical dendrites are covered by precipitations (La ma). Two radiating fibers to the right (Fb r). (C) Microphotograph of area adjacent to A and B. Lack of details, especially in collaterals, is due to difficulty in focusing in 100 μ thick section, $\times$ 250.

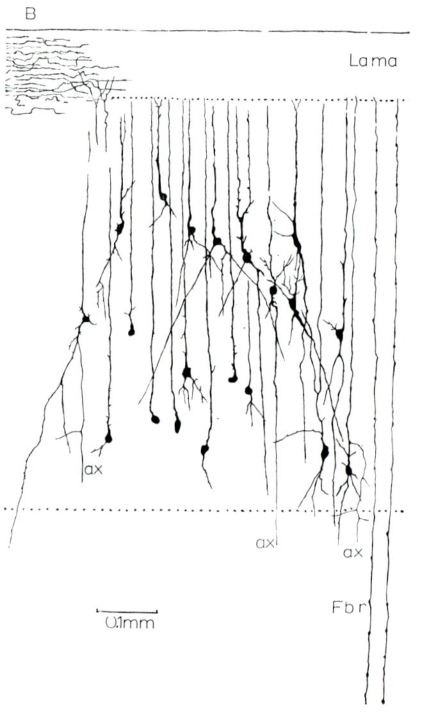
B
Lama
ax
ax
ax
Fbr
0.1mm

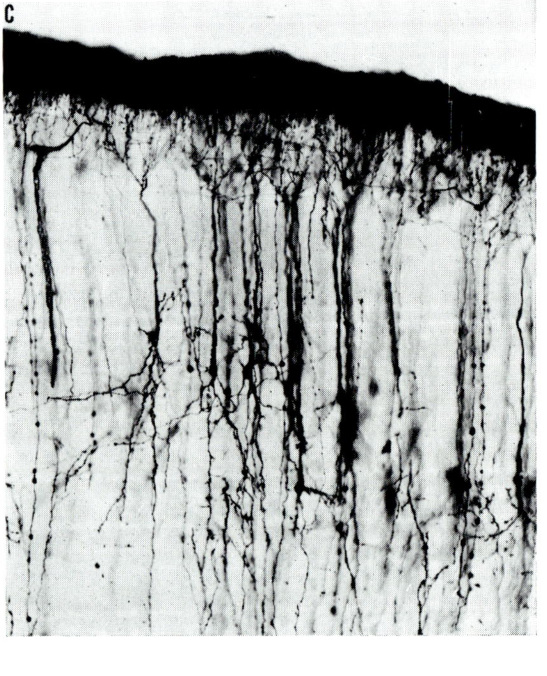
C

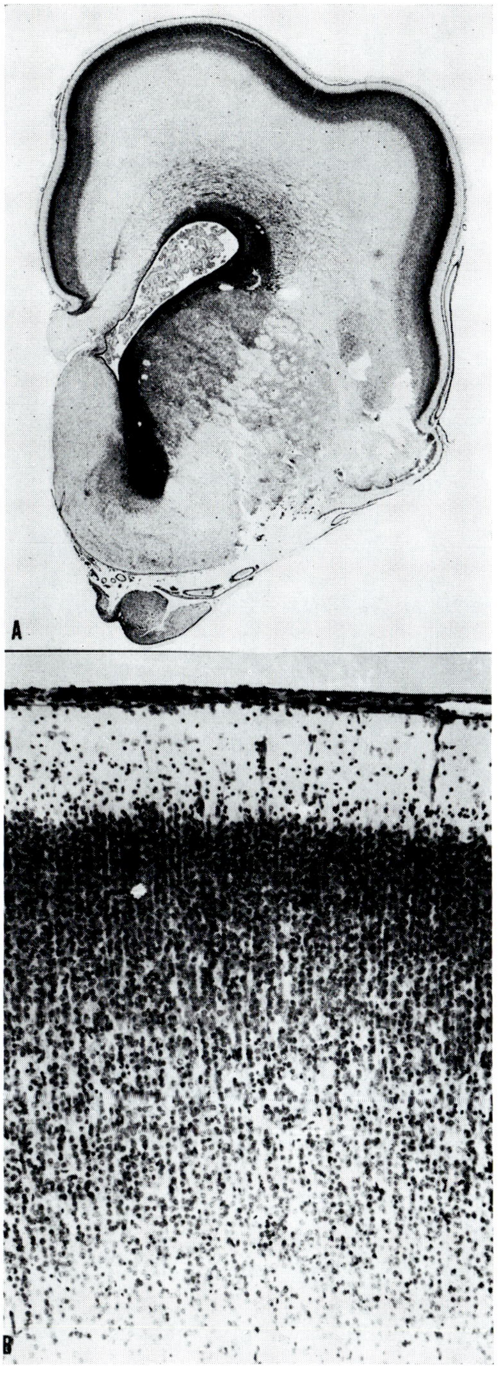

Fig. 21. 180-gram fetus, estimated age 71 days. Cresyl violet. (A) Cross section through one hemisphere at level of anterior limb of internal capsule. Incipient gyration: suprasylvian fissure on dorsal aspect. Cortical stratification more clearly visible than in younger specimens, × 11. (B) Isocortex; detail of (A). Well developed cells in all pyramidal strata except the most superficial one, × 190.

References p. 57–59

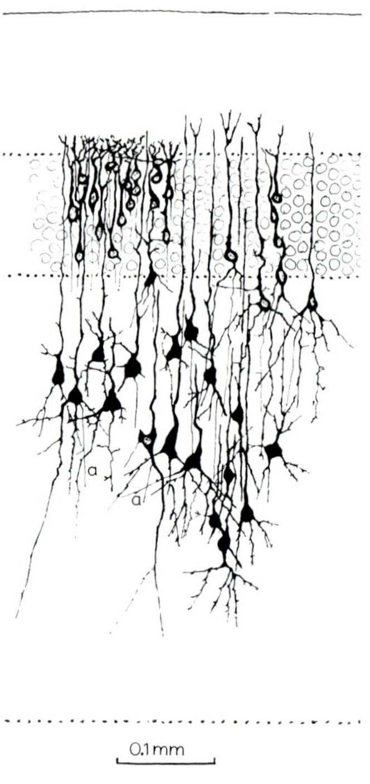

Fig. 22. 187-gram fetus, estimated age 71 days. Superficial cells (enclosed by dotted lines) in pyramidal layer still have an immature bipolar appearance. Cells in middle stratum are more highly developed than in younger specimens. Deep cells not stained. Golgi method.

Nissl bodies. This development is reflected also in the Golgi material (Fig. 24), which shows well differentiated pyramidal cells in all the strata. The more superficial neurons have widely branching apical dendrites. In the middle stratum most pyramidal cells have long descending dendrites. Large, well developed pyramidal cells in the deepest stratum have basal dendrites and apical extensions, which are covered with spines and often ramify widely before termination.

SUMMARY OF SALIENT FINDINGS

Although the neuroembryogenesis is naturally a continuous process the following stages can be recognized.

1.1 g. The evaginated telencephalic vesicles are thin, and an isocortical plate (Co is) has been formed only in their lateral, *i.e.* convex, walls (Figs. 1A and B). The cells in the primordial cortex (Figs. 1C and D) already show signs of differentiation, however, when compared with those in the mantle zone (Mn). The marginal zone (La ma) is most highly developed; it seems to contain horizontal cells. The thin pyramidal layer (La py) is made up of bipolar cells with apical processes which extend into the marginal zone (Fig. 1D).

6.5 g. The pallial wall is thicker, and the formation of the primordial isocortex

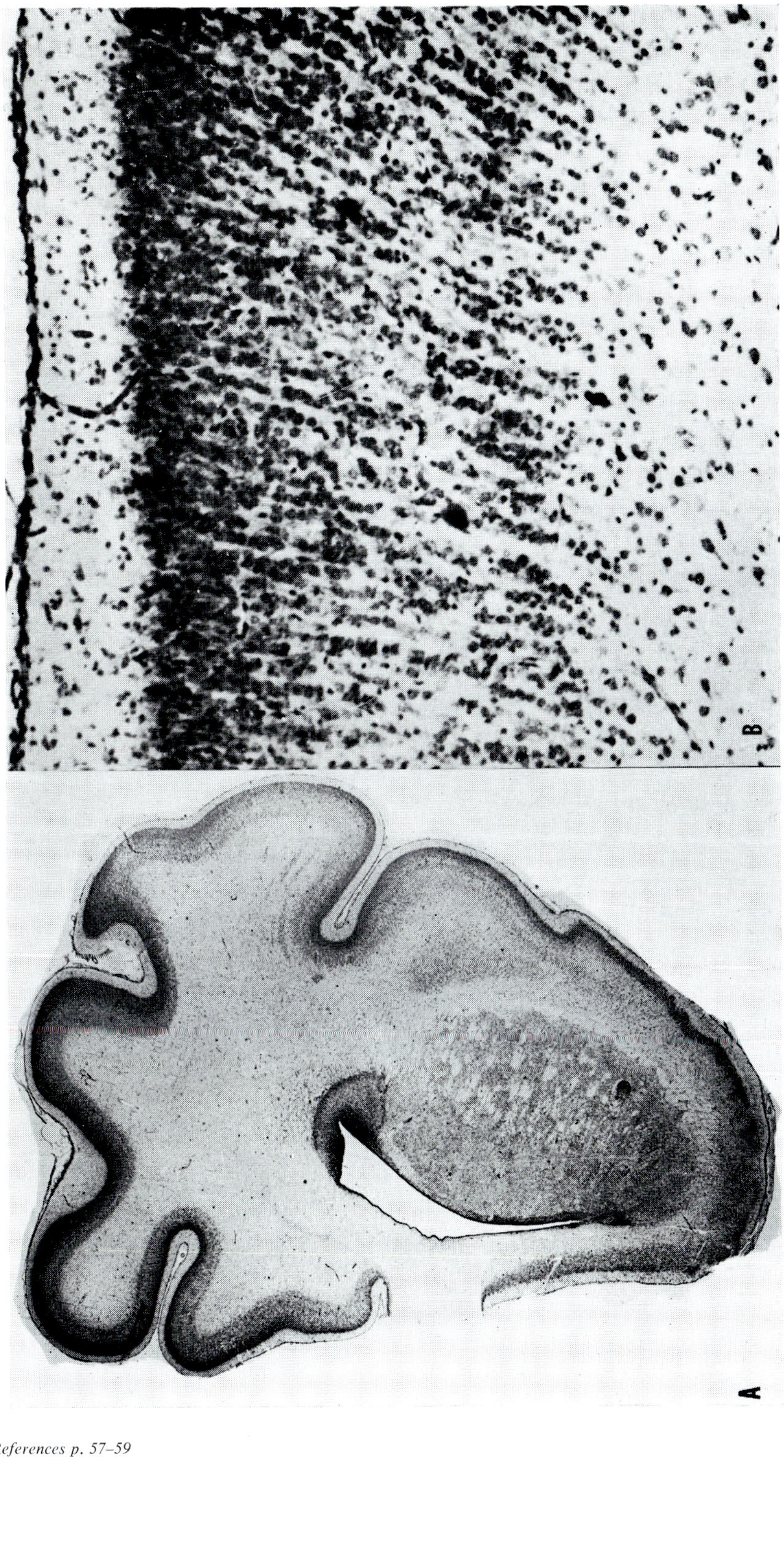

Fig. 23. 450-gram fetus, estimated age 89 days. Cresyl violet. (A) Coronal section through one hemisphere at level of splenium of the corpus callosum. Gyration and cortical striation more evident than in younger specimens, × 11. (B) Isocortex; detail of (A). Immature nerve cells in cortex no longer visible, × 210.

References p. 57–59

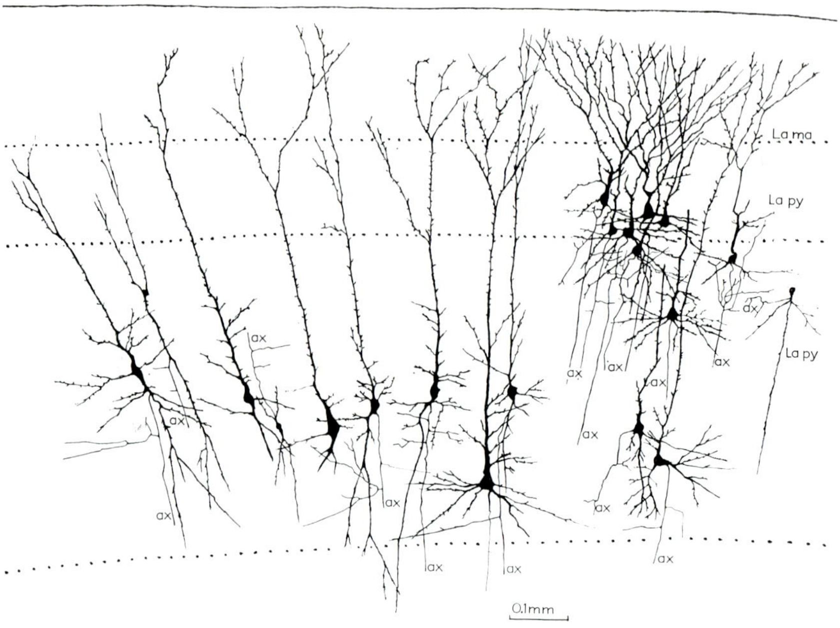

Fig. 24. 468-gram fetus, estimated age 90 days. Mature neurons in cortex. Compare with Fig. 23B. Golgi method.

(Co is) is more complete (Fig. 2A). The 4 layers of the primitive neopallial wall (as defined on p. 4) are recognizable (Fig. 2B); this wall will continue to have the same general appearance until gyration begins. Numerous neuroblasts have migrated into the pyramidal layer (La py), which, consequently, is much thicker than it was previously. The marginal layer (La ma), on the other hand, is comparatively unchanged (Fig. 2D). The intermediate layer (La im), which has replaced the mantle zone, contains numerous fibers. An internal capsule-like structure is visible (Fig. 2A, Cp i).

12 g. A series of Golgi sections have shown that the superficial cells in the pyramidal zone (La py) are of a primitive bipolar type (Figs. 6 and 7), whereas the deeper cells have well developed basal dendrites and axons which emit collaterals to the outer part of the intermediate layer (Figs. 7A, C–E). Neuroblasts were never observed in the cortical plate.

The outer part of the intermediate zone (La im) contains many well differentiated stellate cells with long dendrites which occasionally branch, and with axons that emit collaterals (Fig. 6). These cells will later become incorporated into the pyramidal layer. They should, therefore, be considered as parts of the primordial isocortex even if they appear to be situated in the intermediate layer, which is conventionally regarded as forthcoming white matter.

All cells in the pyramidal layer emit apical dendrites that extend to the deeper part of the marginal layer, where they terminate forming branches of varying length. Furthermore, the marginal zone contains horizontal fibers (Fb h) and cells.

To conclude, at this stage the primordial isocortex already displays 4 different strata: (1) the marginal layer; (2) the primitive bipolar cells in the pyramidal layer; (3) the more deeply situated, pyramidal cells with basal dendrites; and (4) the stellate cells in the intermediate substance. It should be emphasized that there is no indication yet of cortical stratification as seen in the Nissl-stained sections.

The cortical afferent fibers seem to fall into two groups: (1) descending elements from the horizontal fibers in the marginal layer (Fig. 5); and (2) ascending collaterals presumably from thalamic and callosal fibers (Fig. 4C). Both sets of elements, together with collaterals from axons of some deep pyramidal cells (Figs. 7C and D), are directed towards the stellate cells in the outer part of the intermediate zone (Fig. 6). Some branches of the descending collaterals from the horizontal fibers also terminate around the deep (more highly differentiated) pyramidal cells.

No afferent connections from the thalamic or callosal elements were seen to penes trate the cortical plate. It might well be that the marginal cells receive afferent fiber- from the olfactory system, since the olfactory bulbs are covered with bundles which seem to be continuous with the horizontal fibers covering the primordial isocortex.

The internal capsule (Cp i) is made up of elements from the thalamic radiation (R th) and projection fibers (Fb p) which emanate from the cortical cells and proceed further down to lower levels of the neuraxis (Fig. 3). In the telencephalic wall these elements are mainly situated peripherally to the commissural fibers of the corpus callosum (Fb cc) (Fig. 4).

25 g. Many well developed nerve cells are seen in the marginal zone (Figs. 9A and C). The pyramidal layer is thicker but the cells are still rather undeveloped (Fig. 9A). All apical dendrites extend as far as the marginal zone.

The stellate cells in the outer part of the intermediate zone are well differentiated; they form a stratum in the subpyramidal area (Fig. 9B).

The epithelial cells with their radiating fibers predominate in many Golgi sections (Fig. 8).

The intermediate zone is thicker but has the same general structure as that observed in the 12-g specimen.

40 g. All layers have increased in thickness, but the fundamental plan of the hemispherical wall is the same as that observed earlier (Figs. 10 and 11). Numerous neuroblasts migrate through the intermediate layer (Fig. 12) to the pyramidal zone.

The pyramidal layer, when seen in Nissl sections, displays an incipient stratification due to the appearance of a somewhat light band in its middle third (Fig. 13). The impression of a light stratum is due mainly to the more highly developed nuclei and perikarya and to a widening here of the intercellular spaces. Consequently, 5 alternating lighter and darker layers can now be recognized in the cortical plate.

The 'second migration' of glia cells has started, and astrocytes have appeared in the cortical plate (Fig. 15). Hitherto astrocytes were seen only in the matrix. The epithelial cells, with their radiating fibers, are still numerous.

50 g. A new feature is the penetration of afferent fibers into the cortex (Fig. 16). These 'oblique fibers' (according to Cajal) emanate from the thalamic or callosal elements, or, more likely, from both these systems. The fibers terminate mainly in the

References p. 57–59

marginal layer, but a few small collaterals proceed to the middle part of the pyramidal layer.

75 g. The main changes are: (1) the incipient formation of axon collaterals (Fig. 17A, right); and (2) the appearance of single Martinotti cells (C M) in the cortex, which have ascending axons and lack apical dendrites.

The pyramidal neurons, especially those in the middle third of the layer, are more differentiated than they were earlier, but the picture is still largely rather primitive (Fig. 17A). The most highly developed cells have several short basal dendrites and, occasionally, one long process which may descend as far as the deepest part of the zone. The terminal branches of the apical dendrites have now become somewhat more elaborate, and a few short branches are occasionally seen on the shafts. The astrocytes (as) in the cortical plate are more numerous and more highly developed than they were earlier; they dominate the cortical picture in many Golgi sections.

95 g. Two important changes have occurred. (1) The axon collaterals of pyramidal cells in the middle third of the layer have developed considerably. They frequently have a more or less horizontal course and are, therefore, largely distributed within the same stratum as the corresponding cell bodies (Fig. 18B; 4, 5). (2) Numerous stellate cells have appeared in the pyramidal layer (11–14). Many of their axons divide and terminate within the cortex and, consequently, they can facilitate intra-cortical connections, *i.e.* serve as interneurons. Similar cells are seen in the outer part of the intermediate zone (9–10), as they had been from the 12-g stage onward. Well developed Martinotti cells are also present in the pyramidal layer (Fig. 18B; 8).

The basal dendrites of the pyramidal cells, which are situated in the middle part of the layer, are now more highly developed (3–5), and occasional spines are observed on the apical processes. The dendrites and axon collaterals of more deeply situated neurons (6–7) are less well developed, but the most primitive cells are seen now, as earlier, in the most superficial part of the pyramidal layer (Fig. 18B; 1). In all cortical and subcortical areas the astrocytes are numerous and well developed; frequently they are attached to blood vessels (Fig. 19).

A slight indication of the forthcoming gyration was noted.

145 g. The cortical picture (Fig. 20) is fundamentally the same as in the 95-g animal. Recurrent collaterals from the axons of pyramidal cells are now clearly seen to proceed to the marginal layer (Fig. 20A).

180 g. The beginning of a gyration is clearly visible (Fig. 21A). The differentiation of nuclei and cell bodies has progressed further, except in the most superficial part of the pyramidal zone where the cells still have a primitive bipolar appearance (Figs. 21B and 22).

450 g. The gyration of the cerebral hemispheres is more pronounced (Fig. 23A), the stratification of the cortex more evident (Fig. 23B), and the development of nuclear and cytological details more advanced. Golgi-stained sections (Fig. 24) show, *inter alia*, that the superficial neurons in the pyramidal layer have now lost their primitive bipolar appearance and have well developed dendrites, and that there are large pyramidal cells in the deepest stratum of this layer.

DISCUSSION

Formation of the isocortical plate. Differentiation of nerve cells. For a more exact appraisal of the migration of blast cells special methods have to be applied, such as autoradiography, *e.g.* as employed by Sidman *et al.* (1959). Such an analysis was not made in this investigation of the isocortex in the fetal sheep brain, and the following data are, therefore, only approximative.

The migration of neuroblasts in the fetal sheep starts before the 1-g stage (estimated fetal age 20 days) and continues up to at least the 100-g level (estimated age 65 days).

Except for the radiating fibers and rare epithelial cells the intermediate and cortical layers contain only neuroblasts and their derivatives up to the 40-g stage. Astrocytes then appear in increasing numbers. The movement of their precursors, the spongioblasts, constitutes 'a second migration' according to Lorente de Nó (1933). The formation and migration of the spongioblasts probably continues longer than that of the neuroblasts.

At an early stage in development, numerous radiating fibers of the epithelial cells penetrate the telencephalic wall. They appear to serve as scaffolding as suggested by Cajal (1960). From the 100-g stage onward they gradually disappear, *i.e.* when the astrocytes are found in the cortex in increasing numbers and the cortical neurons are becoming more and more mature.

Mitoses were never seen outside the matrix, and, therefore, the isocortical plate seems to be made up exclusively of cells which originated in the germinal zone and migrated through the intermediate layer to cortical areas.

Neuroblasts were never seen in the isocortical plate in the Golgi sections of this material, *i.e.* from the 12-g stage onward. Cajal (1906, 1911) also states that these elements are rare in the fetal cortex in rabbit and mouse. Furthermore, with the exception of stellate cells, differentiated neurons were not seen below the pyramidal layer. Consequently, it seems probable that all neuroblasts in the neopallial wall migrate to predetermined areas in the cortical plate, where differentiation will then start. That differentiated pyramidal cells are able to migrate or even rotate (Rabinowicz, 1964) is inconceivable. Cajal has also refuted the idea of a rotation of cortical neurons (1911). The capacity for migration is the most characteristic quality of the neuroblasts, which also seem to be ideally shaped for that purpose. Levi-Montalcini (1964) has pointed out that the neuroblasts lose this capacity after they have reached the ultimate positions where their transformation into nerve cells will begin. The downward movement of cortical layers (*vide infra*) is different and is not based upon the active migration of individual cells.

The further differentiation of neurons in the cortical plate involves a series of extremely complicated processes.

A *marginal layer* appears earlier than the other layers. Indeed, it can be recognized as soon as a cortical plate has been formed, *i.e.* in the lateral hemispherical wall of the 1.1-g fetus. There were no Golgi sections from this early stage, but Nissl sections reveal, quite clearly, differentiated nerve cells, *i.e.* bipolar cells which are oriented parallel with the surface of the brain. The marginal layer also acquires a mature

References p. 57–59

appearance earlier, *i.e.* within a shorter period of development, than do the other cortical layers. The increase in volume during the subsequent development seems to be due less to the addition of nerve cells than to the invasion of the zone by glia cells, the multiplication of glial fibers, the branching and growth of the endings of the apical dendrites and, possibly, the increase in the horizontal fiber system.

The large Cajal–Retzius cells were rarely seen in this material. This seems to be due partly to the fact that these cells are less common in lower than in higher vertebrates, particularly in man, and partly to technical difficulties; the superficial parts of the brain are frequently covered by precipitates in sections stained according to Golgi's rapid method. A subpial granular layer (Brun, 1965) was never observed.

It is remarkable that, as early as at the 12-g stage, well developed *stellate cells* were observed in the subpyramidal regions. Nissl-stained sections indicate that such cells are present even in the 6-g fetus. They are first scattered in the outer part of the intermediate zone, where they form a stratum. During the subsequent development cell bodies of prospective pyramidal and other cortical neurons, which have developed and migrated later than the stellate cells in question, will occupy positions in the wide extracellular regions of the outer part of the intermediate zone. In other words, the pyramidal zone will extend downwards and incorporate the stellate cells. The wide spaces referred to will also receive assocation and projection fibers as well as glia cells.

The presence of a subpyramidal layer of stellate cells in a very early phase of prenatal development has hardly been appreciated previously. Cajal (1906) recognized in rabbits (Nissl sections?) at term a deep layer of spindle- or ball-formed 'polymorphous' cells, which must be homologous to the formation described here. They can also be seen in Retzius, 1893, Fig. 1 (14-cm dog fetus) and in Lorente de Nó, 1933, Fig. 14 (newborn rat).

In the recently formed cortical plate of the 1.1-g specimen the bipolar cells beneath the marginal zone were referred to as pyramidal. However, the true nature of these cells is not definitely known; it seems conceivable that they will not subsequently develop into pyramidal cells, but will either move further out and become part of the marginal layer, or be transformed into stellate cells.

A well developed *pyramidal layer* was seen, however, in the 6.5-g fetus. The cells here, as seen in Nissl sections, are less well developed than the stellate elements in the outer part of the intermediate zone and the cells in the marginal layer. Golgi sections from the 12-g stage onward show that the subsequent development of the pyramidal cells is also slower than that of the cells in the other cortical layers.

The metamorphosis of bipolar into pyramidal cells of a mature type was found to occur in the same way in sheep as in other aminals such as mice and rabbits, as described by Cajal (see the INTRODUCTION). Thus, the maturation of a pyramidal neuron is measured in terms of the development of its dendrites, axon collaterals and dendritic spines.

The pyramidal layer grows, during a certain period of fetal development, by the successive addition of cells. Consequently, cells of different 'ages' are present, *i.e.* they have appeared here earlier or later. According to Angevine and Sidman, cells that were formed at the same time during neurogenesis are to be found predominantly in the same cortical stratum, and 'younger', *i.e.* more recently formed cells, occupy more superficial strata than do cells that are 'older', *i.e.* that appeared in the germinal zone at an earlier stage.

The least differentiated, pyramidal cell is the bipolar element (see *e.g.* Fig. 7B) whose shape resembles that of a migrating neuroblast (Fig. 17B). Even in the 12-g specimen the apical dendrites of the pyramidal cells were seen to extend to the marginal zone. Consequently, this 'anchoring' is an early and, presumably, fundamental phenomenon.

If cells that were formed most recently in gestation occupy the most superficial stratum of the pyramidal layer, then the perikarya of their predecessors must be depressed to deeper levels, *i.e.* away from the surface, when new cells have reached this stratum. This view implies that the apical dendrites, the terminal branches of which are already fixed in the marginal zone, grow by expansion through the movement of their cell bodies, which is in the direction of deeper levels.

According to Angevine and Sidman there is a relation between the 'age' (as previously defined) of a nerve cell and the distance between its cell body and the hemispherical surface. Let us then assume that all neuroblasts, after having reached their destination in the cortical plate, start to develop immediately, or after the same latency, and that, in maturation, they follow more or less the same time pattern. In a given specimen one would then always expect to find the most developed cells in the deepest stratum of the pyramidal layer and would also expect that maturation would appear to decrease successively towards the surface, so that the most primitive cells are found in the most superficial part of the pyramidal layer. These expectations have been found, at least partly to, be correct: in Golgi sections of fetal sheep weighing between 12 and 187 g, the bipolar, primitive 'pyramidal' cells were always found in the most superficial stratum. A similar observation has been made by other authors, *e.g.* Cajal and Lorente de Nó, on other species. In the 12-g specimen the best developed cells were also found in the deepest stratum of the pyramidal layer. However, Nissl, as well as Golgi, sections from fetal lambs weighing from 39 to 197 g show, contrary to our expectations, that the cells in the middle stratum of the cortical layer are better developed than those in deeper strata (*cf.* strata C and D in Figs. 13 and 18). Cajal's statement (1906) that 'morphological differentiation of the pyramidal cells starts in deeper strata, especially the middle one (with large pyramidal cells), and continues towards the superficial one or the small pyramids, which are the last neurons to develop', seems to be based upon a similar observation. Lorente de Nó (1933) asserts: 'The deep layers are the most advanced and the differentiation is less in the upper layers, *i.e.* the differentiation proceeds from below upwards. The deep pyramids have very long and thick dendrites . . .' 'Deep pyramids' seem to refer to what in the mature cortex corresponds to cells in the 4th and the lower part of the 3rd stratum. He also holds that the light band, which is the first indication of a striation as seen in Nissl sections (Rose's *lamina dissecans*), is due to the development of dendritic and fibrillar plexuses in the 4th and 3rd cortical strata.

The observation that, during a certain phase of development, the cells in the middle

References p. 57–59

part of the pyramidal layer appear more mature than deeper cells can be explained in two ways: (a) the deep cells migrated into the cortical plate later than those in the middle stratum; they would then prove an exception to Angevine and Sidman's concept; or (b) the deep cells did appear earlier in the pyramidal layer but have had a retarded development in comparison with the more superficially situated elements.

Up to the 65-g stage the pyramidal layer proper contains only simple bipolar cells with apical dendrites, which extend to the marginal zone, *i.e.* primitive pyramidal cells; and stellate cells are seen only in the transitional zone. A striking change then occurs: numerous *stellate and Martinotti cells* appear among the pyramidal cells in the deeper part of the layer in the 94-g specimen.

Which route did the non-pyramidal cells follow before coming to their final destinations? Three ways seem possible. (a) After migration into the cortical plate the cell bodies of their precursors are first situated superficially in accordance with Angevine and Sidman's concept. During their subsequent successive descent to lower strata the cells will have the same shape as their neighbors, the precursors of the true pyramidal cells, since all cells during these early phases have a pyramidal shape. After reaching their destination they will change from bipolar to stellate in shape. (b) Some already differentiated stellate cells in the transitional zone have moved further out. (c) The cells derive from neuroblasts which migrate into the cortical plate comparatively late, *i.e.* after the 65-g stage, proceed directly to their final lodging place (without a detour through the most superficial areas), and start to develop shortly after they have come into the cortical plate. The last alternative seems to be the most likely, which again implies that there may be certain exceptions to Angevine and Sidman's view.

Stellate and Martinotti cells in the cortex of embryos and young animals and infants have been described and illustrated by earlier authors, *e.g.* Retzius (1893), Kölliker (1896), Cajal (1906) and Lorente de Nó (1933). However, no one has previously commented upon the time pattern of their appearance in relation to that of the other types of cortical cells.

Presumptive cells of *Golgi's type II* were seen in only one case (a 147-g fetus). According to Cajal (1911), they are scarce also in rodents before, and even after, birth. Scheibel and Scheibel (1964) observed many 'short-axoned stellate or granule-cells' in the 2nd and 4th layers of the newborn cat; these cells were found to continue to develop during subsequent weeks. Noback and Purpura (1961) stated that, in kittens, Golgi II type cells 'are present at birth but more readily observed after the first postnatal week'. The axons of these cells were not described.

Development of afferent cortical connections. The first afferent fibers to appear were the descending collaterals from the horizontal fibers in the marginal layer, and the collaterals from the callosal and other fibers in the outer part of the intermediate zone; both were seen in the 12-g specimen. It is interesting to note that they terminate around the comparatively well differentiated nerve cells in the deeper part of the pyramidal zone and stellate cells in the outer part of the intermediate zone. The descending fibers mentioned are of particular interest: they are of a type which has not been previously described either in prenatal or in postnatal phases of any animal. They were not seen after the 94-g stage, and may possibly degenerate and disappear.

The ascending, afferent, 'oblique' fibers, seen in the cortical plate of the 49-g specimen, are so-called unspecific afferent fibers (Lorente de Nó, 1938). They terminate mainly in the outer part of the cortical plate. Similar elements were observed by Cajal (1906) in the newborn mouse, and by Scheibel (1962) in the newborn cat.

The specific afferent fibers which terminate mainly in the 4th layer of the adult cortex (Lorente de Nó, 1938) were not observed in any of the specimens examined. This point undoubtedly requires more detailed examination since one would expect these elements to appear at or earlier than the 468-g stage. The latter represents the final stage covered by this study. Scheibel and Scheibel (1964) observed endings of specific afferents in the 4th layer of the cortex in a newborn cat.

Cortical development in mammals. In addition to this study on fetal lambs the cortical development has been investigated, *inter alia*, in the following species: the mouse (Cajal, 1906, 1911, 1960; Lorente de Nó, 1933; Kobayashi *et al.*, 1964); the rabbit (Cajal; Noback and Purpura, 1961; Marty, 1962); the rat (Lorente de Nó; Eayrs and Goodhead, 1959; Noback and Purpura); guinea-pig (Cajal); the kitten (Retzius, 1893; Scheibel, 1962; Scheibel and Scheibel, 1964; Purpura *et al.*, 1960; Noback and Purpura, 1961; Purpura *et al.*, 1964; Marty, 1962); the dog (Cajal; Retzius, 1893); and in man (Cajal; Retzius, 1893; Kölliker, 1896; Lorente de Nó; Conel, 1939–1959; Rabinowicz, 1964; Schadé and Van Groenigen, 1961; Schadé *et al.*, 1964). These studies do not allow of comprehensive comparisons, since, among other considerations, they do not cover the very early phases of prenatal development. However, they support the view that the differentiation of cortical cells in the sheep is basically similar to that in other species (*cf.* Noback and Purpura, 1961). Furthermore, it is also clear that development is comparatively more rapid in sheep than in any other of the species mentioned. Thus, the stage of cortical development in mice, rabbits and kittens at term, seems to be approximately comparable to that of a fetal lamb weighing 94 g, which is estimated to correspond to a fetal age of 62 days, *i.e.* approximately 2/5 of the total gestation period. Fig. 18B in this study *e.g.* is comparable to two illustrations in Lorente de Nó's paper (1933) which show the cortical plate in a 12-h-old mouse (Fig. 13) and in a newborn rat (Fig. 14). Fig. 158 in Cajal's monograph, 1960, which illustrates the cortex in a somewhat older animal, *i.e.* a 4-day-old mouse, can also be compared with Fig. 18B.

In human embryos, according to Lorente de Nó (1933), there is a rather advanced differentiation in the 5th month, and he assumes that differentiation is actually established much earlier. The stage of cortical development, as shown in his Fig. 18 (human embryo of the 5th month), may be compared to that of Fig. 18B (lamb, estimated fetal age 62 days).

Stratification in fetal isocortex. Stratification in both fetal and adult animals is due to the aggregation, in horizontal layers, of cells with similar structure and spacing. The following factors are of importance: packing density of perikarya; shape, size and appearance of cell bodies, nuclei and dendrites; distribution of dendrites, axons and collaterals, especially horizontally. Nissl's method for cell staining is, of

References pp. 57–59

course, the classical procedure for studying cytoarchitectonics prenatally and postnatally (Brodman, 1909). It is an expedient way of obtaining an over-all view of cortical structure. However, the Nissl method has disadvantages, as pointed out by Lorente de Nó (1933). The Golgi sections, on the other hand can reveal many details, such as shape and distribution of dendrites, axons and collaterals, which are left unstained in the Nissl sections. The Golgi method is indispensable not only for studying the detailed structure of the cortex but also for comparing stratification in fetal specimens with that in adult animals. In fact, without the aid of Golgi sections, it would be impossible to compare fetal and adult striation as seen in Nissl sections. Therefore, a combination of the Nissl and the Golgi methods is a powerful tool for analyzing fetal, cortical structure.

Stratification during fetal life is a dynamic process and must be understood in terms of cortical genesis. The following aspects of development within the pyramidal layer are of special importance. (a) Development occurs more or less simultaneously among cells in the same stratum. Consequently, these cells are of similar appearance. (b) Cortical strata of nerve cells are of different 'ages'. Various strata seem to be different because their cells are not in the same phase of development. (c) Strata change position in relation to the most superficial stratum as emphasized by Angevine and Sidman. The dark band of cells in the most superficial part of the pyramidal zone in one specimen is not necessarily homologous to a dark band of similar appearance in an older fetus (or to layer II in the adult cortex), since the cells in the specimen first-mentioned may be situated further down in the fetus last-mentioned. (d) The spongioblasts start to migrate later than the neuroblasts. The appearance of glia cells will, naturally, modify striation.

Consequently, caution is necessary when comparison is made of cortical strata in fetuses of different ages, and in adult animals of the same and of other species. Lorente de Nó (1933) has expressed a similar opinion in criticizing Brodman's principle of 'the tectogenetic fundamental type of 6-layers'.

An impression of stratification is evident in the isocortical plate from the very beginning of its formation, when two layers, the marginal and the pyramidal, can be recognized. Further stratification will then occur within the pyramidal layer, mainly through the differential development of the cells here.

No further comments are required when stating that the marginal zone corresponds to the first cortical stratum, and that the stellate cells in the outer part of the intermediate zone will become parts of the 6th stratum (layer VIb according to Lorente de Nó, 1938, or layer 7 according to Cajal, 1911). These strata could already be recognized in the 6.5-g specimen.

In Nissl sections, striation within the pyramidal layer (excluding the stellate-cell layer) is first produced by the appearance of a light band in the middle of the layer (Fig. 13B, C). The impression of lightness is mainly due to the fact that the perikarya and their basal dendrites here are better developed, and the cell bodies further apart from each other, than those above and below this stratum. These cells are presumably the precursors of the large pyramidal cells in layers III and IV of the adult cortex. Lorente de Nó (1933) seems to have reached a similar conclusion (see *e.g.* his Figs. 13

and 14). Differentiation then proceeds gradually from this stratum in the direction of the surface (*cf.* Cajal, 1906; Lorente de Nó, 1933), disregarding for the moment the development below these strata.

When migration of neuroblasts within the neopallial wall has ceased (presumably after the 100-g stage) the most superficially-situated cells in the pyramidal layer will probably remain there. Consequently, these cells must be precursors of the pyramids of layer II in adult animals. They retain a primitive bipolar shape longer than any other pyramidal cells in the cortical plate. Their ultimate maturation occurs between the 265- and 459-g stages (estimated fetal ages 79 and 90 days, respectively).

The intracortical stellate cells, which appeared in the deep part of the pyramidal layer after the 65-g stage, seem to correspond approximately to the 4th (*i.e.* internal granular) layer of the mature cortex.

The development of the pyramidal cells in layers 5 and 6 is retarded compared with that in the 3rd and 4th layers (*vide supra*). It occurs mainly after the 187-g stage (estimated fetal age 71 days and more).

Functional development. The anatomical findings presented here will be correlated to physiological data elsewhere (Bernhard *et al.*, 1967). From a purely anatomical point of view a few comments will be made.

Through its early development, acquisition of relative maturity, and its structure, the marginal zone stands in contrast to the pyramidal layer. Some observations, admittedly incomplete, indicate that the marginal zone develops in relation to, and receives connections from, the olfactory system. Furthermore, the horizontal fibers constitute a powerful system for intracortical connections. It seems well worth while to direct more attention to this layer, which, from an embryological and an anatomical point of view, has hitherto been rather neglected.

The close proximity of the marginal and stellate cell layers in the very young fetuses, the early maturation of these cells and their connection through afferent fibers point to a relationship between them which may or may not disappear during their subsequent evolution.

Some anatomical features, which appear during evolution and may be of importance for understanding the functional development, are shown in the diagrams of Fig. 25. The concept of junctions between fibers and cells, as illustrated, is based upon circumstantial evidence, since the actual synaptic connections were never seen (as they rarely are in Golgi sections). For the younger specimens these connections may not yet exist; on the other hand, when they are established, the actual chains must be much more complicated than those shown in the diagrams.

The stellate cells in the outer part of the intermediate zone have the appearance of interneurons. They can, therefore, form parts of closed and open chains, which are of the same type as those seen in all parts of the central nervous system including the cerebral cortex. The fundamental role of such chains for the correct performance of neurological functions is well known from Lorente de Nó's work (1938). Their presence at a very early stage of development underscores the importance of these structures (Fig. 25A).

The afferent fibers are also of considerable interest. The descending elements from

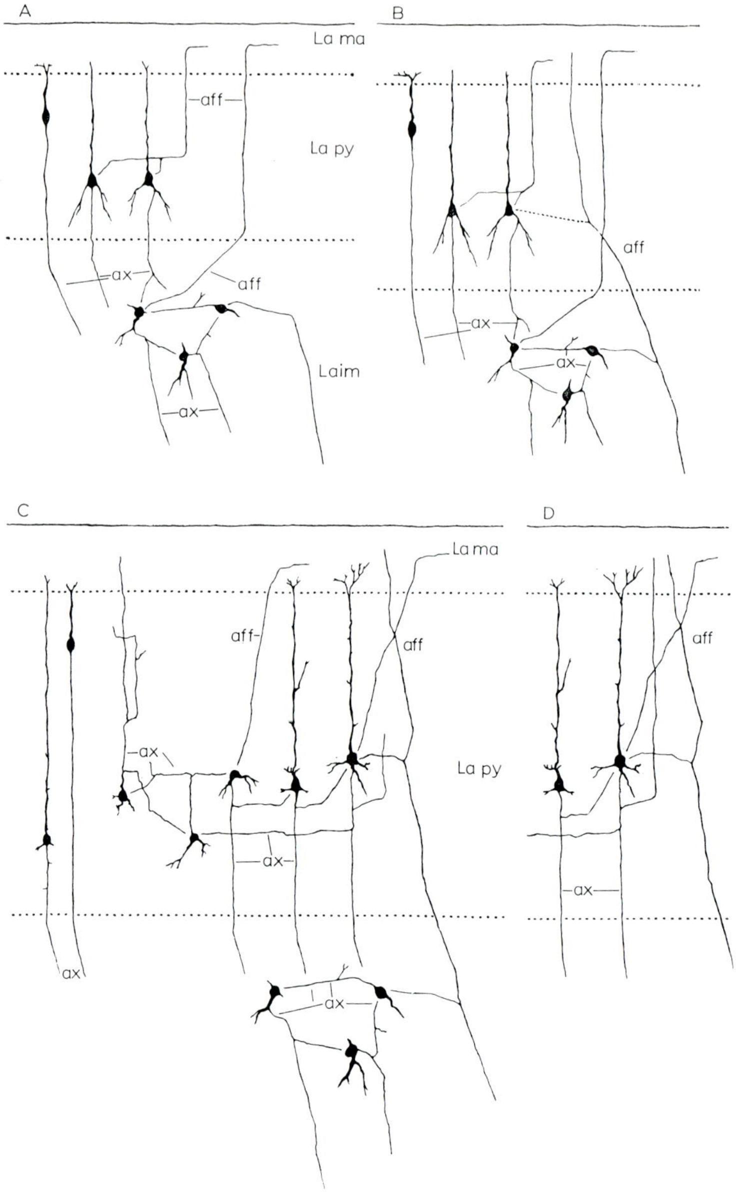

Fig. 25. Diagram showing anatomical features at different stages of development. A = 12-gram stage; B = 50-gram stage; C = 95-gram stage; D = 145-gram stage.

the marginal layer probably have their origin in the horizontal fibers, which in turn seem to emanate from the horizontal nerve cells in this layer. The possible connections between these cells and the olfactory system have already been mentioned. Only the descending fibers can transmit impulses to the pyramidal cells in the early stages, provided synaptic connections exist; ascending, callosal and thalamic collaterals do not appear with certainty in the cortical plate until the 50-g stage. However, the stellate cells could receive impulses from both the descending and ascending collaterals before that stage (Fig. 25A).

At the 50-g stage or possibly earlier, afferent fibers (thalamic or callosal or both) ascend through the cortical plate (Fig. 25B). Some small branches remain in the pyramidal layer, but their main destination is the marginal zone; a fact that again points to the functional importance of this structure during the early phases of development.

The pyramidal cell layer has a rather simple structure before the 65-g stage (estimated fetal age 60 days). Then, between the 65-g and 95-g stages rather dramatic changes occur: the appearance of stellate cells coincides with the incipient development of collaterals on axons of the pyramidal cells which are already precent (Fig. 25C). The purpose of the stellate cells and the collaterals is to provide intracortical connections vertically and horizontally. Some what later (corresponding to a weight of 147 g or less) recurrent collaterals from the pyramidal cells also reach the marginal zone (Fig. 25D). Thus, cells in the marginal, pyramidal, and subpyramidal layers become connected. Although the neuronal connections become increasingly complex they still represent variations on the same fundamental pattern as seen in Fig. 25A.

Thus, within a few days of development the pyramidal layer changes from a rather primitive structure (at 65 g) to a cortex of comparatively mature type (at 95 g). Flexner (1951–1952) has described a corresponding period of rapid biochemical, cytological and functional development in the guinea-pig.

SUMMARY

A histological study was made of the early development of the isocortical plate in the brains of fetal sheep, stained chiefly according to the Golgi and Nissl methods. Forty-four brains were examined in detail; the weight and the estimated fetal age (e.f.a.) of each specimen, and the histological methods used, are given in the Table on p. 75. Fetal age was estimated by weight, according to a curve published by Barcroft, 1946.

The primordial neopallial wall is conventionally divided into 4 concentric zones: the germinal, the intermediate, the pyramidal, and the marginal. Formation of new cells — neuroblasts and spongioblasts — takes place only in the germinal zone. Neuroblasts were never seen in the marginal and the pyramidal layers. Their metamorphosis into nerve cells must begin shortly after they have migrated into the cortical plate.

At an early stage of development the telencephalic wall is penetrated by numerous radiating fibers whereas the corresponding cell bodies (epithelial cells) are situated mainly in the matrix. The fibers, which probably serve as scaffolding, disappear gradually from the 100-g stage onward.

Callosal and projection fibers were seen in the intermediate zone from the 12-g stage onward; the former run chiefly in the inner part and the latter in the outer part of the zone.

An internal capsule was definitely present in a 12-g specimen and probably also in a 6.5-g fetus.

References pp. 57–59

The incipient formation of an isocortical plate was observed in a 1.1-g specimen (e.f.a. 20–25 days). In the neopallium of the 6.5-g fetus (e.f.a. 43 days) the cortical anlage was more completely developed. Subsequently this anlage grows owing to the following factors: the successive addition of neuroblasts (at least up to the 100-g stage), the appearance of astrocytes (beginning approximately at the 40-g stage and continuing up to or beyond the 100-g stage), the growth and differentiation of neurons and glia cells, the penetration of the cortex by projection fibers, etc.

The degree of cortical differentiation increases with fetal age. Neurons of a basically mature type were seen in all strata for the first time in a 450-g specimen (e.f.a. 89 days).

The conclusion that follows from the preceding two paragraphs is that, in sheep, the main cortical development occurs comparatively early in gestation, *i.e.* from an e.f.a. ranging from about 40 days to 90 days. The most dramatic changes were found when a 65-g and a 95-g specimen were compared; the difference in estimated fetal ages was here only 3 days. (The total period of gestation in sheep is about 150 days and the weight at term is usually around 4500 g).

Cortical development in relation to total gestation period proceeds more rapidly in sheep than in other vertebrates. The stage of development in the 94-g specimen (e.f.a. 62 days) was estimated to be approximately comparable to that in mice, rabbits and kittens at term and to human embryos at 5 months.

The development starts earlier in the marginal than in the pyramidal layer; well differentiated neurons were already seen in the former layer in a 1.1-g specimen. The zone also becomes mature more rapidly.

An incipient formation of a pyramidal layer possibly occurs as early as in the 1.1-g fetus and is clearly visible in the 6.5-g specimen.

Well differentiated stellate cells were observed in the outer part of the intermediate zone of the 12-g fetus; such cells are probably already present in the 6.5-g specimen. This layer, which will subsequently become incorporated into the pyramidal zone, is the homolog of stratum VIB in the adult isocortex.

The primitive, undifferentiated, pyramidal cells are bipolar and oriented radially, *i.e.* perpendicularly towards the hemispherical surface. All of them have well developed apical dendrites, which extend into the marginal zone. During their transformation into pyramidal neurons, the various cell components appear in approximately the following order: terminal branches of the apical dendrites; descending and basilar dendrites from the cell body; branches on the apical dendrites; axon collaterals; spines on the apical dendrites.

Development occurs more or less simultaneously in cortical neurons at the same level but differs in cells in various cortical strata. This forms, *inter alia*, the basis for the stratification within the isocortical plate which, in the Golgi sections, is recognizable at an early stage. In the 12-g specimen (e.f.a. 48 days), *e.g.* the deep pyramidal cells are more fully developed than the superficial ones. Thus, even at this early stage in development there are already 4 cortical strata, *i.e.* the marginal, the superficial pyramidal, the deep pyramidal, and the stellate cell layers.

Up to the 60-g stage there are only pyramidal cells and their precursors in the pyramidal layer (excepting the stellate cells). Then, between the 65-g and 95-g stages, stellate and Martinotti cells become visible therein. These cells appear when axon collaterals start to develop. The purpose of these elements, which signify a rather advanced degree of cortical maturation, is apparently to provide intracortical connections.

The fetal homologs of cortical cells and strata in the adult animal become differentiated in approximately the following order: (1) The marginal, plexiform layer, (2) the deep stellate cells in layer VIB, (3) the large pyramids in layer IV and in lower layer III, (4) the stellate cells in the deep part of the cortex, *i.e.* the internal granular layer, (5) the pyramids in layers V and VI, (6) the medium-sized pyramids in layer III, (7) the small pyramids in layer II, (8) the external granular layer.

Afferent collaterals to the cortical cells appear in the following order. (1) Descending collaterals from the horizontal layer to the deep pyramidal cells and the stellate cells in the outer part of the intermediate zone (prospective layer VIB). Ascending elements from projection fibers (callosal and thalamic?). Stage: 12 g (e.f.a. 48 days). (2) Ascending, 'oblique' fibers (unspecific afferent fibers) to the marginal layer and — to a lesser degree — to the pyramidal zone. Stage: 49 g (e.f.a. 59 days). (3) Collaterals on axons from the pyramidal cells start to develop at the 94-g stage (e.f.a. 62 days). Recurrent axon collaterals reach the marginal layer in a 147-g specimen (e.f.a. 66 days). (4) Ascending axons from Marinotti cells were first seen in a 66-g specimen (e.f.a. 60 days), but were more numerous in the 94-g fetus (e.f.a. 62 days).

Specific afferent fibers were not seen in this series.

Some comments concerning the functional development are made in the DISCUSSION, *inter alia*, in relation to the diagrams in Fig. 25.

ACKNOWLEDGEMENT

This work was supported by a grant from the Association for the Aid of Crippled Children.

REFERENCES

ANGEVINE, J. B., Jr., AND SIDMAN, R. L., (1961); Autoradiographic study of cell migration during histogenesis of cerebral cortex in the mouse. *Nature*, **192**, 766–768.

ANTHONY, R., AND DE GRZYBOWSKI, J., (1937); Le néopallium du mouton. *J. Anat. (Lond.)*, **71**, 41–53.

ÅSTRÖM, K. E., (1953); On the central course of afferent fibers in the trigeminal, facial, glossopharyngeal, and vagal nerves and their nuclei in the mouse. *Acta physiol. scand.*, Suppl. 106, **29**, 211–320.

BARCROFT, J., (1946); *Researches on Pre-natal Life*. Oxford, Blackwell.

BERNHARD, C. G., KAISER, I. H., AND KOLMODIN, G. M., (1959); On the development of cortical activity in fetal sheep. *Acta physiol. scand.*, **47**, 333–349.

BERNHARD, C. G., KOLMODIN, G. M., AND MEYERSON, B. A., (1967); On the prenatal development of function and structure in the somesthetic cortex of the sheep. This volume, pp. 60–77.

BRODMAN, K., (1909); *Vergleichende Lokalisationslehre der Grosshirnrinde*. Leipzig, Barth.

BRUN, A., (1965); The subpial granular layer of the foetal cerebral cortex in man. *Acta path. et microbiol. scand., Suppl. 179*, **65**, 1–98.

CAJAL, S. RAMÓN Y, (1894); *Les Nouvelles Idées sur la Structure du Système Nerveux*. Paris, Reinwald.

CAJAL, S. RAMÓN Y, (1906); *Studien über die Hirnrinde des Menschen*. Vol. 5, Leipzig, Barth.

CAJAL, S. RAMÓN Y, (1911); *Histologie du Système Nerveux de l'Homme et des Vertébrés*. Vol. 2, Paris, Maloine.

CAJAL, S. RAMÓN Y, (1960); *Studies on Vertebrate Neurogenesis*. L. Guth, Translater, Springfield, Thomas.

CONEL, J. L., (1939–1959); *The Postnatal Development of the Human Cerebral Cortex*. Vols. I–VI. Cambridge, Mass. Harvard University Press.

EAYRS, J. E., AND GOODHEAD, B., (1959); Postnatal development of the cerebral cortex in the rat. *J. Anat. (Lond.)*, **93**, 385–402.

EIDELBERG, E., KOLMODIN, G. M., AND MEYERSON, B. A., (1965); Ontogenesis of steady potential and direct cortical response in fetal sheep brain. *Exptl. Neurol.*, **12**, 198–214.

FLEXNER, L. B., (1951–1952); The development of the cerebral cortex: a cytological, functional, and biochemical approach. *Harvey Lect.*, **47**, 156–179.

HIS, W., (1904); *Die Entwicklung des menschlichen Gehirns während der ersten Monate*. Leipzig, Hirzel.

KOBAYASHI, T., INMAN, O. R., BUNO, W., AND HIMWICH, H. E., (1964); Neurohistological studies of developing mouse brain. W. A. Himwich and H. E. Himwich, Editors. *The Developing Brain. Progress in Brain Research, Vol. 9*, Amsterdam, Elsevier (pp. 87–88).

KÖLLIKER, A., (1896); *Handbuch der Gewebelehre*. Vol. 2, 6th Ed. Leipzig, Engelmann.,

KOLMODIN, G. M., AND MEYERSON, B. A., (1966); Ontogenesis of cortical paroxysmal activity in foetal sheep. In course of publication in *Electroencephalog. Clin. Neurophysiol.*

LANDACRE, F. L., (1930); The major and minor sulci of the brain of the sheep. *Ohio J. Sci.*, **30**, 36–51.

LEVI-MONTALCINI, R., (1964); Events in the developing nervous system. D. P. Purpura and J. P. Schadé, Editors. *Progress in Brain Research, Vol. 4, Growth and Maturation of the Brain*. Amsterdam, Elsevier (pp. 1–26).

LORENTE DE NÓ, R., (1933); Studies on the structure of the cerebral cortex. *J. Psychol. Neurol. (Lpz.)*, **45**, 381–438.

LORENTE DE NÓ, R., (1938); Architectonics and structure of the cerebral cortex. J. F. Fulton, Editor. *Physiology of the Nervous System*. Oxford University Press. Ch. 15.

MARTY, R., (1962); Développement post-natal des réponses sensorielles du cortex cérébral chez le chat et le lapin. Aspects physiologiques et histologiques. *Arch. Anat. micr. Morph. exp.*, **51**, 129–264.

MARTY, R., AND SCHERRER, J., (1964); Critères de maturation des systèmes afférents corticaux. D. P. Purpura and J. P. Schadé, Editors. *Progress in Brain Research, Vol. 4, Growth and Maturation of the Brain*. Amsterdam, Elsevier (pp. 222–234).

MEYERSON, B. A., (1964); The effect of asphyxia on induced cortical activity in fetal sheep. *Acta physiol. scand.*, **62**, 489–490.

MOLLIVER, M. E., (1967); An ontogenetic study of evoked somesthetic cortical responses in the sheep. This volume, pp. 78–90.

NOBACK, C. R., AND PURPURA, D. P., (1961); Postnatal ontogenesis of neurons in cat neocortex. *J. comp. Neurol.*, **117**, 291–307.

PURPURA, D. P., CARMICHAEL, M.W., AND HOUSEPIAN, E. M., (1960); Physiological and anatomical studies of development of superficial axodendritic synaptic pathways in neocortex. *Exp. Neurol.*, **2**, 324–347.

PURPURA, D. P., SHOFER, R. J., HOUSEPIAN, E. M., AND NOBACK, C. R., (1964); Comparative ontogenesis of structure-function relations in cerebral and cerebellar cortex. D. P. Purpura and J. P. Schadé, Editors. *Progress in Brain Research, Vol. 4, Growth and Maturation of the Brain*. Amsterdam, Elsevier (pp. 187–221).

RABINOWICZ, TH., (1964); The cerebral cortex of the premature infant of the 8th month. D. P. Purpura and J. P. Schadé, Editors. *Progress in Brain Research, Vol. 4, Growth and Maturation of the Brain*, Amsterdam, Elsevier (pp. 39–86).

RETZIUS, G., (1891); Ueber den Bau der Oberflächenschicht der Grosshirnrinde beim Menschen und bei den Säugethieren. *Verh. biol. Ver. (Stockh.)*, **3**, 90–102.

RETZIUS, G., (1893); Die Cajal'schen Zellen der Grosshirnrinde beim Menschen und bei Säugethieren. *Biol. Untersuch. (Stockh.)*, **5**, 1–8.

ROMANES, G. J., (1947); The prenatal medullation of the sheep's nervous system. *J. Anat. (Lond.)*, **81**, 64–81.

ROSE, J., (1942); A cytoarchitectural study of the sheep cortex. *J. comp. Neurol.*, **76**, 1–55.

ROSE, M., (1926); Ueber das histogenetische Prinzip der Einteilung der Grosshirnrinde. *J. Psychol. Neurol.*, **32**, 97–160.

SCHADÉ, J. P., VAN BACKER, H., AND COLON, E., (1964); Quantitative analysis of neuronal parameters in the maturing cerebral cortex. D. P. Purpura and J. P. Schadé, Editors. *Progress in Brain Research, Vol. 4, Growth and Maturation of the Brain.* Amsterdam, Elsevier (pp. 150–175).

SCHADÉ, J. P., AND VAN GROENIGEN, W. B., (1961); Structural organization of the human cerebral cortex. I. Maturation of the middle frontal gyrus. *Acta anat. (Basel)*, **47**, 74–111.

SCHEIBEL, A., (1962); Neural correlates of psychophysiological development in the young organism. B. Wortis, Editor. *Recent Advances in biological Psychiatry.* New York, Plenum Press (pp. 313–327).

SCHEIBEL, M., AND SCHEIBEL, A., (1964); Some structural and functional substrates of development in young cats. W. A. Himwich and H. E. Himwich, Editors. *Progress in Brain Research, Vol. 9, The developing Brain.* Amsterdam, Elsevier (pp. 6–25).

SIDMAN, R. L., MIALE, I. L., AND FEDER, N., (1959); Cell proliferation and migration in the primitive ependymal zone; an autoradiographic study of histogenesis in the nervous system. *Exp. Neurol.*, **1**, 322–333.

VIGNAL, W., (1888); Recherches sur le développement des éléments des couches corticales du cerveau et du cervelet chex l'homme et les mammifères. *Arch. Physiol. norm. path.*, **2**, 228–254 (Quoted by S. Ramón y Cajal, 1960).

VON LENHOSSÉK, M., (1895); *Der feinere Bau des Nervensystems im Lichte neuester Forschungen.* Berlin, Kornfeld.

On the Prenatal Development of Function and Structure in the Somesthetic Cortex of the Sheep

C. G. BERNHARD, G. M. KOLMODIN AND B. A. MEYERSON

Department of Physiology, Karolinska Institutet, Stockholm (Sweden)

INTRODUCTION

In recent years there has been an increasing interest in the ontogenetic functional development of the mammalian central nervous system. The development of excitatory and inhibitory mechanisms of *spinal* reflex functions has been studied electrophysiologically in prenatal sheep (Änggård, *et al.* 1961) and guinea-pig (Bergström, 1962; Bergström *et al.*, 1961, 1962a and b), in pre- and peri-natal cat (Naka, 1964a and b) and in postnatal cat (Malcolm, 1953, 1955; Skoglund, 1960a–e; Wilson, 1962; Eccles and Willis, 1962).

Investigations on the development of *cortical* mechanisms have also been made on different species. The electrophysiological studies on the functional development of cortical mechanisms have been focused on cortical responses evoked by direct stimulation and via afferent pathways. Investigations in which the changes in these responses were correlated to developmental changes in the cortical morphology have been made on newborn rabbits (Hunt and Goldring, 1951; Do Carmo, 1960; Laget and Delhaye, 1962; Marty, 1962) and newborn cats (Scherrer and Oeconomos, 1955; Ellingson and Wilcott, 1960; Purpura *et al.*, 1960; Purpura, 1961 and 1964; Marty, 1962; Scheibel, 1962; Schadé and Pascoe, 1964). The studies by Purpura *et al.* (1964) provide extensive material on the structural and functional aspects of the cortical ontogeny of the parietal cortex in the cat.

All the investigations on the cortical mechanisms were made during the *postnatal* period. It is true that the brains of the rabbit and the cat are still at a relatively early stage of development at birth, and there occurs a considerable postnatal cortical development which makes it possible to study the relation between developmental, structural and functional changes during the first weeks after birth. However, the fact that one can evoke cortical responses in these animals shows that synaptic activity in the cortical systems studied is already established at birth, that is, at this stage the initial developmental phase of synaptic transmission has already passed.

The aim of this paper is to present a review of a series of investigations made in this department during recent years on the *prenatal* development of cortical mechanisms within the parietal cortex. These investigations have been made on sheep which have a relatively long gestation time (140–150 days) in comparison with the cat (63 days) and the rabbit (31 days). It should be mentioned that the newborn sheep is behaviorally much more mature than the newborn cat which may indicate that in sheep the cortical functions have reached a higher degree of maturation at birth than in cats. As will be shown, the maturity of some basic cortical mechanisms of the newborn cat corresponds to that of a 65–70 days old sheep fetus, *i.e.* at a fetal age of about half the gestation period. Analogously the sheep fetus shows several cortical mechanisms during the second half of the prenatal period which appear several days after birth in the cat. The investigations to be reviewed cover a prenatal period from ages at which there is cortical 'silence' and unresponsiveness up to ages in the fetal sheep corresponding to the postnatal period of the cat. It was therefore possible to catch the relatively early stage at which cortical excitability and cortical synaptic activity first appear. In this paper special attention will be given to the relation between structure and function during this important phase of development.

All the experiments to be reviewed were made on unanesthetized externalized sheep fetuses in placental contact with the decerebrate ewe which was maintained on artificial respiration (for details see Bernhard *et al.*, 1959). The various results to be reviewed were obtained on material ranging in fetal age from about 35 days (weight 1–2 g) to full term (140–150 days; weight about 4000 g).

Specimens taken from the fetal brains were used for a histological investigation on the structural development of the cortex in sheep made by Åström (1967). In the present paper reference will be made to this study when comparing the functional and structural development.

It should be emphasized that in the present review all the ages were estimated on a weight basis using the table relating weight and age presented by Joubert (1956).

I. STAGES IN THE FUNCTIONAL AND MORPHOLOGICAL DEVELOPMENT

(A) Period of unresponsiveness to electrical stimulation of the cortex

The initial prenatal period is characterized by cortical unresponsiveness to direct electrical stimulation. Neither single shocks nor repetitive stimuli are followed by any electrical sign of cortical activity even when the stimulus strength is 10–12 times higher than that giving *e.g.* direct cortical response (DCR) in older fetuses and adult animals. This period of unresponsiveness ends at the prenatal age of 65 days when the first detectable response to cortical stimulation can be obtained (Eidelberg *et al.*, 1965; see below).

(1) Anatomical characteristics

This prenatal period is characterized by a lissencephalic brain; and according to Åström (1967), the development of cortical structures during the period pertinent for our discussion may be described as follows.

At an age of 32 days there is a thin layer of cells (3–5 cells in depth) with a bipolar appearance — precursors to pyramidal cells — whose outer processes run towards the marginal zone. Within this zone there are scattered bipolar cells having dendrites running parallel to the surface.

References p. 75–77

At an age of 47 days the superficial part of the *marginal layer* contains numerous horizontal fibers which send collaterals to the pyramidal layer. The deep part receives pyramidal apical dendrites which do not extend to the surface. The superficial cells of the *pyramidal layer* whose apical dendrites terminate in the deep part of the marginal layer are less developed than the more deeply situated pyramidal cells whose apical dendrites also end in the deep marginal zone. These pyramidal cells have basal dendrites with lengths varying from 10 to 300 μ some of which continue to the underlying *intermediate zone* where they are seen together with the dendrites of stellate cells. The pyramidal axons descend through the intermediate zone where some of them emit collaterals. There are also afferent fibers presumably of thalamic origin which, however, end in the intermediate zone. It should be noted that at this stage no afferent fibers were seen to penetrate the cortical plate.

During the following days up to an age of 58 days (Fig. 1) the pyramidal layer

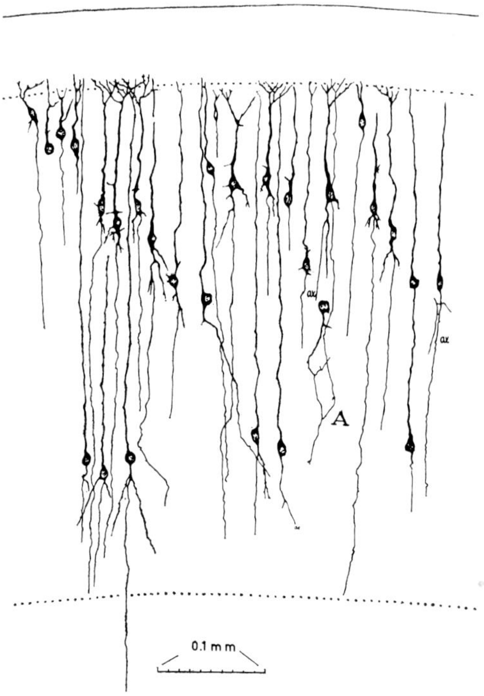

Fig. 1. 66-g fetus, estimated age 58 days. Composite picture of pyramidal cells. Cells in superficial stratum of pyramidal layer have immature bipolar appearance. Cells in middle part are more highly developed than those in deeper stratum of the layer; some of them have long descending basal dendrites. Martinotti cell with ascending axon (A). Short axon collaterals (ax) on cell at right. (From Åström, 1967.)

increases in thickness. All apical dendrites tend to extend into the marginal zone where they emit short ramifications. The basal dendrites, 1–2 in number, develop somewhat in length and run inwards. Astrocytes now also appear in the cortical plate. Towards the end of this period the afferent fibers penetrate into the cortex and reach the marginal layer where the terminal branches run horizontally. There are only a few afferents which end in the middle part of the pyramidal layer. In the underlying intermediate zone the stellate cells develop dendrites which form a subpyramidal stratum.

(2) Functional characteristics

A recent study of the *steady potential* (SP) made on 32 fetuses ranging from 35 to 120 days of fetal age shows that in general, as in the adult, the cortex is positive in relation to a reference electrode on the intact skull (Fig. 2). The results indicate

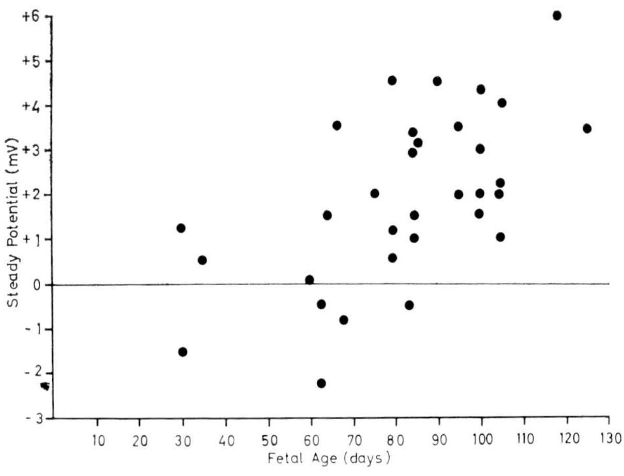

Fig. 2. Steady potential in fetuses of different gestational ages. Recording immediately after exposure of the cortex about 15 min after delivery. (From Eidelberg *et al.*, 1965.)

a trend of increasing values with fetal age although this is not of the same order of magnitude as that found during postnatal life in guinea-pig and rat (Bureš, 1957). Attention should be given to a recent observation on the effect of asphyxia on the fetal SP compared with that of the adult (Eidelberg *et al.*, 1966). There is for instance a marked difference with regard to the rate of decrease in the SP during asphyxiation, the rate of decrease being 5 times less in the fetal brain. It should also be mentioned that in sheep fetuses old enough to exhibit a continuous EEG activity this activity is far more susceptible to asphyxia than the SP in fetuses of the same age. The fetal SP seems to be a reflection of basic biophysical and biochemical processes that obviously are less dependent upon oxygen than the neuronal mechanisms underlying the EEG activity.

As to the question of *cortical cell membrane potentials*, Kolmodin and Meyerson have made a preliminary series of intracellular microelectrode measurements on fetuses belonging to this fetal period. From these intracellular measurements on cortical cells within the parietal region it is evident that a transmembrane potential is present in the early prenatal period. Further material has to be collected before conclusions can be drawn concerning a possible increase in the optimal membrane potential

References p. 75–77

values with age, and the relation to *e.g.* the size of the cell soma (*cf.* Haapanen *et al.*, 1958).

The only *spontaneous cortical activity* seen during this early period is the so-called PN I activity described by Bernhard *et al.* (1959). It can be recorded with surface electrodes and on an extended material it was obtained on fetuses from 60 days of age. The PN I activity consists of waxing and waning, regional spindle-like bursts with a frequency of 8–14 per sec (Fig. 3). In order to obtain this type of activity a high amplification has to be used since the amplitude usually does not exceed 20 μV.

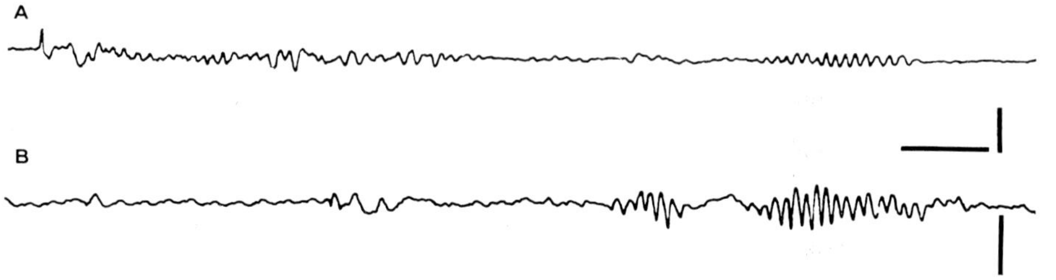

Fig. 3. Early type of cortical activity (PN I) recorded from 2 fetuses. A, gestational age 60 days; B, gestational age 65 days. Horizontal bar 1 sec; vertical bar 50 μV.

When recorded from separate regions the potentials do not always occur in synchrony. They are influenced by asphyxia as may be seen after temporary occlusion of the ewe's aorta. During a short period of asphyxiation the spindles often appear more frequently and increase in amplitude. The PN I activity has also been found in young fetuses of the guinea-pig (Bergström *et al.*, 1962b).

Recent investigations on the appearance and shape of the *cortical response to afferent stimulation* are of great interest in this context. From early experiments made by Barcroft and Barron (1939) on reflex movements in fetal sheep it is known that skin receptors on the nose and their central connections to the bulbar level are functionally mature at a gestational age of 40 days since electrical as well as natural stimulation of the nose is followed by reflex movements of both head and forelegs. As to the functional projection of the afferent inflow from these skin receptors to the cortex, Molliver (1967) found no response until the 48–50th day. At this time an electrical response could be recorded with a surface electrode within a discrete region of the lissencephalic brain (see Fig. 1 in the paper of Molliver, p. 80 this Volume).

At this early fetal stage the response was found to be surface positive. As mentioned above, ascending fibers extend only to the intermediate zone at the fetal age of 45–48 days. At a later time they penetrate the cortical plate and reach the marginal layer in the 58–60th day of fetal life. A comparison of the appearance of the somesthetic cortical response and the histological data favors the view that the surface positive response obtained within this early developmental period signals depolarization of the afferent presynaptic terminals, the surface structures serving as a source in relation to the sink in the deeper structures. The possibility, on the other hand, that the surface positivity represents deep postsynaptic activity has been discussed by Molliver (1967).

The ascending fibers which are seen at this fetal age seem to be of the non-specific type (Åström, 1967) originally described by Lorente de Nó (1933). The conclusion would be that the evoked positive cortical response to tactile stimulation which appears in this early period signals activity in non-specific afferents. In this context it should be mentioned that in the visual afferent system of the cat the non-specific system has been claimed to develop earlier than the specific (Rose and Lindsley, 1965).

Finally, it has been shown that it is possible to obtain *metrazol induced activity* (intravenous or intraperitoneal administration) during this early prenatal period. In the initial study by Bernhard *et al.* (1962) on the epileptogenic properties of the fetal brain, the youngest fetus tested which exhibited metrazol activity had an age of 75 days, *i.e.* an age which falls within the later prenatal period characterized by more highly developed cortical structures (see below). However, in later experiments (Kolmodin and Meyerson, 1965) we have found that trains of metrazol induced potentials can be recorded from the cortical surface after large doses as early as at an age of 48 days (Fig. 4), *i.e.* the same age at which the somesthetic surface positive response is first obtained. Since at this age there is synaptic activity both at the bulbar and thalamic levels as shown by the classical reflex studies and the experiments on the evoked cortical response, respectively, the appearance of metrazol induced activity in subcortical structures may not be unexpected at this fetal age.

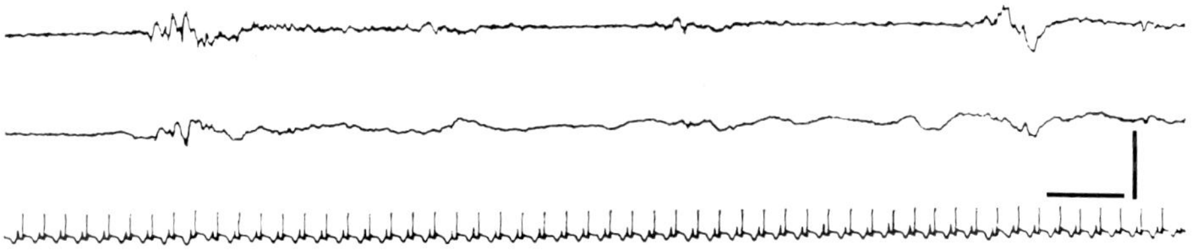

Fig. 4. Effect of metrazol in a 48-day fetus. Records from left (upper row) and right (middle row) hemisphere after 40 mg of metrazol intraperitoneally. Lower row EKG of fetus. Horizontal bar 1 sec; vertical bar 50 μV.

That, at this stage, the metrazol induced activity is initiated from subcortical structures is indicated by the following: (1) that seizure activity obtained from deeper structures precedes that recorded from the surface of the cortex, and (2) that the metrazol activity in the two hemispheres appears in synchrony at this early stage, when the transcallosal system is not likely to function. This activity recorded from the cortical surface may thus have its origin in subcortical structures. The metrazol induced bursts of activity recorded, and which incidently in some respects resemble the PN I activity, may represent fluctuating depolarizations of the afferent terminals radiating towards the cortical plate, and the PN I activity could have the same origin.

The observation that repetitive electrical cortical stimulation does not elicit any post-stimulatory discharge at this fetal age is included in the definition of this prenatal period. The relevance of these findings in the discussion of convulsive disorders has been considered elsewhere (Bernhard *et al.*, 1962).

Table I shows the time during prenatal life when the various electrical signs of activity appear.

References p. 75–77

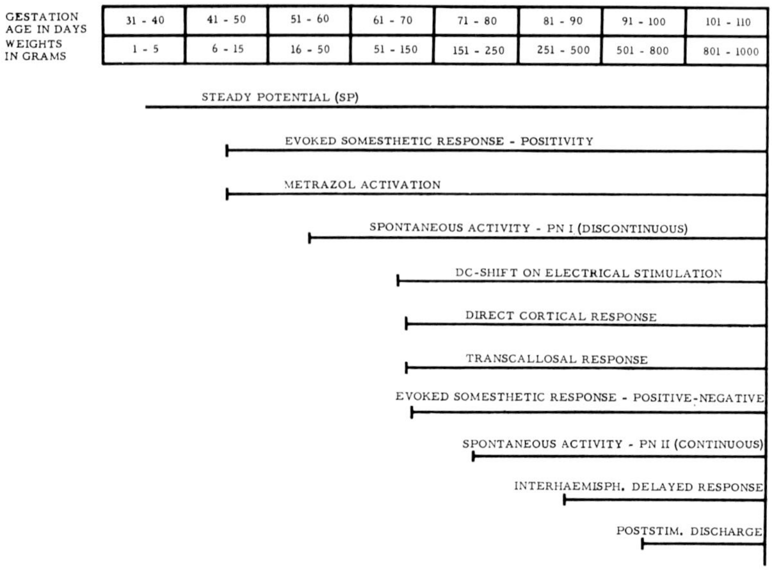

(B) Period of responsiveness to electrical stimulation of the cortex

At the fetal age of about 64 days a direct cortical response (DCR) can be evoked, and a DC shift can be built up with repetitive cortical stimulation (Eidelberg *et al.*, 1965). At about the same age a short latency interhemispheric transcallosal response to cortical stimulation is also obtained (Meyerson, 1964). The delayed interhemispheric response appears later in this period (Meyerson, unpublished observation) as does the post-stimulatory discharge in response to repetitive cortical stimulation (Bernhard *et al.*, 1962).

(1) Anatomical characteristics

The brain surface of the 60-day-old fetus is still lissencephalic but at the 66th day there is a shallow impression representing the future site of the suprasylvian gyrus.

According to Åström (1967) dramatic histological changes occur at this age mainly in the *pyramidal layer* which within a few days 'changes from a rather primitive structure to a cortex of comparatively mature type'. In the 65-day fetus (Fig. 5) the axons of the pyramidal cells in the middle stratum have several collaterals (up to 300 μ in length) which mainly runs horizontally forming a primitive band of Baillager. Recurrent collaterals are occasionally seen which, however, do not reach the marginal zone. The cells in the middle layer now have a true pyramidal shape and the basal dendrites are numerous and may extend to the lower part of the pyramidal layer. Their apical dendrites which have proximal branches are thick and have 'indications of spines'. Stellate and Martinotti cells appear for the first time *in* the pyramidal layer. The stellate cells which may serve as interneurons have axons ramifying within the pyramidal layer. Most of them terminate within the pyramidal zone while some descend to lower levels. From the *marginal layer* fibers descend to the pyramidal

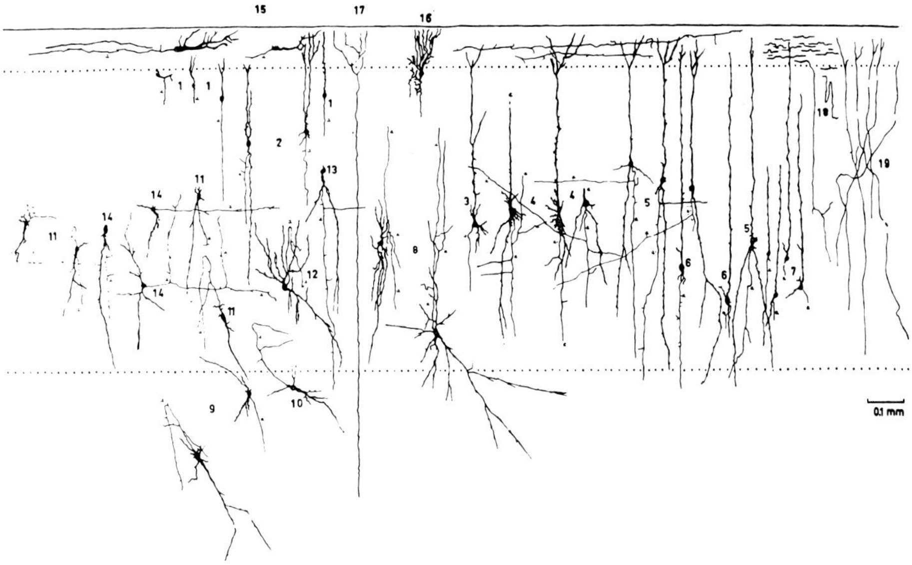

Fig. 5. 94-g fetus, estimated age 62 days. Golgi method. 1, simple bipolar cells in superficial part of pyramidal layer; 2, somewhat deeper and more highly developed cell, its axon having short collaterals; 3, 4, 5, pyramidal cells in middle part of layer; some have long axon collaterals, basal and apical dendrites are more highly developed; 6, 7, deep pyramidal cells are less well developed than those in middle stratum; 8, Martinotti cells with ascending axons; 9, 10, stellate cells in subpyramidal zone of the type seen in younger specimens; 11, 12, 13, 14, stellate cells in pyramidal layer, not seen in younger specimens; 15, horizontal cells in marginal layer; 16, astrocyte; 17, radiating fiber; 18, descending afferent fibers to pyramidal layer; 19, ascending "oblique" afferent fibers. (From Åström, 1967.)

layer where they terminate in the middle part. The *ascending fibers* cross the pyramidal layer, and end in the marginal zone. Some of their collaterals terminate in the middle part of the pyramidal layer. The histological picture indicates that neurons of the marginal, pyramidal and subpyramidal layers may become connected at this time.

(2) Functional characteristics

When the direct cortical response (DCR) recorded close to the stimulating electrodes first appears at the fetal age of 65 days it has a high threshold. The sequence of negative and positive deflections of the response which can be obtained is essentially of the same type as those which have been described in the mature animal, although at this fetal stage there are great variations. Fig. 6A shows a direct cortical response recorded from a 66-day-old fetus and consisting of an early negativity, the primary potential, followed by a slow negativity. With increasing fetal age the threshold decreases considerably and there develops a closer relationship between the different phases of the response and the stimulus parameters, characteristic for the mature cortex. At the earliest stage the primary potential is extremely sensitive to repetitive stimulation, and may be depressed even at a stimulus frequency of 0.2/sec. In contrast the following slow negativity may be succsessively built up by repetitive stimulation, a phenomenon which is also observed in the mature brain (Ochs, 1962; Eidelberg *et al.*, 1965).

References p. 75–77

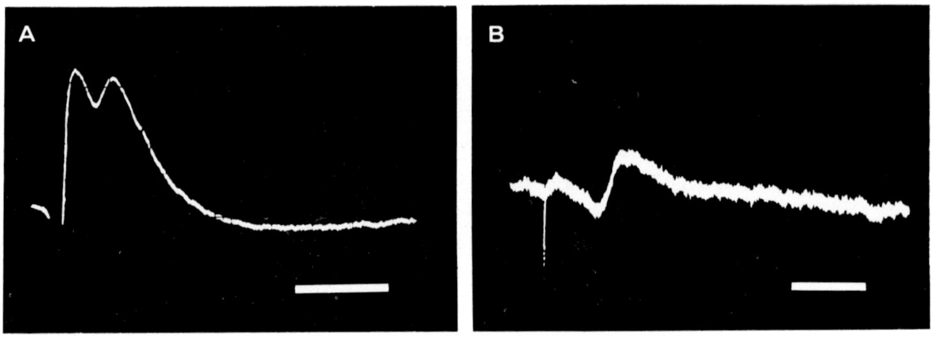

Fig. 6. (A) Direct cortical response (DCR) in a 66-day fetus. Horizontal bar 50 msec. (B) Transcallosal response (TCR) in a 78-day fetus. Horizontal bar 100 msec. Negativity upwards.

From the histological studies reviewed above it is evident that when the fetus enters the period of cortical responsiveness to direct electrical stimulation a very marked development of the neuronal network has taken place especially within the pyramidal layer. There is thus a close temporal correlation between the structural and functional cortical maturation within a short period of time. As mentioned above there is for instance a marked step in the development of the pyramidal cells and their apical dendrites, and this step also occurs in the neurons serving as presynaptic elements of the pyramidal cells. According to Purpura and Grundfest (1957) and Purpura (1959), the primary negative potential of the direct cortical response represents a postsynaptic excitatory potential of the apical dendrites. The appearance of this response would thus indicate that the apical dendrites are now synaptically activated by electrically stimulated presynaptic neurons. Analogously the surface positive wave following upon the primary potential which also can be recorded at this fetal age may be taken as an indication that more deeply situated neurons can also be synaptically activated (Adrian, 1936).

Contrary to Purpura and Grundfest (1956), who claim that dendrites are electrically unexcitable, Clare and Bishop (1955) considered them to be directly excitable, a view recently supported by Merlis (1965). In this context observations on the effect of asphyxia on the cortical functions in the sheep fetus are of interest (Meyerson, 1964). It was found that the primary potential in fetal sheep is far more resistant to asphyxia than in the adult animal. Furthermore the DCR seems to be more resistant to asphyxia than the transcallosal response which appears at about the same fetal age (see below) and which in all probability is of postsynaptic origin (see *e.g.* Grafstein, 1963). The remarkable resistance of the fetal direct cortical response indicates that it is much less dependent on oxygen than one would expect from a response generated by synaptic mechanisms. The possibility should be taken into account that this resistance to asphyxia may indicate that the primary potential is recorded from the neurons which are directly stimulated unless one does not assume that in the fetus this particular synaptic link has special characteristics. One could thus argue that the primary potential is a sign of basic primitive functions, like the steady potential, and that it signals activity of presynaptic origin which is more resistant to asphyxia than

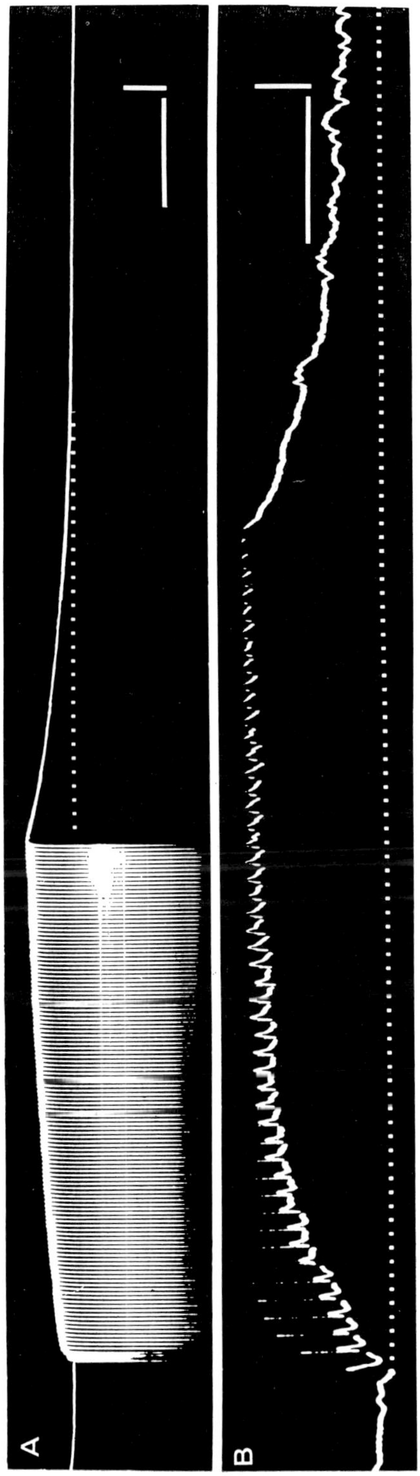

Fig. 7. Steady potential shift induced by repetitive stimulation. (A) 60-day fetus. Stimulus repetition rate 25/sec. Horizontal bar 1 sec, vertical bar 1 mV. (B) 100-day fetus. Stimulus repetition rate 15/sec. Horizontal bar 0.5 sec; vertical bar 200 μV.

responses of postsynaptic origin such as that evoked by transcallosal stimulation. Another alternative would be that the primary potential consists of one presynaptic and one postsynaptic fraction (Kandel *et al.*, 1958) the former being resistant to asphyxia.

The negative shift of the steady potential induced by repetitive cortical stimulation which has been thoroughly studied in the adult animal (*cf.* O'Leary and Goldring, 1964) is another sign of cortical response that is regularly obtained in the sheep fetus after the 65th day. Actually, such an induced SP shift seems to be the very first sign of cortical response to direct electrical stimulation during fetal life, since in 3 fetuses out of 15 between 50 and 65 days old repetitive stimulation with frequencies above 10/sec evoked a negative shift (Fig. 7A), whereas in the same fetuses no direct cortical response could be recorded (Eidelberg *et al.*, 1965). The finding that after asphyxiation, induced by clamping the cord, for about 15 min no shift could be obtained shows that this phenomenon is dependent on physiological conditions. The shift generally outlasts the stimulation period also in older fetuses which exhibit a direct cortical response (Fig. 7B), as is also the case in adult animals. The fact that a negative shift can be induced at a fetal age when no direct cortical response is obtained indicates that the electrically induced SP shift is not to be regarded as a result of a temporal summation of individual DCR negativities as has been proposed (see Goldring *et al.*, 1959). This conclusion is supported by the observation that in older fetuses exhibiting a slow negativity to single shocks the SP shift induced by repetitive stimulation may even be positive. Irrespective of the genesis of the electrically induced SP shift it constitutes an introduction into the fetal period of cortical responsiveness to direct stimulation.

In close temporal relation to the appearance of the direct cortical response an interhemispheric response can be elicited. Its characteristics indicate that it represents a transcallosal response, the main components being a positive–negative potential sequence followed by a second positivity (Meyerson, 1964; Fig. 6B). Like the direct cortical response the transcallosal response is at its first appearance variable, has a high threshold and follows a slow temporal course. During development it becomes more stable and the threshold decreases. There is also a shortening of the latency of this response with age. This shortening is however much less in fetal sheep than that found in cats during the postnatal period (Grafstein, 1963). Among the characteristics of the fetal transcallosal response so far investigated it should be mentioned that it is obtained from symmetrical points on the cortical surface of the hemispheres, and that it first appears within a discrete region near the vertex in which the suprasylvian gyrus is found in the more developed brain (Meyerson, unpublished observations). The interesting difference in susceptibility to asphyxia between the direct and transcallosal response during fetal life has already been mentioned, the sensitivity of the transcallosal response being referred to its supposedly postsynaptic origin.

As described above, an evoked cortical response to tactile stimulation of the skin can be obtained during the first fetal period. It consists at that stage of a surface-positive response indicating depolarization of the afferents which are entering the cortical plate but which do not yet evoke any postsynaptic activity. In the beginning

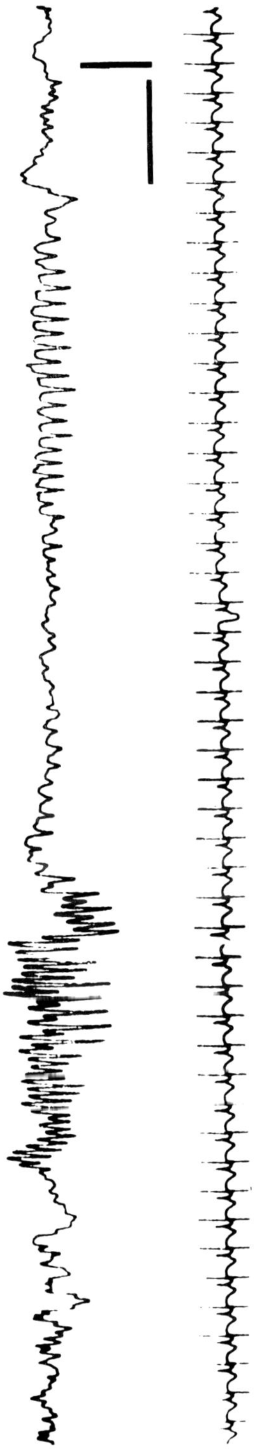

Fig. 8. Spontaneous cortical activity in a 75-day fetus. Lower row EKG of fetus. Horizontal bar 1 sec; vertical bar 50 μV. Negativity upwards.

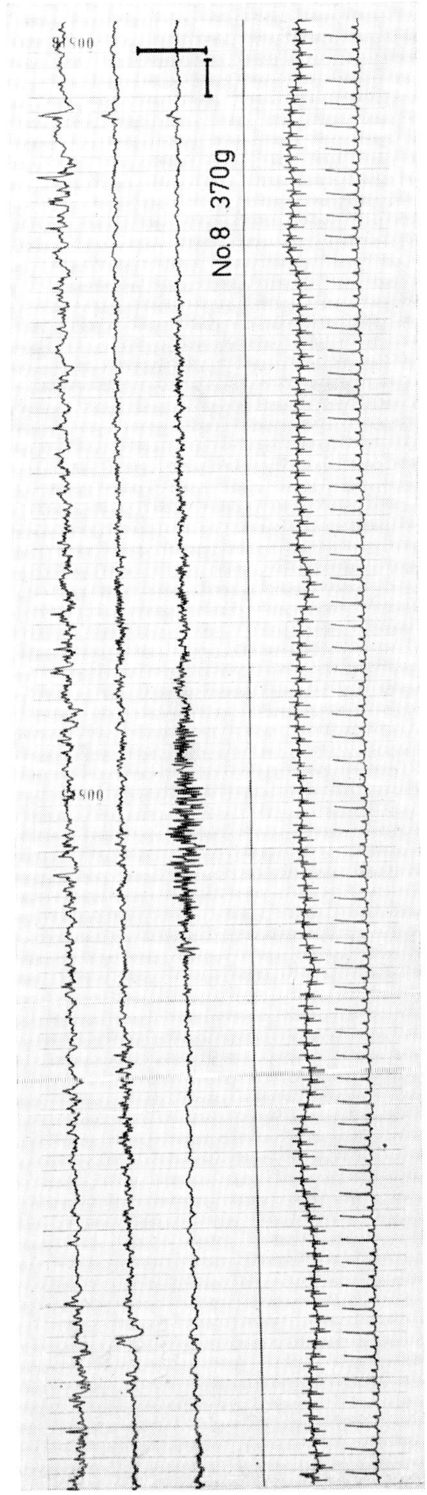

Fig. 9. Spontaneous activity from an 87-day fetus recorded from three different cortical points within the parietal region. Horizontal bar 1 sec; vertical bar 200 μV. (From Bernhard *et al.*, 1959.)

of the second fetal period a surface negativity appears following upon the initial positivity (Molliver, 1967). During a period of 10–15 days the initial positivity increases. The following negative wave also increases with age and appears earlier on the preceding positive phase. The result is that after an additional 10–15 days the response is dominated by the negative phase (see Fig. 5 in the paper of Molliver, p. 86, this Volume).

As mentioned above, the histological studies show that at the beginning of the second fetal period a marked step occurs in the structural development of the pyramidal neurons and their apical dendrites. There is thus a striking temporal correlation between these structural changes and the appearance of the surface-negative wave of the evoked response indicating that depolarization now takes place in the apical dendrites as a result of axodendritic synaptic activation. As mentioned above the afferent terminals which were found in the cortical plate during this fetal period seem to be of the non-specific type (Åström, 1967), which would mean that the response obtained is the result of activity induced via the non-specific afferent system. At the age of about 110 days the response changes, and now displays a shorter duration and a shortening of the latency (Molliver, 1967). It is possible that these changes may represent the appearance of cortical activation by the specific afferent system. However, further investigations are needed to answer this question.

Finally, some data concerning the appearance of other electrical signs of cortical activity which appear later in the second fetal period may be mentioned. The spontaneous cortical activity recorded with surface electrodes is still of the primitive PN I type during the initial phase of this fetal period (see Table I). As illustrated in Fig. 8, two types of spontaneous PN I activity can be obtained at this stage. The record shows a train of the typical 14–15/sec PN I activity described earlier followed by a sequence of surface-positive waves which regularly have a frequency of 8 per sec. Not until about the 87th day is a continuous wide-spread spontaneous activity obtained. The records in Fig. 9 are from different cortical points, and it should be noticed that there is more continuous activity in the upper record (more frontal) than in the two lower, the lowest mainly showing spindles of PN I activity. Thus, during development the continuous EEG activity in different cortical regions may appear at different ages as observed by Verley (1959) on rabbits during postnatal development. In the sheep there is an interval of about a week between the appearance of the first signs of cortical synaptic activity and responsiveness to direct stimulation on the one hand, and on the other the appearance of the continuous wide-spread spontaneous activity of the more mature type which develops further during the last third of the prenatal period (see Bernhard *et al.*, 1959).

Electrically evoked seizure activity (post-stimulatory after-discharge) cannot be obtained until the 85–90th day of fetal life (Kolmodin and Meyerson, 1966). The delayed interhemispheric response which is dependent on extracallosal connections (Rutledge and Kennedy, 1960) also appears in the second period, around the 80th day (Meyerson, unpublished observations).

The authors are aware that the data so far obtained are too sparse to allow a meaningful comparison of the development of the last mentioned types of cortical

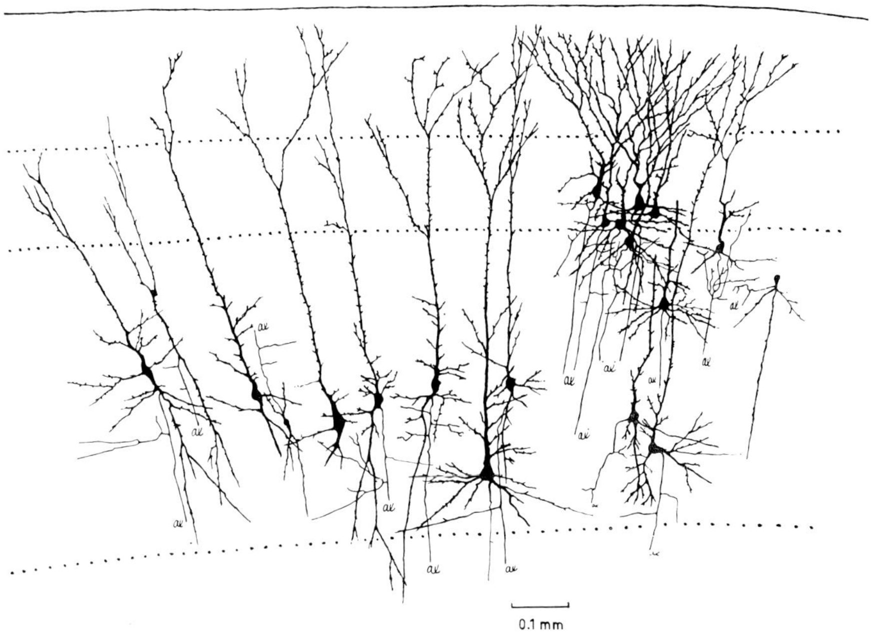

Fig. 10. 450-g fetus, estimated age 84 days. Golgi stained section. See text. (From Åström, 1967.)

acitivity with the morphological data. Suffice it to say that during the period from about the 65th to the 86th day the 5 pyramidal zones develop. In the middle zone the pyramidal cells have recurrent collaterals which reach the marginal layer. Most typical for this period is the development of the superficial pyramidal cells and the basilar dendrites. The superficial pyramidal neurons which are the last to develope now show widely branching apical and basilar dendrites (Fig. 10), and the numerous basilar dendrites of the middle and deep pyramidal cells which are covered with spines show extensive ramifications. It should be added that the corresponding structural development takes place during the postnatal period in cats (Noback and Purpura, 1961; Marty, 1962; Scheibel, 1962; Scheibel and Scheibel, 1963), rabbits (Noback and Purpura, 1961; Laget and Delhaye, 1962), rat (Lorente de Nó, 1933; Noback and Purpura, 1961) and mouse (Lorente de Nó, 1933; Kobayashi *et al.*, 1963). Electrophysiological studies show that corresponding changes in the spontaneous cortical activity also take place after birth in cats (Grossman, 1955; Scheibel, 1962; Scheibel and Scheibel, 1963), rabbits (Schadé, 1960; Laget and Delhaye, 1962) and mouse (Kobayashi *et al.*, 1963).

II. COMMENTS AND CONCLUSIONS

A comparison of the morphological data from the sheep's somesthetic area obtained at different prenatal ages (Åström, 1967) with data from the postnatal cat (see Noback and Purpura, 1961; Marty, 1962) show that the stage of development of the above described cortical structures in the middle of the sheep's fetal life corresponds

References p. 75–77

in most details to the developmental stage of the newborn cat. The interest is thereby focused on the cells in the marginal layer, the superficial and deep pyramidal cells and their axon collaterals, apical and basilar processes as well as the stellate cells. It may be added that electron microscopic studies on the newborn cat show the existence of axodendritic synaptic structures (Voeller *et al.*, 1963; Pappas and Purpura, 1964). The cortex of the newborn cat is electrically excitable, and exhibits direct cortical responses (see *e.g.* Purpura *et al.*, 1960), transcallosal responses (Grafstein, 1963) and surface-negative evoked responses to afferent stimulation (see *e.g.* Scherrer and Oeconomos, 1955; Marty, 1962). This is so also in the 65–70 day sheep fetus, the only difference being that the negativity of the evoked response to tactile stimulation at this stage is preceded by a positivity, the possible genesis of which has been discussed above. The initial period in which the functions mentioned appear for the first time was never investigated in the cat or rabbit since no prenatal studies were made on these animals.

The electrophysiological investigations on the prenatal cortical development in sheep fetuses show that there is a period before the 65th day during which the cortex is electrically inexcitable, and during which no definite sign of synaptic activity can be obtained. A steady potential as well as cortical cell membrane potentials were found. At the end of this period the cortical structures have a relatively primitive appearance. The precursors of the pyramidal cells are still of bipolar type, the apical dendrites are slender and have short ramifications in the lowest part of the marginal layer and no collaterals, there are few basal dendrites, the dendrites have no spines and there are no stellate or Martinotti cells in the pyramidal layer. Up to the 45–48th day the afferent fibers only extend to the intermediate zone and do not penetrate into the cortical plate until the 58th to 60th day. The surface-positive response to tactile stimulation obtained at the 48–50th day thus seems to indicate a depolarization of these afferents which have not reached the relatively thin pyramidal layer. The primitive PN I and metrazol waves which appear at about the same time seem to be the result of subcortical activity which may engage the same afferent terminals.

At the 65th day the cortex becomes electrically excitable (SP shift to repetitive cortical stimulation, direct cortical response and transcallosal response) and fractions of the responses to cortical stimulation as well as the growing negativity of the evoked response to tactile stimulation represent signs of the appearance of postsynaptic activation. At this fetal stage a definite step (between the 58th and 65th day) in the morphological maturation has taken place especially within the pyramidal layer. Axons of the pyramidal cells have several horizontal collaterals, and the apical dendrites, which are now thick and have proximal branches, show indications of spines. Stellate and Martinotti cells appear in the pyramidal layer, and have axons which ramify in this zone. Descending fibers from the marginal zone end in the middle pyramidal layer and ascending fibers crossing the pyramidal zone and ending in the marginal layer send collaterals to the middle pyramidal zone. Thus, at this stage the fibers which ascend and descend into the pyramidal layer as well as the extensions of the 'interneurons' in this layer run towards the pyramidal cells, and appear to provide conditions for an extended presynaptic transmission. In addition, the marked step in the development of the apical dendrites of the pyramidal cells indicates that they have reached a degree of maturity which would enable them to participate in synaptic activity.

The investigations on sheep fetuses thus show that there is a close temporal correlation between the significant step in functional development in terms of electrical cortical excitability and synaptic activation and the very marked histological changes that occur within a short time which obviously represents an important period in the ontogeny of the parietal cortex.

ACKNOWLEDGEMENTS

The investigations were supported by grants from the Association for the Aid of Crippled Children, Statens Medicinski Forskningsråd, Stiftelsen Therese och Johan Anderssons Minne and Stiftelsen Gustaf och Thyra Svenssons Minne and Expressens Prenatalforskningsfond.

REFERENCES

ADRIAN, E. D., (1936); The spread of activity in the cerebral cortex. *J. Physiol.*, **88**, 127–161.

ÄNGGÅRD, L., BERGSTRÖM, R., AND BERNHARD, C. G., (1961); Analysis of prenatal spinal reflex activity in sheep. *Acta physiol. scand.*, **53**, 128–136.

ÅSTRÖM, K. E., (1967); On the early development of the isocortex in fetal sheep. This volume, pp. 1–59.

BARCROFT, J., AND BARRON, D. H., (1939); Movement in the mammalian foetus. *Ergebn. Physiol.*, **42**, 107–152.

BERGSTRÖM, R. M., (1962); Prenatal development of motor functions. *Ann. Chir. Gynaec. Fenn.*, **51**, 112.

BERGSTRÖM, R. M., HELLSTRÖM, P.-E., AND STENBERG, D., (1961); Prenatal stretch reflex activity in the guinea-pig. *Ann. Chir. Gynaec. Fenn.*, **50**, 458–466.

BERGSTRÖM, R. M., HELLSTRÖM, P.-E., AND STENBERG, D., (1962a); Studies in reflex irradiation in the foetal guinea-pig. *Ann. Chir. Gynaec. Fenn.*, **51**, 171–178.

BERGSTRÖM, R. M., HELLSTRÖM, P.-E., AND STENBERG, D., (1962b); Über die Entwicklung der elektrischen Aktivität im Grosshirn des intrauterinen Meerschweinchen-Fetus. *Ann. Chir. Gynaec. Fenn.*, 51 fasc. **4**, 466–474.

BERNHARD, C. G., KAISER, I. H., AND KOLMODIN, G. M., (1959); On the development of cortical activity in fetal sheep. *Acta physiol. scand.*, **47**, 333–349.

BERNHARD, C. G., KAISER, I. H., AND KOLMODIN, G. M., (1962); On the epileptogenic properties of the fetal brain. An electrophysiological study on the electrically and chemically induced convulsive brain activity in sheep fetuses. *Acta paediat.*, **51**, 81–87.

BUREŠ, J., (1957); The ontogenetic development of steady potential differences in the cerebral cortex in animals. *Electroenceph. clin. Neurophysiol.*, **9**, 121–130.

CLARE, M. H., AND BISHOP, G. H., (1955); Properties of dendrites; apical dendrites of the cat cortex. *Electroenceph. clin. Neurophysiol.*, **7**, 85–98.

DO CARMO, R. J., (1960); Direct cortical and recruiting responses in postnatal rabbit. *J. Neurophysiol.*, **23**, 496–504.

ECCLES, R. M., AND WILLIS, W. D., (1962); Presynaptic inhibition of the monosynaptic reflex pathway in kittens. *J. Physiol.*, **165**, 403–420.

EIDELBERG, E., KOLMODIN, G. M., AND MEYERSON, B. A., (1965); Ontogenesis of the steady potential and the direct cortical response in fetal sheep brain. *Exp. Neurol.*, **12**, 198–214.

EIDELBERG, E., KOLMODIN, G. M., AND MEYERSON, B. A., (1965); In preparation.

ELLINGSON, R. J., AND WILCOTT, R. C., (1960); Development of evoked responses in visual and auditory cortices of kittens. *J. Neurophysiol.*, **23**, 363–375.

GOLDRING, S., O'LEARY, J. L., WINTER, D. L., AND PEARLMAN, A. L., (1959); Identification of a prolonged post-synaptic potential of cerebral cortex. *Proc. Soc. exp. Biol. (N.Y.)*, **100**, 429–431.

GRAFSTEIN, B., (1963); Postnatal development of the transcallosal evoked response in the cerebral cortex of the cat. *J. Neurophysiol.*, **26**, 79–99.

GROSSMAN, C., (1955); Electro-ontogenesis of cerebral activity. *Arch. Neurol. Psychiat. (Chic.)*, **74**, 186–202.

HAAPANEN, L., KOLMODIN, G. M., AND SKOGLUND, C. R., (1958); Membrane and action potentials of spinal interneurons in the cat. *Acta physiol. scand.*, **43**, 315–348.

HUNT, W. E., AND GOLDRING, S., (1951); Maturation of evoked response of the visual cortex in the postnatal rabbit. *Electroenceph. clin. Neurophysiol.*, **3**, 465–471.

JOUBERT, D. M., (1956); A study of prenatal growth and development in the sheep. *J. Agr. Sci.*, **47**, 382–428.

KANDEL, E. R., BRINLEY, F. J., AND MARSHALL, W. H., (1958); Some properties of the direct cortical response. *Electroenceph. clin. Neurophysiol.*, **10**, 765.

KOBAYASHI, T., INMAN, O., BUNO, W., AND HIMWICH, H. E., (1963); A multidisciplinary study of changes in mouse brain with age. *Recent Advan. biol. Psychiat.*, **5**, 293–308.

KOLMODIN, G. M., AND MEYERSON, B. A., (1966); Ontogenesis of paroxysmal activity in fetal sheep. Submitted for publication.

LAGET, P., AND DELHAYE, N., (1962); Etude du développement néonatal de diverses activités électriques corticales chez le lapin. *Actualités neurophysiol.*, **4**, 259–284.

LORENTE, DE NÓ, R., (1933); Studies on the structure of the cerebral cortex. *J. Psychol. Neurol.*, **45**, 381–438.

MALCOLM, J. L., (1953); Some observations on dorsal root potentials. *The Spinal Cord. Ciba Found. Symp.*, London, Churchill (pp. 84–91).

MALCOLM, J. L., (1955); The appearance of inhibition in the developing spinal cord of kittens. *Biochemistry of the Developing Nervous System.* New York, Academic Press (pp. 104–109).

MARTY, R., (1962); Développement post-natal des résponses sensorielles du cortex cérébral chez le chat et le lapin. *Arch. Anat. micr. Morph. exp.*, **51**, 129–264.

MERLIS, J. K., (1965); Excitability cycle of the direct cortical response studied with minimal stimuli and response averaging. *Electroenceph. clin. Neurophysiol.*, **18**, 118–123.

MEYERSON, B. A., (1964); The effect of asphyxia on induced cortical activity in fetal sheep. *Acta physiol. scand.*, **62**, 489–490.

MOLLIVER, M., (1967); An ontogenetic study of evoked somesthetic cortical responses in the sheep. This volume, pp. 78–90.

NAKA, K. I., (1964a); Electrophysiology of the fetal spinal cord. I. Action potentials of the motoneuron. *J. gen. Physiol.*, **47**, 1003–1022.

NAKA, K. I., (1964b); Electrophysiology of the fetal spinal cord. II. Interaction among peripheral inputs and recurrent inhibition. *J. gen. Physiol.*, **47**, 1023–1038.

NOBACK, C. R., AND PURPURA, D. P., (1961); Postnatal ontogenesis of neurons in cat neocortex. *J. comp. Neurol.*, **117**, 291–307.

OCHS, S., (1962); Analysis of cellular mechanisms of direct cortical responses. *Fed. Proc.*, **21**, 642–647.

O'LEARY, J., AND GOLDRING, S., (1964); DC potentials of the brain. *Physiol. Rev.*, **44**, 91–125.

PAPPAS, G. D., AND PURPURA, D. P., (1964); Electron microscopy of immature human and feline neo, cortex. *Growth and Maturation, Vol. 4, Progress in Brain Research.* J. P. D. P. Purpura and Schadé-Editors, Amsterdam, Elsevier (pp. 176–186).

PURPURA, D. P., (1959); Nature of electrocortical potentials and synaptic organizations in cerebral and cerebellar cortex. *International Review of Neurobiology, Vol. 1.* C. C. Pfeiffer and J. R. Smythies, Editors, New York, Academic Press (pp. 47–163).

PURPURA, D. P., (1961); Morphophysiological basic of elementary evoked response patterns in the neocortex of the newborn cat. *Ann. N.Y. Acad. Sci.*, **92**, art. 3, 840–859.

PURPURA, D. P., (1964); Relationship of seizure susceptibility to morphologic and physiologic properties of normal and abnormal immature cortex. *Neurological and Electroencephalographic Correlative Studies in Infancy.* New York, Grune and Stratton.

PURPURA, D. P., CARMICHAEL, M. W., AND HOUSEPIAN, E. M., (1960); Physiological and anatomical studies of development of superficial axodendritic synaptic pathways in neocortex. *Exp. Neurol.*, **2**, 324–347.

PURPURA, D. P., AND GRUNDFEST, H., (1956); Nature of dendritic potentials and synaptic mechanisms in cerebral cortex of cat. *J. Neurophysiol.*, **19**, 573–592.

PURPURA, D. P., AND GRUNDFEST, H., (1957); Physiological and pharmacological consequences of different synaptic organizations in cerebral and cerebellar cortex. *J. Neurophysiol.*, **20**, 494–522.

PURPURA, D. P., SCHOFER, R. J., HOUSEPIAN, E. M., AND NOBACK, C. R., (1964); Comparative ontogenesis of structure-function relations in cerebral and cerebellar cortex. *Growth and Maturation of the Brain, Vol. 4, Progress in Brain Research.* D. P. Purpura, and J. P. Schadé Editors. Amsterdam, Elsevier (pp. 187–221).

ROSE, G. H., AND LINDSLEY, D. B., (1965); Visually evoked electrocortical responses in kittens. *Science*, **148**, 1244–1246.

RUTLEDGE, L. T., AND KENNEDY, T. T., (1960); Extracallosal delayed responses to cortical stimulation in chloralosed cat. *J. Neurophysiol.*, **23**, 188–196.

SCHADÉ, J. P., (1960); Origin of the spontaneous electrical activity of the cerebral cortex. *Recent Advan. biol. Psychiat.*, **2**, 23–42.

SCHADÉ, J. P., AND PASCOE, E. G., (1964); Maturational changes in cerebral cortex III. Effects of methionine sulfoximine on some electrical parameters and dendritic organisation of cortical neurons. *The Developing Brain, Vol. 9, Progress in Brain Research.* W. A. and H. E. Himwich, Editosr. Amsterdam, Elsevier (pp. 132–154).

SCHEIBEL, A. B., (1962); Neural correlates of psychophysiological developments in the young organism. *Recent Advan. biol. Psychiat.*, **4**, 313–327.

SCHEIBEL, M. E., AND SCHEIBEL, A. B., (1963); Some structuro-functional correlates of development in young cats. *Electroenceph. clin. Neurophysiol.*, Suppl. **24**, 235–246.

SCHERRER, J., AND OECONOMOS, D., (1955); Réponses évoquées corticales somesthétiques des mammifères adultes et nouveau-nés. *Les Grandes Activités du Lobe Temporal.* Paris, Masson (pp. 249–268).

SKOGLUND, S., (1960a); On the postnatal development of postural mechanisms as revealed by electromyography and myography in decerebrate kittens. *Acta physiol. scand.*, **49**, 299–317.

SKOGLUND, S., (1960b); The spinal transmission of proprioceptive reflexes and the postnatal development of conduction velocity in different hindlimb nerves in the kittens. *Acta physiol. scand.*, **49**, 318–329.

SKOGLUND, S., (1960c); The activity of muscle receptors in the kitten. *Acta physiol. scand.*, **50**, 203–221.

SKOGLUND, S., (1960d); Central connections and functions of muscle nerves in the kitten. *Acta physiol. scand.*, **50**, 222–237.

SKOGLUND, S., (1960e); The reactions to tetanic stimulation of the two-neuron arc in the kitten. *Acta physiol. scand.*, **50**, 238–253.

VERLEY, R. L., (1959); Développement des activités électrocorticales, motrices et neurovégétatives des mammifères nouveau-nés. *Thèse.* Paris,EditionsA.G.E.M.P.

VOELLER, K., PAPPAS, G. D., AND PURPURA, D. P., (1963); Electron microscope study of development of cat superficial neocortex. *Exp. Neurol.*, **7**, 107–130.

WILSON, V. J., (1962); Reflex transmission in the kitten. *J. Neurophysiol.*, **26**, 263–276.

An Ontogenetic Study of Evoked Somesthetic Cortical Responses in the Sheep

MARK E. MOLLIVER*

Department of Physiology, Karolinska Institutet, Stockholm (Sweden)

INTRODUCTION

The literature of the last decade demonstrates an increasing interest in the functiona and morphological development of the central nervous system, especially in regard to the nature of spontaneous and evoked cortical activity.

Prenatal spontaneous cortical activity has been demonstrated in the guinea-pig (Jasper *et al.*, 1937) and in the human fetus (Borkowski and Bernstine, 1955), but no developmental sequence was clearly described until Bernhard *et al.* (1959) reported the maturing cortical activity of the sheep fetus from 65 days of gestation to full term at 150 days. The latter authors suggested that peripheral stimulation may produce a widespread cortical disturbance after 100 days of gestation, and that an arousal pattern could be seen at 144 days in fetal sheep.

The cortical response evoked by stimulation of peripheral sensory receptors during the early postnatal period has been described for rabbit and cat (Hunt and Goldring, 1951; Oeconomos and Scherrer, 1953; Scherrer and Oeconomos, 1955; Grossman, 1955; Ellingson and Wilcott, 1960) and the human (Maternal Infant Health, 1962). The neonatal evoked response in all of these studies was distinguished by a markedly prolonged response latency and by a diminished capacity to respond to repetitive stimulation. It was also shown that the response latency gradually diminished in the days following birth.

The evoked cortical responses in the newborn are further distinguished from the mature response by wave-form. The earliest responses were described as being purely surface-negative deflections until one to two weeks after birth at which time an initial surface positivity first appeared and later increased in amplitude (Scherrer and Oeconomos, 1955; Marty, 1962).

In more recent studies of the neonatal cat, electrical stimulation of the ventrolateral thalamic nuclei produced cortical responses that were predominantly surface-negative preceded by a small initial surface positivity (Purpura, 1961a, b and c). The initial positive wave became more prominent during the early weeks of life. The evoked response was attenuated at stimulus rates of 0.5 per sec and disappeared at rates of

* On leave of absence from Harvard Medical School, Boston, Mass. Supported by a Research Fellowship PX-322-11 from the Division of General Medical Sciences, U.S. Public Health Service. Present address: The Johns Hopkins University School of Medicine, Baltimore, Maryland 21205.

10 per sec. Application of GABA to the cortical surface eliminated the surface negativity, and only a small positive wave was seen (Purpura and Carmichael, 1959). Histological studies of the neonatal cat brain showed well developed apical dendrites arising from cortical pyramidal cells, but few and poorly developed basilar dendrites (Noback and Purpura, 1961). Electron micrographs showed numerous synapses on the apical dendrites alone (Purpura, 1961a). Sections of brains from 8-to 20-day-old kittens showed rapid flowering of the basilar dendritic network during this later period.

On the basis of these functional and morphological data plus the results of direct cortical stimulation (Purpura *et al.*, 1960), the hypothesis was suggested that the surface negativity of the evoked response arises from postsynaptic activity in the apical dendrites, and the surface positivity arises from the later developing basilar dendrites (Purpura, 1961a, b and c).

All the above studies of evoked potentials have focused on the neonatal period as a period of relative physiological immaturity. There has been little attention paid to what may have preceded the neonatal state and to where the neonatal period fits into the ontogenetic continuum. The problem also arises as to whether it may be meaningful to compare neonatal functions in different species with gestation periods of different lengths and varying rates of development. It is also unclear whether peripheral stimulation produces cortical activity that is more widespread in the immature organism than in the adult (Bernhard *et al.*, 1959; Scherrer and Oeconomos, 1955).

The present paper reports a longitudinal investigation of the prenatal development of evoked somatosensory cortical responses from early fetal life to full term in sheep. Special attention is given to the early fetal period during which the evoked somesthetic response is first obtained.

MATERIAL AND METHOD

The experiments were performed on 18 fetuses of 17 ewes. Three of the fetuses were not included in the results because of cerebral cyanosis and circulatory collapse. The weights of the 15 fetuses tested ranged from 16 g to 1690 g. The estimated gestational age has been calculated for each fetus from the equations of Hugget and Widdas (1951) and ranged from 55 to 120 days (total gestation time 140–150 days).

An intravenous catheter was introduced into a superficial foreleg vein of the ewe under local procaine anesthesia, and then general anesthesia was induced by the slow infusion of approximately 35 mg/kg of Thiogenal (methylthioethyl-2-pentylthiobarbituric acid - Na), a rapidly eliminated barbiturate. A tracheotomy and gastrostomy were performed. The common carotid arteries were ligated bilaterally, and a polyethylene catheter leading to a Grass blood pressure transducer was placed in one carotid. The ewe was then decerebrated. A dose of 0.5 mg/kg of D-tubocurarine was given intravenously, and the tracheotomy tube connected to a respirator.

Approximately 1 h after decerebration the uterus was exposed, a transverse uterine incision was made between cotyledons and the fetus was gently delivered. Great care was taken to avoid trauma to the umbilical vessels.

References p. 90–91

The fetus was mounted in a mass of cotton previously soaked in mineral oil at 39°, the cotton being firmly shaped to act as a support completely enclosing the fetus except for the skull. The fetal preparation was then placed on a small weighted table, mechanically isolated from the table on which the ewe was lying. The support of oil soaked cotton was used in place of the more conventional head stand with ear bars. The exposed uterus and umbilical cord were also covered with mineral oil and cotton.

Unilateral craniotomy was carefully performed on the fetus, and the left fronto-parietal cortex was widely exposed. The dura over this area was incised and reflected. The exposed cortex was covered with mineral oil at 38°, which was replenished every 10 min.

Skin temperature of the fetus and rectal temperature of the ewe were measured by thermocouple and maintained at 38°. The carotid blood pressure and heart rate of the

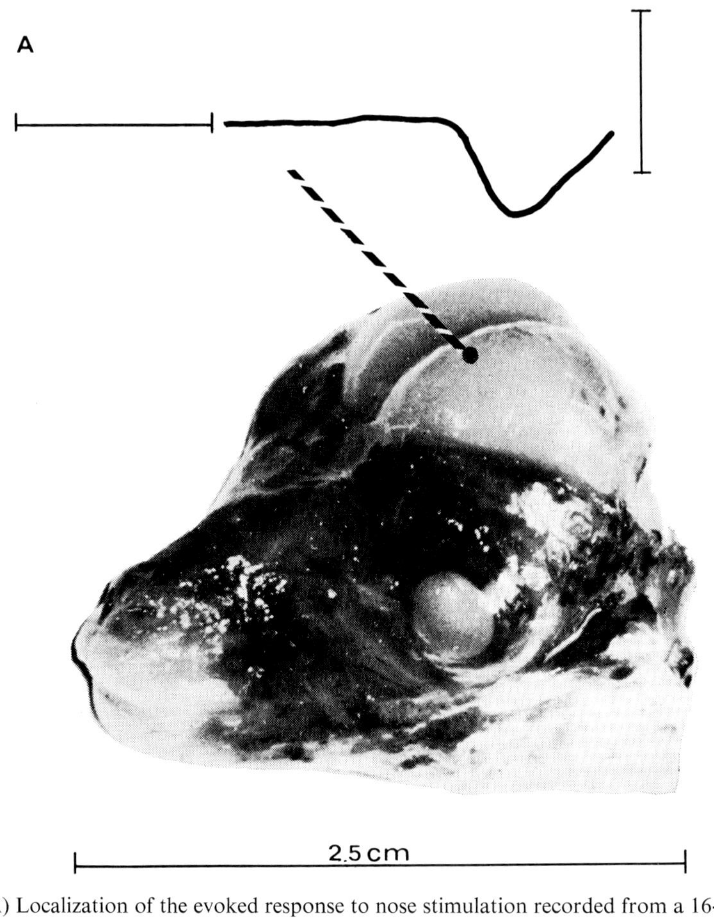

Fig. 1. (A) Localization of the evoked response to nose stimulation recorded from a 16-g sheep fetus (calculated age 55 days). The horizontal time bar equals 100 msec. The vertical bar equals 100 μV.

ewe were continuously monitored on a direct writing polygraph; the fetal electrocardiogram was intermittently observed.

Each recording session was begun no earlier than 3 h after the ewe had been anesthetized, and the recording was thus made on unanesthetized fetuses. Before recording, 1 mg/kg of D-tubocurarine was given intramuscularly.

Experimental procedure. Monopolar differential a.c. recording was used throughout. Recording electrodes consisted of chlorided silver wires with 0.5 mm ball tips and were mounted in Grass electrode holders. The indifferent electrode was placed on the resected edge of the skull. The recording electrode was placed in gentle contact with the pial surface. The electrodes were connected to the cathode follower input of a Grass P 5 preamplifier which drove a 5-inch oscilloscope. Permanent recordings were made with a Grass kymograph camera.

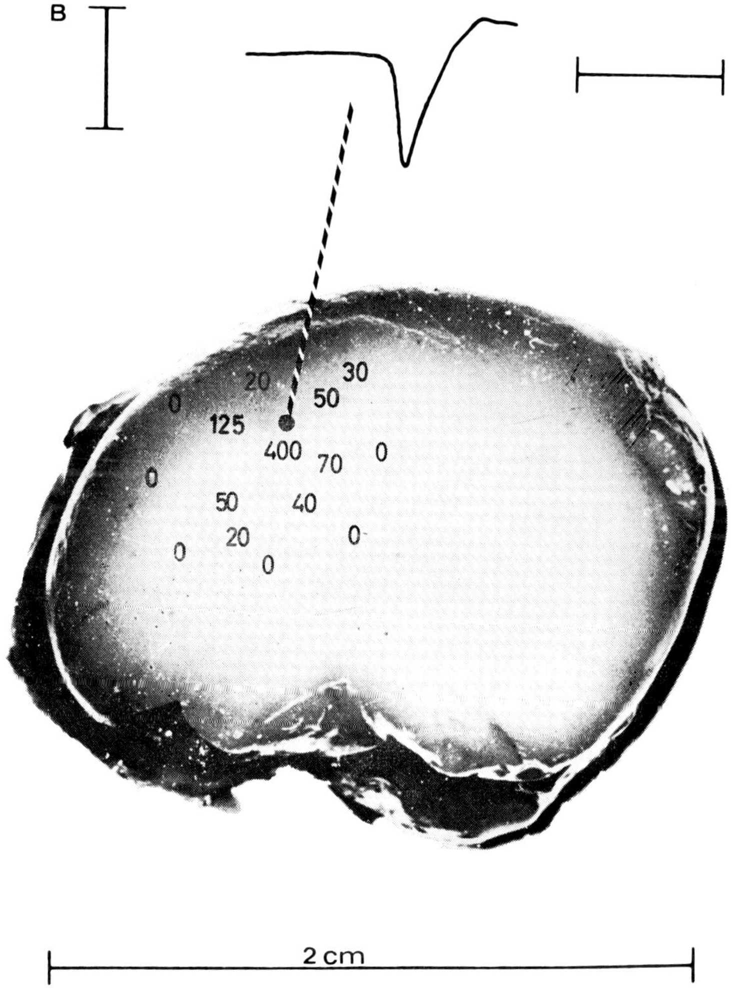

(B) Distribution of evoked cortical activity in a 132-g sheep fetus (calculated age 73 days). Numbers on the cortex represent amplitude in microvolts of the positive wave. Vertical bar, 100 μV; horizontal bar, 100 msec. Polarity = positive down.

References p. 90–91

Only the results of mechanical stimulation are reported in this paper. Stimulation was produced by a cat whisker cemented to a lever arm that extended from the armature of a shielded electromagnetic relay. The relay coil was energized with the output of a Grass stimulator. This stimulating device could be accurately positioned by a three-dimensional micromanipulator.

The stimulating end of the whisker moved a distance of 1 mm in 0.9 msec and then gradually returned to its resting position over a period of 10 msec. The mechanism was well damped, and it was difficult to detect oscillation or after-vibration of the stimulating whisker. The end of the whisker was placed just in contact with the lower lateral aspect of the nares at the muco-cutaneous junction. Mechanical stimulation and cortical recording were done on ipsilateral sides (Adrian, 1943; Hamuy *et al.*, 1950).

In order to delineate the cortical area activated by afferent impulses from a small peripheral area, the recording electrode was moved in small steps over the entire cortex while tactile stimulation was repetitively applied to the nostril. The mechanical stimulator was fixed in position and single stimuli were presented at 30-sec intervals. At least 10 responses were recorded at each electrode position so that artefacts or spontaneous potentials could be eliminated.

RESULTS

(A) Localization in the sensory cortex

The cortical responses induced by tactile stimulation of the ipsilateral nose are presented for 5 sheep fetuses of different gestational ages (Figs. 1 and 2). The smallest sheep fetus studied had a calculated age of 55 days. In this fetus a response could be obtained from one position only (Fig. 1A). An electrode displacement of over 1 mm in any direction resulted in the disappearance of the response. This response was of long latency and duration, and was monophasic surface positive. No spontaneous cortical activity was observed.

Fig. 1B shows the cortex of a 73-day-old fetus. As may be seen, the response recorded from this fetus was still dominated by an initial positivity. The numbers refer to amplitude in microvolts of the positive response recorded from the cortical surface. As the recording electrode was moved away from the area of peak response amplitude, a gradient of diminishing response height was seen. A few millimeters away from the peak response, no activity could be recorded.

Figs. 2A, B and C show the left hemispheres from 3 fetuses respectively of 85, 92 and 110 days of age. The increasing gross anatomical differentiation of the brains is apparent. The primary somatosensory area and adjoining cortex is included within each rectangle. The line drawing beneath each brain is an enlargement of the rectangular area. The distribution of evoked cortical activity is shown on each drawing.

The brains of the 55- and 73-day fetuses are lissencephalic, but in the 85-day fetal brain, sulci have appeared outlining the suprasylvian gyrus, which is more readily discernible in the 92- and 110-day fetuses. The evoked cortical responses reproduced

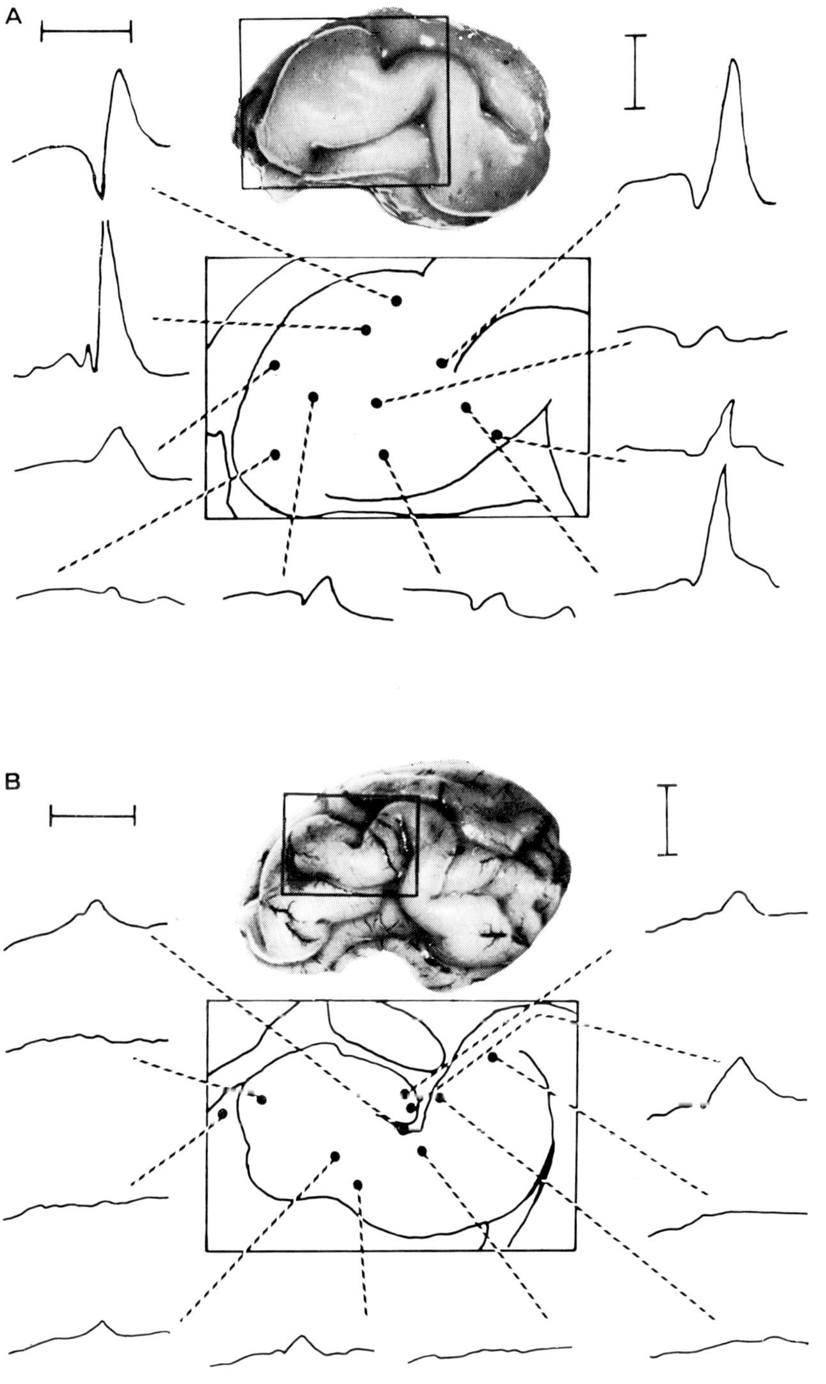

Fig. 2. Distribution of evoked cortical responses. A, from a 388-g sheep fetus (calculated age 85 days); B, from a 468-g sheep fetus (calculated age 92 days); C, from a 1170-g sheep fetus (calculated age 110 days). In all diagrams vertical line marks 100 μV and horizontal bar marks 100 msec. Polarity = positive down.

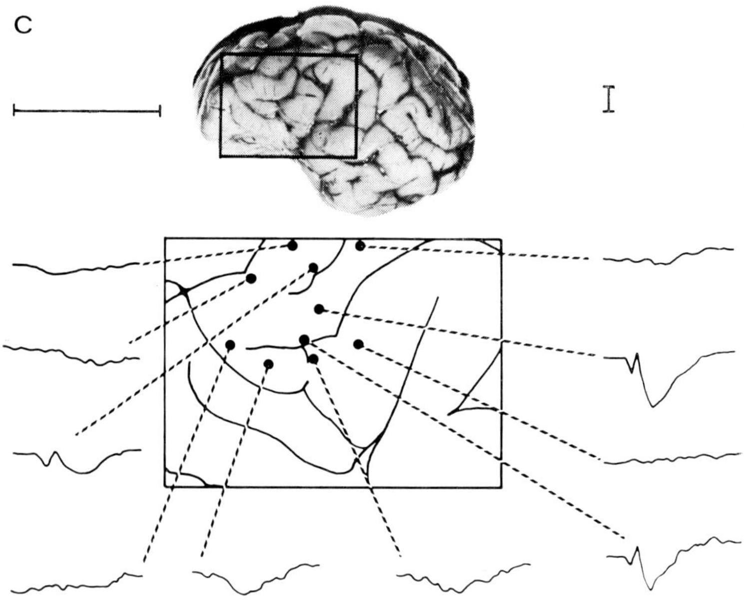

Fig. 2c. Legend on p. 83.

in Fig. 2A, B and C are localized to a small region of the suprasylvian gyrus. The 'active' cortical regions in these latter 3 fetal brains represent corresponding anatomical areas. The active cortical regions in the 55- and 73-day fetuses (Fig. 1A and B) also lie in an area corresponding to the expected position of the suprasylvian gyrus.

(B) The latency of the evoked response

The time delay between a peripheral stimulus and its cortical response was found to be much greater in the young fetuses than it was in the adult sheep. The term latency as used in this paper refers to the time between the onset of the peripheral stimulus and the *peak* of the surface positivity. A latency of 140 msec was observed in the

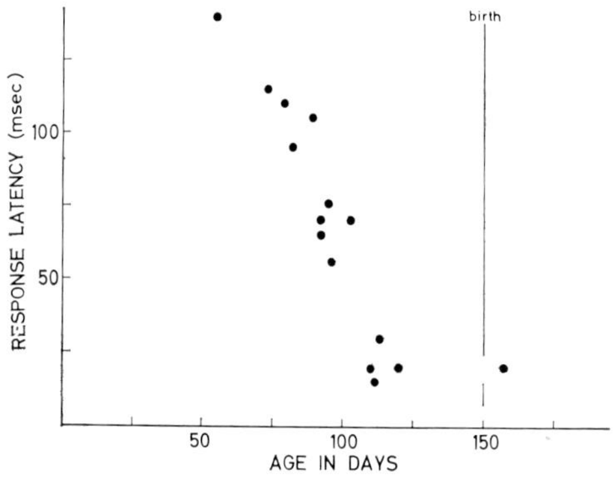

Fig. 3. Response latency during maturation of fetal sheep. Abscissa: calculated age in days from conception. Ordinate: latency in msec. from onset of peripheral stimulus to peak of initial surface positivity.

55-day-old fetus. This is compared with a latency of 10 to 20 msec in the adult sheep (Woolsey and Fairman, 1946). The response latencies of all fetuses studied in this series are plotted as a function of age in Fig. 3. The latency falls sharply from about the 80th to the 110th day of fetal life and then gradually levels off. This function may be viewed as a continuous one or as composed of two separate processes with their discontinuity at 110 days.

(C) The response to repetitive stimulation

The maximum rate of peripheral stimulation that will continue to produce a detectable cortical response was shown to increase with age (Fig. 4). Sheep fetuses of

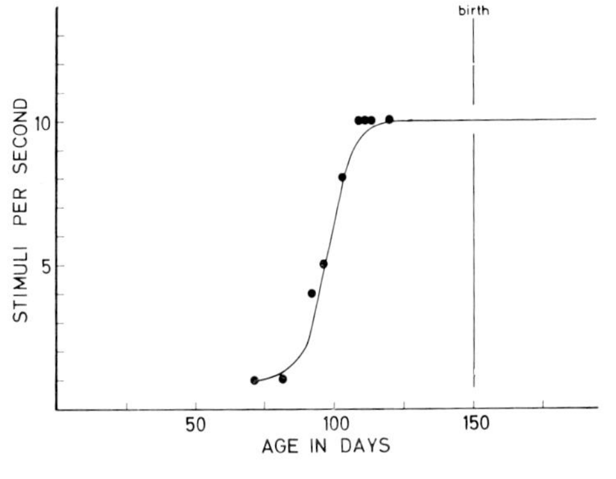

Fig. 4. Relationship between fatigability to repetitive stimulation and developmental age in the sheep fetus. Abscissa: calculated age in days from conception. Ordinate: maximum rate of peripheral stimulation to be followed by evoked responses. The continuation of the curve beyond the last point is based on maximum frequencies of 10 per sec found in adult sheep.

70–80 days gestational age could follow a stimulus frequency of up to 1 per sec, whereas a 110-day fetus followed at a rate of 10 per sec. It was shown in another series of experiments that adult sheep were able to follow the same type of stimulus up to a maximum rate of 10 per sec (Molliver and Änggård, unpublished).

(D) The wave form of the evoked cortical potential

The wave-form of evoked cortical responses of fetal and neonatal animals differed in a systematic way from the classical response (Bard, 1938) composed of an initial surface positivity followed by a negativity, which was also demonstrated in the adult sheep.

The first responses obtainable in fetal life were predominantly surface positive and of relatively long duration (50–100 msec). With advancing fetal age, the responses became more clearly diphasic with an initial surface positivity followed by a marked negativity (Fig. 5). As gestation proceeded, the negative deflection increased to amplitudes much greater than the initial positivity. From the 90th to the 100th day the evoked cortical response may be described as a predominantly negative wave preceded

References p. 90–91

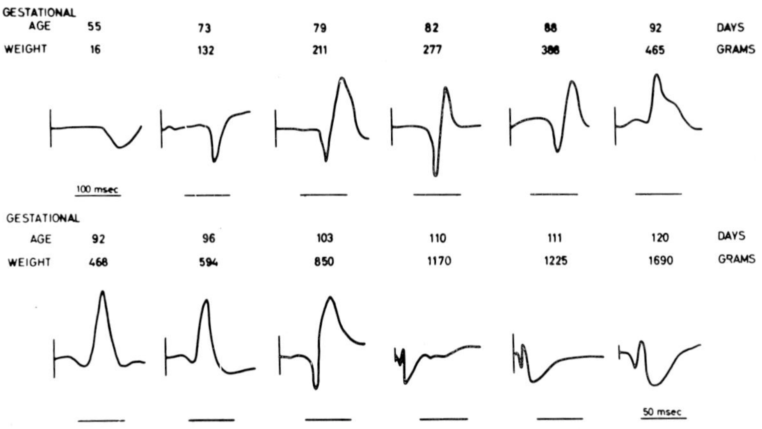

Fig. 5. The wave form of evoked cortical responses recorded from a series of fetal sheep. Upper row of figures shows calculated gestational ages; lower row shows body weights. Vertical markers at start of each response designate 100 μV. Horizontal bars mark 100 msec except where otherwise noted. Polarity = positive down.

by a small positive deflection. During the subsequent developmental period the negative component diminished in amplitude, and the response assumed the adult form of an initially and predominantly positive diphasic response. Three fetal sheep during the latter part of gestation showed a peculiar triphasic positive–negative–positive sequence. A response indistinguishable from that of the adult was not observed before 7 days postpartum, when an initially and predominantly positive response was found.

(E) Spontaneous cortical activity

Before evoked potentials were recorded in any fetus, the surface of the cortex was explored for spontaneous activity. No such activity was recorded from the youngest fetus in which a cortical response was evoked (55 days). The remaining fetal sheep all showed spontaneous activity which was qualitatively identical to that previously described (Bernhard *et al.*, 1959). The spontaneous cortical activity outside of the sensory area was unaffected by peripheral stimulation throughout the period under study.

(F) Effect of anesthesia on the evoked response

After all recordings had been completed on 4 fetal sheep ranging from 110–120 days of gestational age, a slow intravenous infusion of barbiturate anesthetic was given to the ewes. Two were given pentobarbital and two given Thiogenal. From time to time during the infusion both spontaneous and evoked cortical activity was examined. As the infused dosage approached the anesthetic level, spontaneous cortical activity gradually decreased in amplitude and disappeared beneath the noise level. At that time, the evoked somatosensory response was unchanged in latency, amplitude, configuration and capacity to follow repetitive stimulation.

As the barbiturate infusion continued the evoked response remained unaltered until the maternal blood pressure began to fall sharply, both maternal and fetal heart rate increased, and the fetus became deeply cyanotic. Then the amplitude of the evoked cortical response decreased until the response was no longer obtainable — a few minutes before the fetal heart slowed and stopped.

DISCUSSION

Earlier investigations on the evoked cortical response to afferent stimulation made on cats and rabbits during the *postnatal* period show that in both *newborn* cat and rabbit the somesthetic response is already present (see Hunt and Goldring, 1951; Scherrer and Oeconomos, 1955; Ellingson and Wilcott, 1960; Purpura, 1961a, b; Laget and Delhaye, 1962; Marty, 1962). Thus the initial ontogenetic phase of the somesthetic response has never previously been studied. A comparison of the structural and functional characteristics of the somesthetic cortical region in the newborn cat and in fetal sheep of different ages shows that the developmental stage of the newborn cat corresponds to that of the 65–70-day fetal sheep (see Bernhard *et al.*, 1965). The present investigations on *prenatal* sheep were made on fetuses from 50 days of age and included the initial developmental period of the somesthetic response.

The cortical distribution of evoked somesthetic responses was found to be sharply localized from the time of the first recorded potentials, and there was no functional reorganization during development of cortical topographic projection of the nose area. The anatomic connections for the cortical afferent projection thus seem to be fixed early in prenatal development.

The latencies of the earliest evoked responses are strikingly prolonged, and slow peripheral and central conduction velocities must be primarily implicated. Electron microscopic studies of fiber diameters in peripheral nerve in fetal sheep showed that the largest fibers in the sciatic nerve increased from 0.96 μ diameter at 52 days gestational age to 3.95 μ diameter at 95 days (Änggård and Ottoson, 1963). This degree of fiber diameter change would be sufficient to explain the prolonged latencies on the basis of decreased conduction velocities (Gasser and Grundfest, 1939). It should also be mentioned that a rapid myelination of peripheral nerves of fetal sheep has been found during a period from 90–105 days of gestational age as demonstrated by X-ray diffraction studies (Höglund and Ringertz, 1961).

Although slow conduction velocity in nerves and tracts may be adequate to explain the long response latencies, as yet obscure cortical factors may also be involved. Intimately tied up with the prolonged latency of evoked responses during neurological development is the phenomenon of decreased responsiveness to repetitive stimulation. Clearly, the refractory period of nerve fibers must be prolonged in proportion to the delayed conduction. That synaptic factors are also involved has been indicated by the prolonged absolute unresponsive time following an evoked superficial cortical response in the newborn cat. It has been hypothesized that presynaptic refractoriness plus delayed transmitter synthesis may be important factors in preventing rapid recovery of the immature synapse (Purpura *et al.*, 1960). Inhibition and immaturity of postsynaptic structures are factors also to be considered.

References p. 90–91

The cortical response in the adult animal evoked by peripheral stimulation is comprised of an initial surface positive wave followed by a negative wave. The changing relative amplitudes of the positive and negative components constitute the most remarkable developmental feature of the evoked response. The present investigation on sheep shows that when the evoked potential first appears during development it is surface positive. Later in gestation a biphasic positive-negative potential develops and its negative phase increases in amplitude during the subsequent 30 days. This same phenomenon has been demonstrated in the fetal dog at 40–50 days of gestation (Molliver, 1966). Although appearing to be in conflict with recent descriptions of predominantly negative 'immature' cortical potentials (Marty, 1962; Purpura *et al.*, 1964), this demonstration of the predominantly positive prenatal cortical surface potentials merely extends previous observations to an earlier ontogenetic period. In fetal sheep the initial positivity of the evoked response grows in amplitude until 82 days of gestation when it then decreases steadily until 100 days whereupon it again increases (Fig. 5). Histologic investigations on fetal sheep made in parallel with the present experiments (Åström, 1967) have demonstrated 'presumably afferent fibers' extending as far as the outer part of the intermediate zone in the 12- to 20-g fetus (gestational age 50–60 days). In this subpyramidal region lies a dense network of dendrites of relatively well differentiated stellate cells plus basal dendrites descending from deep pyramidal cells. It is tentatively suggested that the slow surface positive potential found at this early ontogenetic stage may reflect the summation of postsynaptic potentials in stellate cells and basal dendrites lying at the junction of intermediate and pyramidal zones. Evidence that positive surface potentials may be the electrical sign of deep postsynaptic potentials has been presented for the adult cat (Mountcastle *et al.*, 1957). This is an hypothesis which will be investigated in fetal animals by deep microelectrode penetrations and by a microscopic search for functional contacts near the junction of the pyramidal and intermediate zones. Subsequent developmental changes in the immature initially positive phase may result from movement of this deep lying 'dipole' closer to the surface recording electrode, the movement being adpial migration of these stellate cells and maturation of basal dendrites of more superficial pyramidal cells. Alternatively, that the early surface postive wave may arise from synchronous depolarization of presynaptic afferent terminals has not been disproven (Li *et al.*, 1956; Bernhard *et al.*, 1967).

The appearance and growth of the negative phase of the surface potential coincide with marked developmental changes in the pyramidal layer of the sheep cortex, particularly maturation of the apical dendrites of pyramidal cells (Åström, 1967), a course which closely resembles that described in the newborn cat (Noback and Purpura, 1961). These microscopic observations are consistent with the hypothesis that the surface negative potential may arise in part from postsynaptic activation of apical dendrites, as has been concluded for newborn cats (Purpura *et al.*, 1964). At the developmental stage when surface negative potentials become prominent, 'corticopetal fibers' are seen obliquely traversing the cortex and ending primarily in the marginal layer (Åström, 1967). It may be postulated that some of these afferent fibers synapse with the large Cajal–Retzius cells and that the postsynaptic potentials thereby produced adjacent to the pial surface are betrayed by a high amplitude surface negativity that is demonstrable only as long as Cajal–Retzius cells remain. Investigations are planned to determine the existence of synapses on Cajal–Retzius cells and to describe their electrical activity.

It has been suggested that the corticopetal fibers described above may be nonspecific afferents by the histologic criteria derived from Entorhinal Cortex (Lorente de Nó, 1933). The sharp localization of cortical responses in fetal sheep plus the absence of a generalized effect of stimulation on spontaneous cortical activity do not support this hypothesis.

Near the end of fetal life in the sheep, the evoked somesthetic cortical potential acquires a complex triphasic form prior to assuming the classical mature pattern (Fig. 5). At this period the microscopic structure of the cortex has achieved a complexity that approaches that of the adult and defies meaningful structure-function correlations.

The electrical activity of fetal cortex reflects a morphologic organization that is peculiar to the immature nervous system and hypotheses based on their relationship may not be applicable to mature cerebral cortex. The value of such hypotheses resides in their potential contribution to an understanding of the mechanisms of ontogenesis.

SUMMARY

The ontogenetic development of the evoked cortical response to tactile stimulation of the nose was studied in unanesthetized sheep fetuses kept in placental contact with the decerebrate ewe.

The first detectable evoked cortical response obtained at a fetal age of 55 days was a surface positive potential. Reference to the structural characteristics of the sheep cortex at this fetal age suggests that this first surface positive response may reflect postsynaptic potentials in stellate cells and basal dendrites residing at the junction of pyramidal and intermediate zones. Later in gestation the positivity was followed by a negative deflection which increased with age and dominated the surface response at a fetal age of 90–95 days. This negative phase may result from postsynaptic activation of developing apical dendrites and of Cajal–Retzius cells, which lie close to the pial surface. Experimental results are also presented on the cortical distribution of the evoked response as well as on its latency and fatigability at different fetal ages. The results indicate a rapid development of this projection system between the fetal ages of 60–110 days.

ACKNOWLEDGEMENTS

The investigations were supported by a grant from the Assocation for the Aid of Crippled Children. I am grateful to Prof. C. G. Bernhard for his hospitality and encouragement during this investigation. I want to thank L. Änggård and K. Theorell for their help and suggestions. I am indebted to H. van der Loos for criticisms of the manuscript.

References p. 90–91

REFERENCES

ADRIAN, E. D., (1943); Afferent areas in the brain of ungulates. *Brain*, **66**, 89–103.

ÄNGGÅRD, L., AND OTTOSON, D., (1963); Observations on the functional development of the neuromuscular apparatus in fetal sheep. *Exp. Neurol.*, **7**, 294–304.

ÅSTRÖM, K. E., (1967); On the early development of the isocortex in fetal sheep. *Developmental Neurology*. This volume, pp. 1–59.

BARD, P., (1938); Studies on the cortical representation of somatic sensibility. *Harvey Lect.*, **33**, 143–169.

BERGSTRÖM, R., BERNHARD, C. G., AND ÄNGGÅRD, L., (1960); Analysis of some prenatal reflex functions in sheep. *Acta physiol. scand.*, Suppl. 175, **50**, 23–24.

BERNHARD, C. G., KAISER, I. H., AND KOLMODIN, G. M., (1959); On the development of cortical activity in fetal sheep. *Acta physiol. scand.*, **47**, 333–349.

BERNHARD, C. G., KOLMODIN, G. M., AND MEYERSON, B. A., (1967); On the prenatal development of function and structure in the somesthetic cortex of the sheep. *Developmental Neurology*. This volume, pp. 60–77.

BORKOWSKI, W. J., AND BERNSTINE, R. L., (1955); Electroencephalography of the fetus. *Neurology*, **5**, 362–365.

ELLINGSON, R. L., AND WILCOTT, R. C., (1960); Development of evoked responses in visual and auditory cortices of kittens. *J. Neurophysiol.*, **23**, 363–375.

GASSER, H. S., AND GRUNDFEST, H., (1939); Axon diameters in relation to the spike dimensions and the conduction velocity in mammalian A fibers. *Amer. J. Physiol.*, **127**, 393–414.

GROSSMAN, C., (1955); Electro-ontogenesis of cerebral activity. *Arch. Neurol. Psychiat. (Chic)*, **74**, 186–202.

HAMUY, T. P., BROMILEY, R. B., AND WOOLSEY, C. N., (1950); Somatic areas I and II of the dog's cerebral cortex. *Amer. J. Physiol.*, **163**, 719–720.

HÖGLUND, G., AND RINGERTZ, H., (1961); X-ray diffraction studies on peripheral nerve myelin. *Acta physiol. scand.*, **51**, 290–295.

HUGGET, A. ST. G., AND WIDDAS, W. F., (1951); The relationship between mammalian foetal weight and conception age. *J. Physiol.*, **114**, 306–317.

HUNT, W. E., AND GOLDRING, S., (1951); Maturation of the evoked response of the visual cortex in the post natal rabbit. *Electroenceph. clin. Neurophysiol.*, **3**, 465–471.

JASPER, H. H., BRIDGMAN, C. S., AND CARMICHAEL, L., (1937); An ontogenetic study of cerebral electrical potentials in the guinea pig. *J. exp. Psychol.*, **21**, 63–71.

LAGET, P., AND DELHAYE, N., (1962); Etude du développement néonatal de diverses activités électriques corticales chez le lapin. *Actualités neurophysiol.*, **4**, 259–284.

LI, C., CULLEN, C., AND JASPER, H., (1956); Laminar microelectrode studies of specific somatosensory cortical potentials. *J. Neurophysiol.*, **19**, 113–130.

LORENTE DE NÓ, R., (1933); Studies on the structure of the cerebral cortex. *J. Psychol. Neurol. (Lpz.)*, **45**, 381–438.

MARTY, R., (1962); Développement post-natal des réponses sensorielles du cortex cérébral chez le chat et le lapin. *Arch. Anat. micr. Morph. exp.*, **51**, 129–264.

MATERNAL INFANT HEALTH. A primer of EEG in the newborn. Nat. Inst. Health, Bethesda, 1962, privately dist.

MOLLIVER, M., (1966); On the development of the somesthetic cortical response in fetal dog. In course of publication.

MOUNTCASTLE, V. B., DAVIES, P. W., AND BERMAN, A. L., (1957); Response properties of neurons of cat's somatic sensory cortex to peripheral stimuli. *J. Neurophysiol.*, **20**, 374–407.

NOBACK, C. R., AND PURPURA, D. P., (1961); Postnatal ontogenesis of neurons in cat neocortex. *J. comp. Neurol.*, **117**, 291–307.

OECONOMOS, D., AND SCHERRER, J., (1953); Etude des potentiels évoqués corticaux somesthétiques chez le chat nouveau-né. *C.R. Soc. Biol. (Paris)*, **147**, 1229–1232.

PURPURA, D. P., (1961a); Structure and function of cortical synaptic organizations activated by corticopetal afferents in new born cat. *Brain and Behavior*, **1**, 95–138. Amer. Inst. Biol. Sci., Wash. D.C.

PURPURA, D. P., (1961b); Morphological basis of elementary evoked response patterns in the neocortex of the newborn cat. *Ann. N.Y. Acad. Sci.*, **92**, 840–859.

PURPURA, D. P., (1961c); Analysis of axodendritic synaptic organizations in immature cerebral cortex. *Ann. N.Y. Acad. Sci.*, **94**, 604–654.

PURPURA, D. P., AND CARMICHAEL, M. W., (1959); Characteristics of blood-brain barrier to systemic GABA in newborn cat. *Science*, **131**, 410–412.

PURPURA, D. P., CARMICHAEL, M. W., AND HOUSEPIAN, E. M., (1960); Physiological and anatomical studies of development of superficial axodendritic synaptic pathways in neocortex. *Exp. Neurol.*, **2**, 324–347.

PURPURA, D. P., SCHOFER, R. J., HOUSEPIAN, E. M., AND NOBACK, C. R., (1964); Comparative ontogenesis of structure-function relations in cerebral and cerebellar cortex. *Growth and Maturation of the Brain, Vol. 4, Progress in Brain Research*. J. P. Schadé and D. P. Purpura, Editors. Amsterdam, Elsevier, pp. 187–221.

SCHERRER, J., AND OECONOMOS, D., (1955); Réponses évoquées corticales somesthétiques des mammifères adultes et nouveau-nés. *Les Grandes Activités du Lobe Temporal*. Paris, Masson (pp. 249–268).

WOOLSEY, C. N., AND FAIRMAN, D., (1946); Contralateral, ipsilateral and bilateral representation of cutaneous receptors in somatic areas I and II of the cerebral cortex of pig, sheep and other mammals. *Surgery*, **19**, 684–702.

Electron Microscopy of Neuronal and Glial Differentiation in the Developing Brain of the Chick

WOLFGANG WECHSLER AND KARL MELLER

Max-Planck-Institut für Hirnforschung, Abteilung für Allgemeine Neurologie, Köln - Merheim und Institut für Histologie und Experimentelle Neuroanatomie, Göttingen (Deutschland)

I. INTRODUCTION

The electron microscopical technique avoids the use of different staining methods for revealing different cytological components and enables a simultaneous demonstration of all the tissue compartments and cells present. It is therefore possible to study more precisely — in contrast to the techniques of classical neurohistology — the successive stages of cellular differentiation in tissue sections of different developmental stages, and to follow up special regional cytoarchitectural differentiation. However, this great advantage is to some extent reduced by the very minute areas available for observation in electron microscopy. The relations between histogenesis and cytoarchitectural differentiation, therefore, have to be examined by classical methods as well.

Studies of cytological differentiation lend themselves favourably to EM investigations as we assume that the process of cytodifferentiation is basically the same for all regions of the CNS. This synopsis deals with two aspects of neurocytology in the developing brain of the chick embryo. Emphasis is placed upon the salient features of the cytology of differentiating cells (I) and upon some general aspects of neurohistogenesis (II). Under I we will deal with (1) matrix cells, (2) neurons, (3) neuroglia, (4) ependyma and plexus epithelium, under II with problems related to the extracellular space, the development of neuropil and the neurovascular relationship.

II. MATERIAL AND METHODS

Chick embryos ranging from stage 7–44 (Hamburger and Hamilton, 1951) were used. The embryos were incubated for 2, $2\frac{1}{2}$, 4, $4\frac{1}{2}$, 5, 6, $6\frac{1}{2}$, 7, $8\frac{1}{2}$, 9, 13, 16 and 18 days. Telencephalon and tectum opticum mesencephali were divided into small blocks and fixed for 2–4 h (Wohlfarth-Bottermann, 1957). A short prefixation in glutaraldehyde was seldom used. Occasionally reference will be made to findings on embryonic spinal cord of the chick.

The tissue was dehydrated in ascending ranges of acetone, and a further contrast obtained by treatment with phosphormolybdic acid and uranylacetate (Wohlfarth-Bottermann, 1957). Vestopal W was the embedding medium and the photographs were taken with a Zeiss EM 9. For comparison of the EM results chick embryo series of equal developmental stages were used. These sections were stained with a variety of methods, *e.g.* H. and E., cresylviolet, Luxol-fast blue, PAS; Golgi impregnations were available for the 7th and 14th day of incubation.

References p. 141–144

III. GENERAL COMMENTS

The wall of the primitive brain vesicles consists of undifferentiated cells, generally referred to as matrix cells. From these neuroectodermal cells develop neurons, astrocytes, oligocytes, ependymal cells and the epithelium of the plexus. Diagram 1 represents the different stages of cytogenesis in the CNS of vertebrates (Wechsler, 1966f). The origin of microglia will not be discussed.

Diagram 1: Cytogenetic stages of development in the CNS. We distinguish 3 main phases of cytological development:

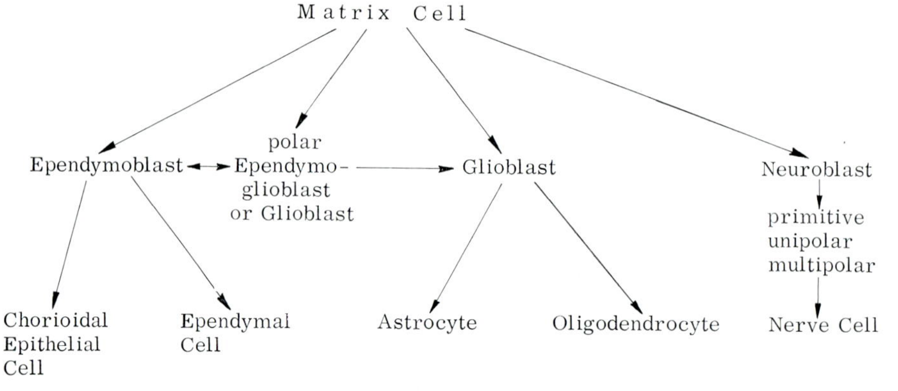

Phase I: The stage of undifferentiated matrix cells,
Phase II: The stage of primordial or early cellular differentiation,
Phase III: The stage of final differentiation and maturation.

During cerebral development cytological and histogenetical processes overlap. As long as the primitive brain vesicles do not show cytoarchitectural or myeloarchitectural differentiation, proliferation of cells is the dominant picture. After a relatively short stage of primordial or early cellular differentiation, characterised by discrete structural and ultrastructural changes, the 3rd and longest phase of brain development is apparent. In this maturation stage typical cellular and fine structural characteristics become obvious and allow the identification of cells.

'Since differentiation (of vertebrate cells) affects the cells in many ways and at many levels, there are a number of sets of criteria for identifying and characterizing a differentiated state. Since they are not always concordant, it becomes important to recognize the significance of each, and to specify criteria when one is characterizing differentiation. Cells may be said to be differentiated by morphological, behavioral, chemical, or developmental criteria ..... With improved microscopy and particularly with the heightened resolution of the electron microscope, morphological description has become increasingly detailed and precise' (Grobstein, 1959).

Publications based on classical staining methods emphasize that cellular differentiation is mainly an alteration in the shape of cells. These alterations have been described in detail, and phylogenetic and ontogenetic points of view have been stressed in relation to neurons and other cells (Fig. 1). Attempts have been made to observe

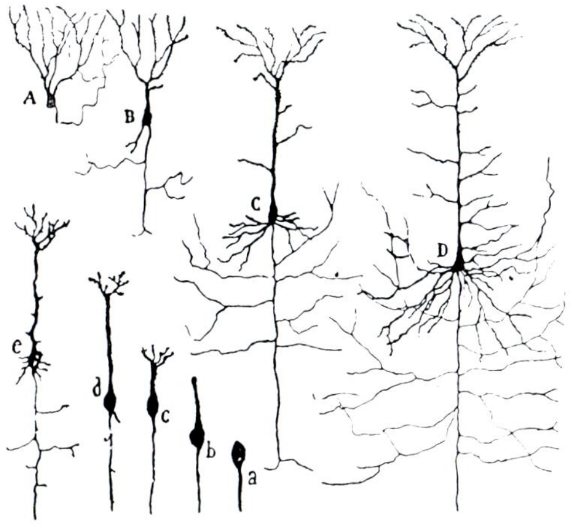

Fig. 1. General principles of the development of cortical pyramidal neurons in ontogeny and phylogeny (Cajal, 1952). A, Frog; B, Reptile; C, Mouse, D; Man. In the lower left the ontogenetic development of nerve cells: a = primitive neuroblast; b = bipolar neuroblast; c = unipolar neuroblast; d + e = progressive differentiation of cortical nerve cells with dendritic proliferation and formation of collaterals.

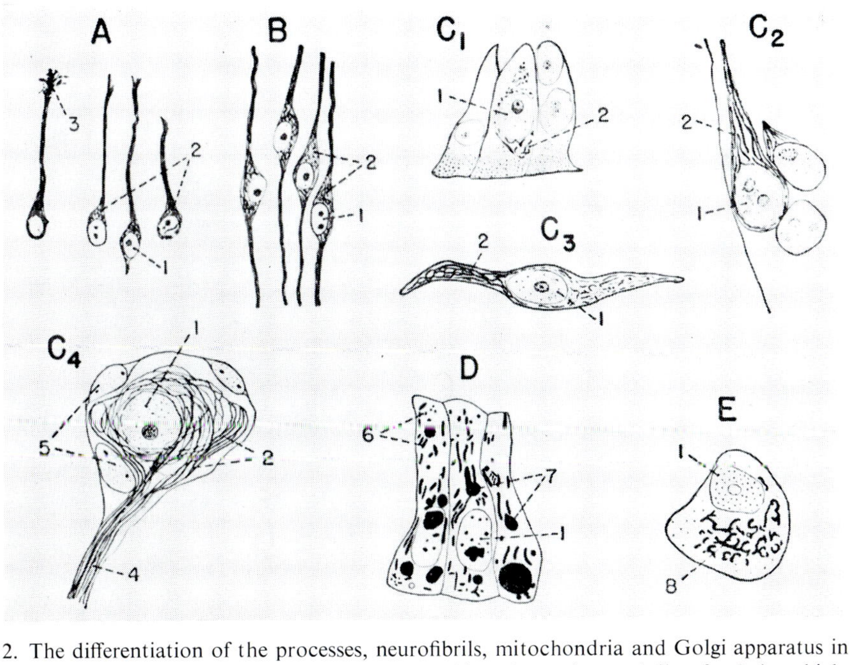

Fig. 2. The differentiation of the processes, neurofibrils, mitochondria and Golgi apparatus in the neuroblast (Romanoff, 1960). A, Monopolar neuroblast from the medulla of a 3-day chick embryo; B, Early bipolar neuroblast, dorsal root ganglion of a 5-day chick embryo. C1–C4, Progressive neurofibrillar formation in neuroblasts: C1 and C2, 40-h chick embryos; C3, 65-h chick embryo; C4, 8-day chick embryo; D, Mitochondria in the undifferentiated cells of the medullary plate of a 24-h chick embryo. E, Golgi apparatus in a cell of the spinal ganglion. 1 = nucleus; 2 = neurofibrils; 3 = growing tip of prospective axon; 4 = axon; 5 = nucleus of sheath or capsular cell; 6 = mitochondria; 7 = yolk granules; 8 = Golgi apparatus.

References p. 141–144

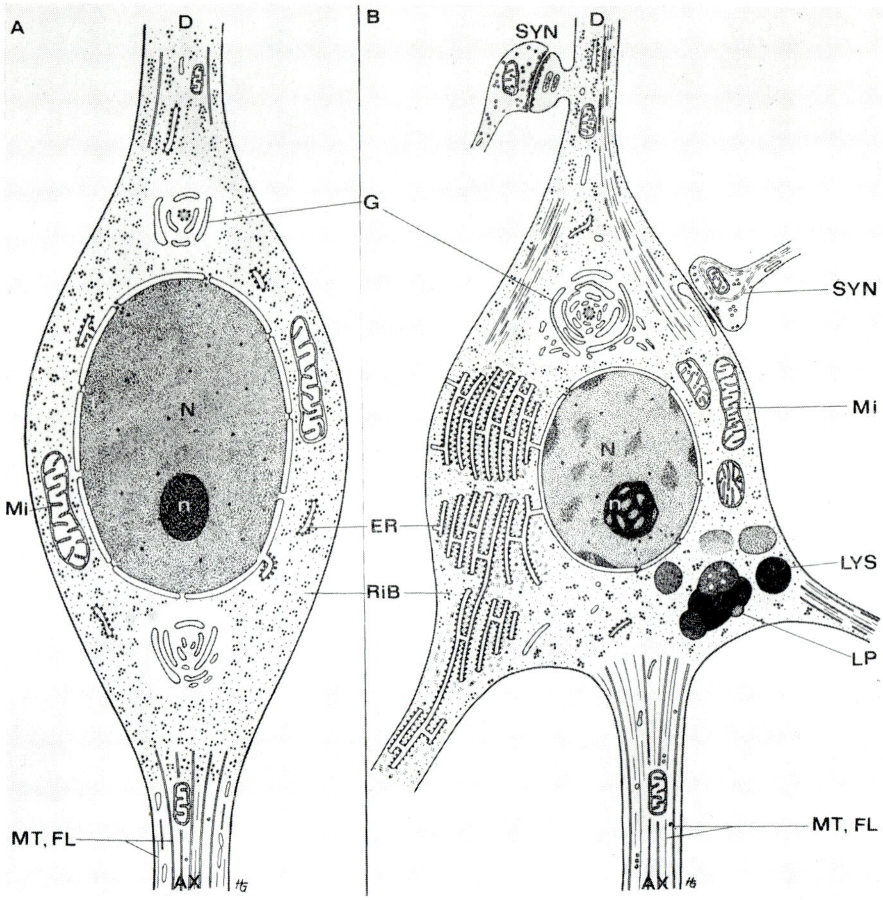

Fig. 3. Diagrammatic representation of the ultrastructure of a neuroblast (A) and of one mature multipolar nerve cell (B). For explanation see text. N = nucleus; n = nucleolus; ER = endoplasmic reticulum; RiB = free ribosomes; Mi = mitochondria; G = Golgi apparatus; FL and MT = neurofilaments and microtubules; SYN = synapses; AX = axon; D = dendrites; LP = lipofuscin; LYS = Lysosomes.

changes in different intracellular structures, *e.g.* nuclei, neurofibrillae, Nissl bodies, neurosomes and the Golgi complex (Fig. 2). To illustrate these, the work of Ramón y Cajal (1929, 1952) should be consulted. Electron microscopy, however, provides the means of establishing a proper cytological basis for cellular differentiation. Although nuclear changes are less obvious, alterations in the cytoplasmic ultrastructure serve as a measure of the progressive degrees of cellular differentiation (Fig. 3a and b). With the latter criteria in mind we would like in this report to summarize both previously published work, and recent results, in order to present a more general concept of cytogenesis and cytodifferentiation in the central nervous system.

IV. NEUROECTODERMAL MATRIX CELLS

The wall of the telencephalon and mesencephalon is made up of undifferentiated cells

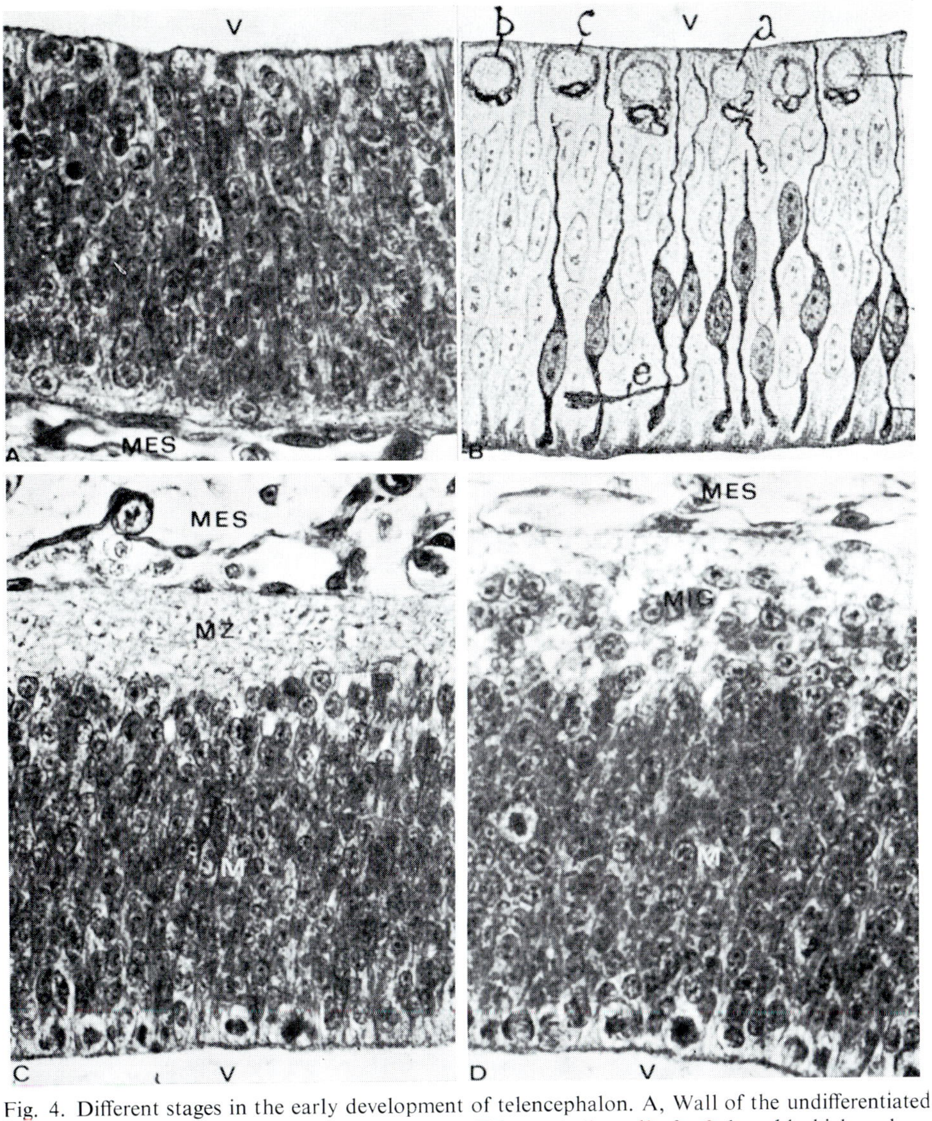

Fig. 4. Different stages in the early development of telencephalon. A, Wall of the undifferentiated primitive brain vesicle of a 2-day-old embryo; B, Telencephalic wall of a 3-day-old chick embryo (a–c = germinative cells after His, e = neuroblasts). Cajal's impregnation method (1952); (C) Wall of the telencephalon showing broader matrix and smaller nucleus-free marginal zone (MZ), 3-day-old embryo; D, Initial phase of migratory zone formation (MIG), 4.5-day-old embryo. V = ventricle; MES = perineural mesenchyme; M = matrix.

up to the 4th and 5th day of incubation: for this reason the designation of a 'matrix' is justified (Fig. 4A–D). This does not contradict older morphological studies which describe apolar, bipolar and unipolar cells, within the matrix zones. We are certain, however, that it is impossible to distinguish between neuroblasts and glioblasts in the matrix layers (Fig. 4B). It can be shown, that all cells of the matrix are still undifferentiated and capable of division (Fujita, 1963, 1965; Källén, 1962; Sauer and Walker, 1959; Sidman and Angevine, 1962; Watterson *et al.*, 1956). The apolar cells

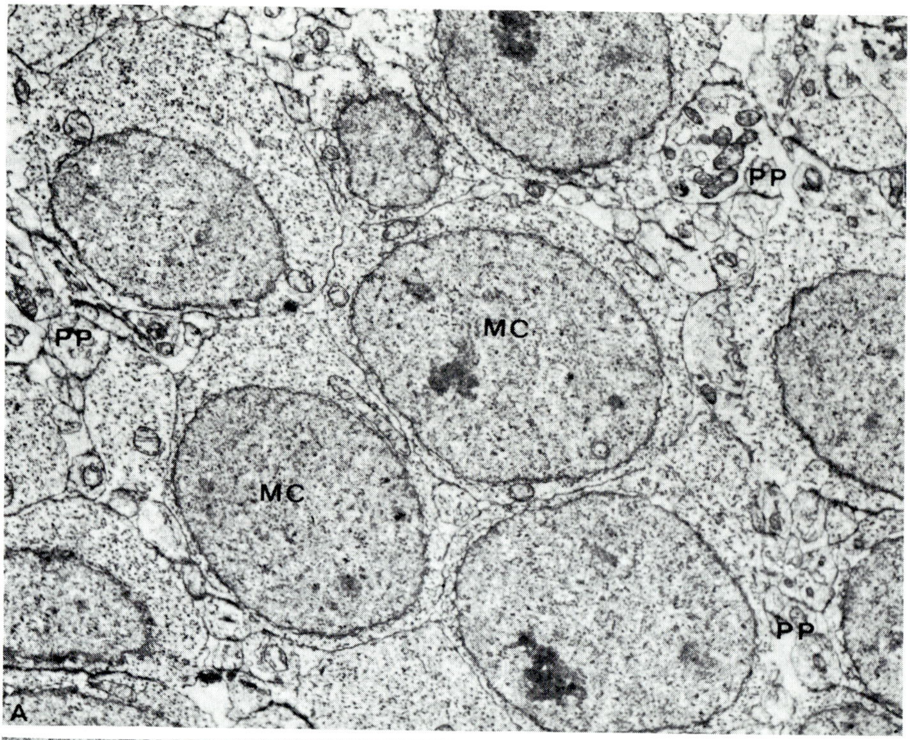
PP
PP
MC
MC
PP
A

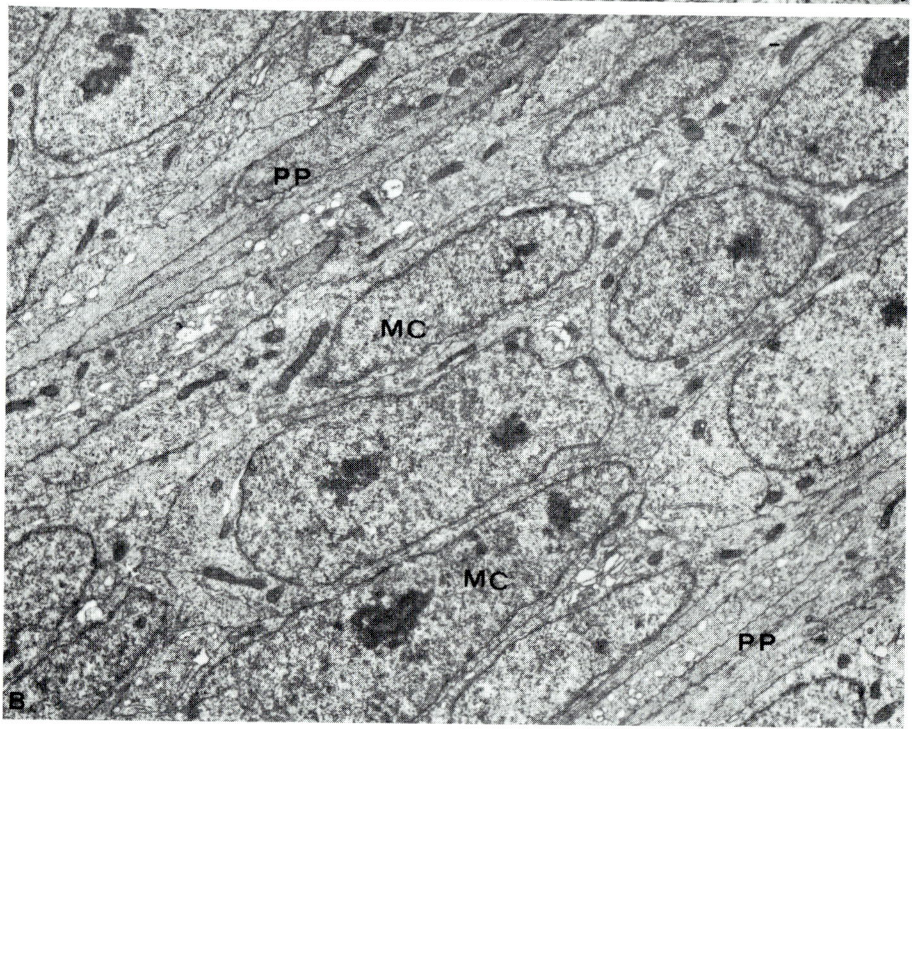
PP
MC
MC
PP
B

(so-called Germinativzellen of His, 1889) are only matrix cells undergoing mitotic division. Within the matrix zones the cells show an intense activity and migrate for the purpose of cell division, towards the inner surfaces.

Our electron microscopical findings of the cerebral matrix zones can be summarized as follows: the cells of the matrix present a uniform and embryonic type of cell as far as their ultrastructure is concerned. In early stages of brain development, it is impossible to separate matrix cells from primitive neuro- and glioblasts. Matrix cells are individual cells and are not connected in a syncytial manner. Bridges of

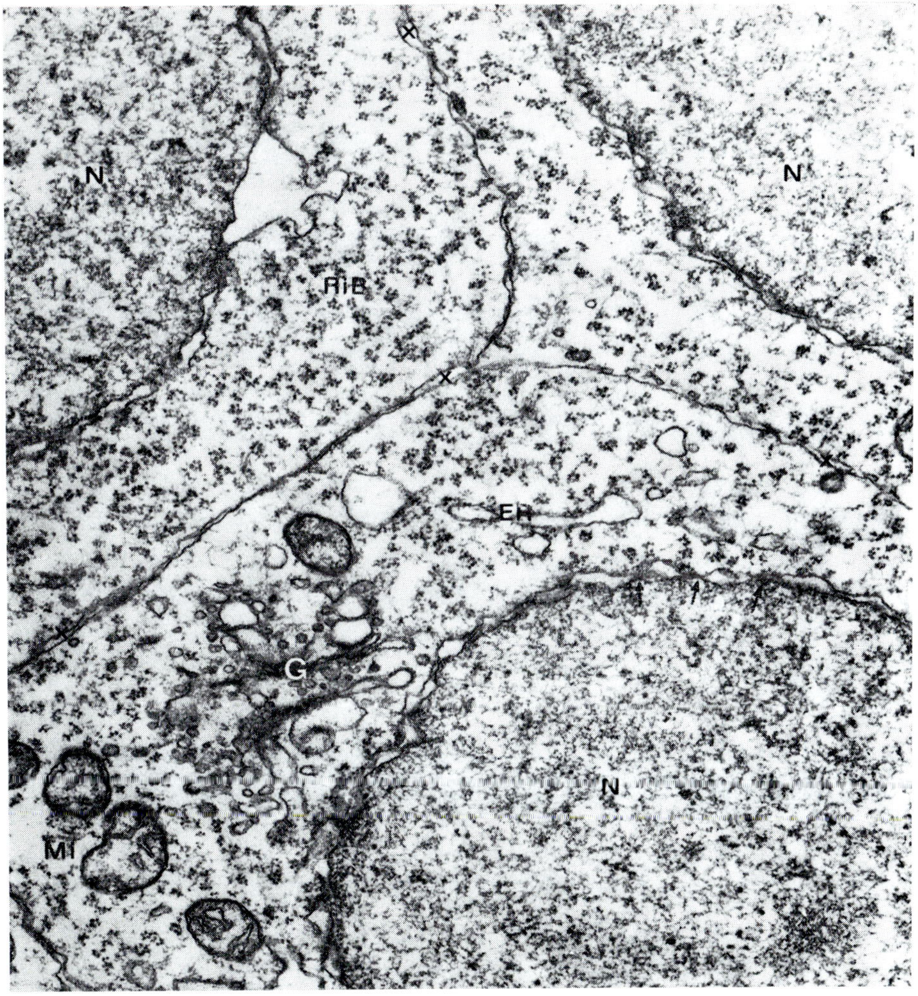

Fig. 6. Ultrastructure of the matrix cells, telencephalon, 4.5-day-old embryo. N = nucleus; G = Golgi apparatus; MI = mitochondria; ER = endoplasmic reticulum; RIB = free ribosomes; x = extracellular space (40,000 ×).

Fig. 5. Matrix zones of telencephalon. A, Cross section, 7-day-old embryo, primary osmic acid fixation (8000 ×); B, Longitudinal section, 8-day-old embryo, glutaraldehyde prefixation (6500 ×). MC = Matrix cells; PP = primitive processes.

References p. 141–144

cytoplasm are present only in those cells that are in the process of mitosis. Matrix cells of the telencephalon and mesencephalon form an epithelial complex at all stages of development, both in the phase of proliferation and in the subsequent stages where numerical reduction and emigration of matrix cells occur. The extracellular space is

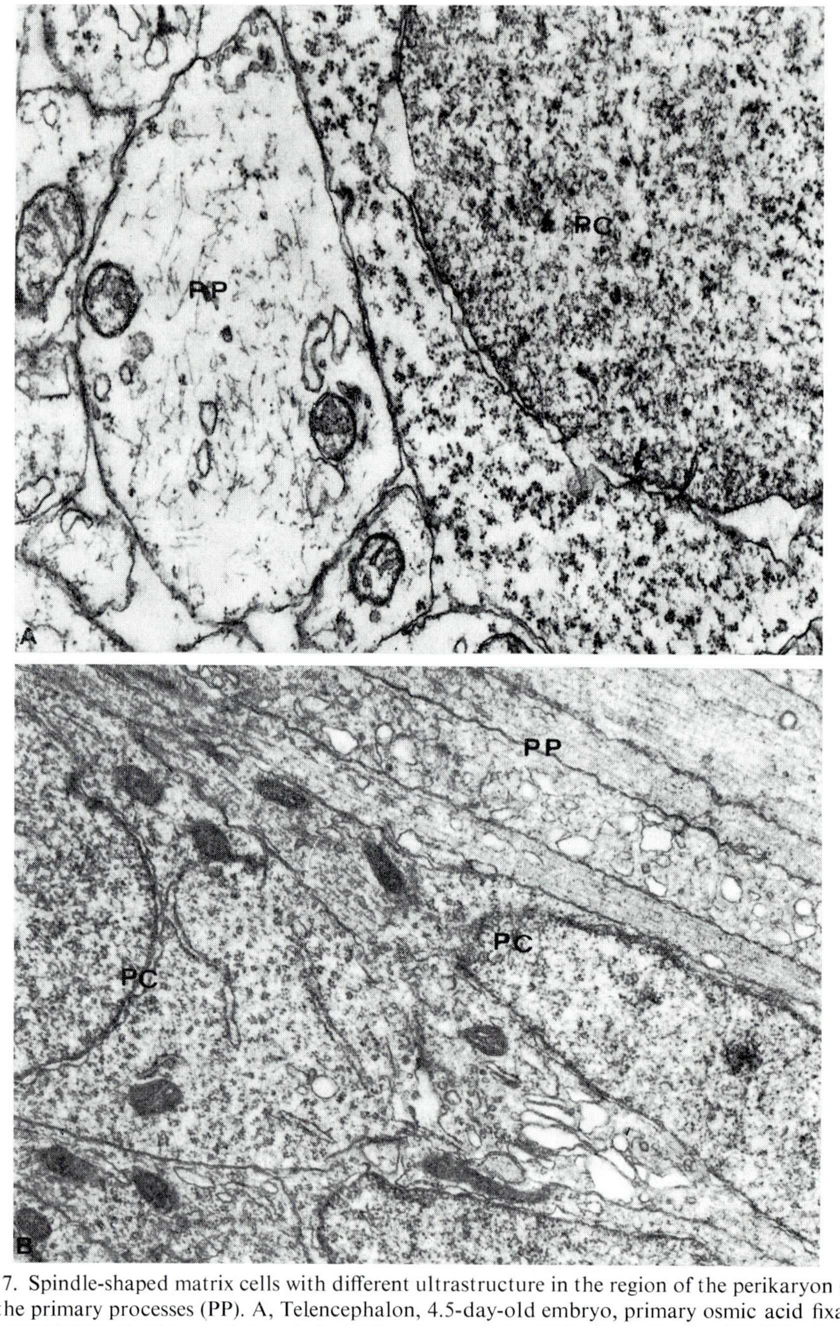

Fig. 7. Spindle-shaped matrix cells with different ultrastructure in the region of the perikaryon (PC) and the primary processes (PP). A, Telencephalon, 4.5-day-old embryo, primary osmic acid fixation (30,000 ×). B, Telencephalon, 8-day-old embryo, glutaraldehyde prefixation (18,000 ×).

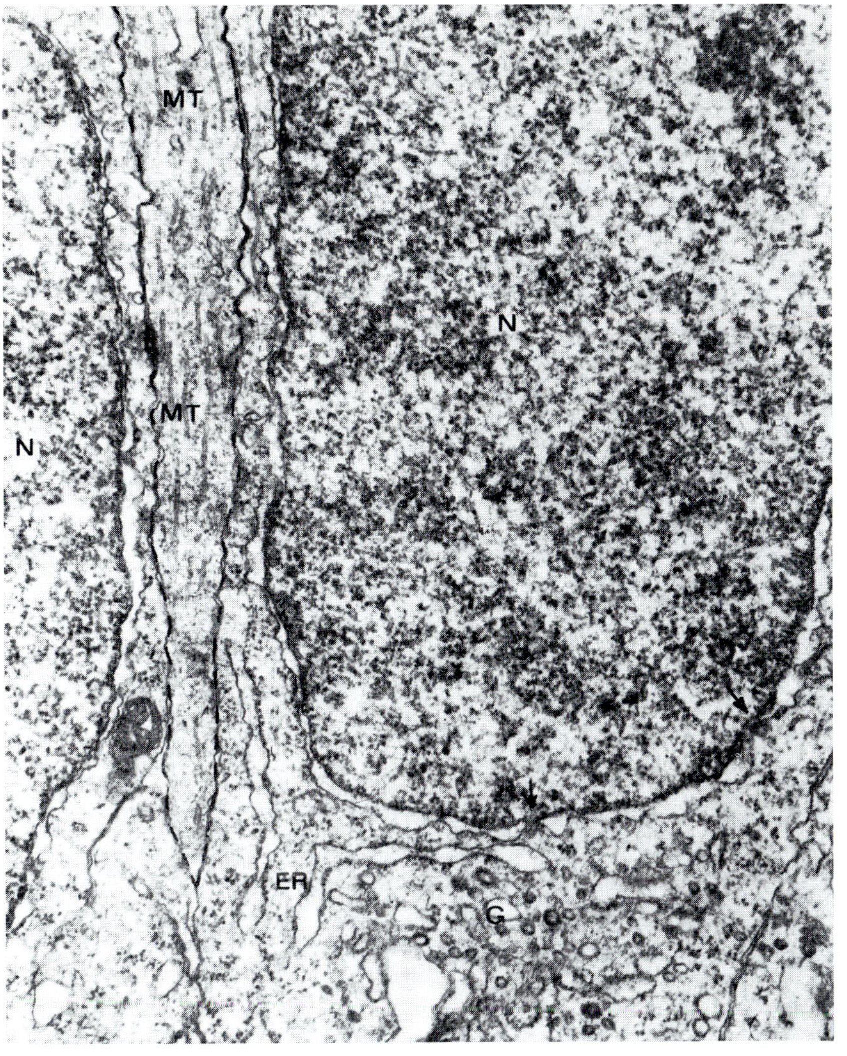

Fig. 8. Ultrastructure of the matrix cells in the region of the perikaryon and the primary processes, telencephalon, 8-day-old embryo: glutaraldehyde prefixation. N = nucleus; ER = endoplasmic reticulum; G = Golgi apparatus; MT = numerous microtubuli in a primary process, shown by hatched lines (40,000 ×).

small; 200 Å is the mean diameter of this intercommunicating system (Figs. 5 and 6).

The ultrastructure of the matrix cells clearly classifies them as embryonic cells (Fujita and Fujita, 1963; Wechsler, 1966a). The evidence for this can be found in the great number of free ribosomes and in the lack of tubes and vesicles of the endoplasmic reticulum (Figs. 6–8). The Golgi complex is relatively small, while well differentiated mitochondria are numerous. The nuclei of matrix cells are ovoid, containing large dense nucleoli and have a round nuclear envelope showing many pores. The karyoplasm is relatively dense. The differences in ultrastructure between cell body and primary processes deserve special consideration, particularly when glutaraldehyde

References p. 141–144

prefixation has been used (Fig. 7A and B). In contrast to the perikaryon, the primary processes contain numerous elongated profiles of microtubuli but fewer ribosomes and mitochondria (Figs. 7 and 8).

When the central processes of matrix cells reach the inner surface of the ventricle, morphological features appear which are characteristic for primitive epithelial cells, viz. microvilli, cilia, apical interdigitations, desmosomes (Meller and Wechsler, 1964; Wechsler, 1966a). These features remain even when the matrix cells become rounded and enter mitosis (Fig. 9). Mitotic stages can be easily followed during the dissolution of the nuclear membrane and redistribution of chromosomal material, while cellular organelles are pushed to the periphery (Figs. 9 and 10). The peripheral primary processes of matrix cells can be studied in the region of the outer wall of the primitive brain vesicles. No special ultrastructural features can be seen. The outer border of the brain vesicle is covered by a continuous basement membrane. In later stages of brain development, processes of polar glioblasts take over the function of neuroglia marginalis primitiva (Fig. 11), a point which will be discussed later.

In conclusion, the ultrastructure of matrix cells is determined by their neuroectodermal nature, as well as by their structural and ultrastructural embryonic features. It is important to realize that these cells develop and maintain a primordial bipolarity,

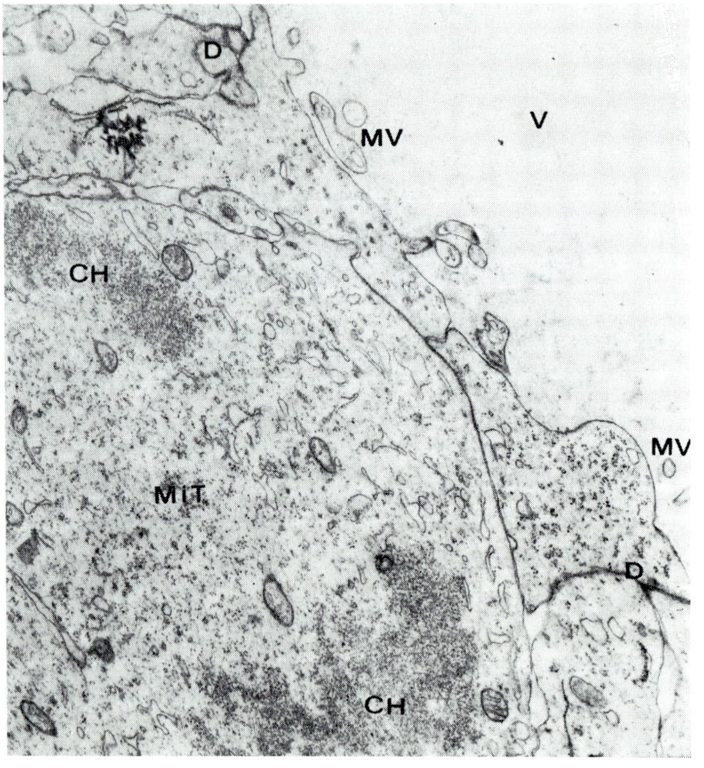

Fig. 9. Epithelial nature of the internal surface of the hemispheric vesicle, 6-day-old embryo. V = ventricle; MV = microvilli; D = desmosomes and apical interdigitations; MIT = mitosis; CH = chromosomes of the diaster (16,000 ×).

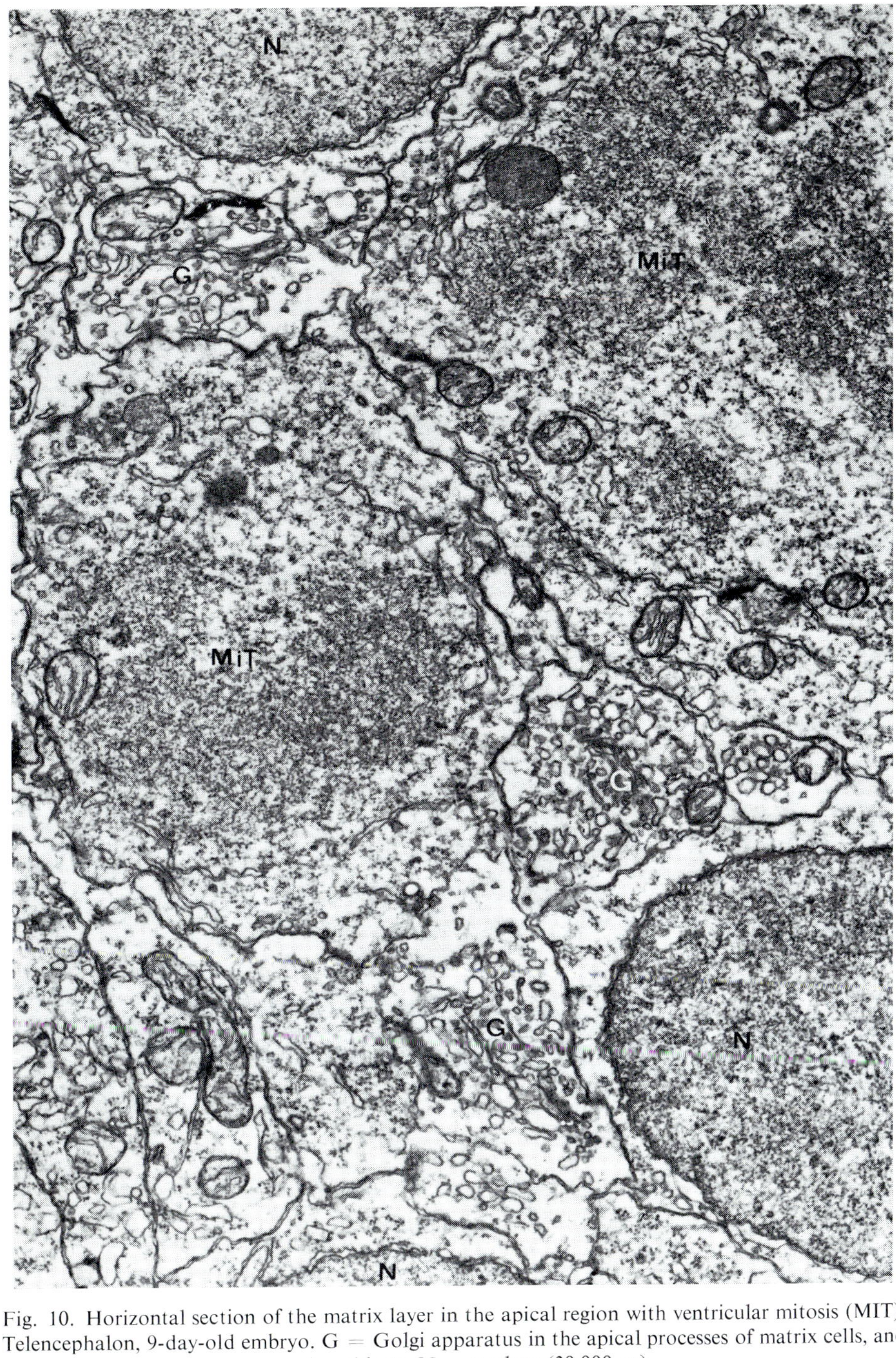

Fig. 10. Horizontal section of the matrix layer in the apical region with ventricular mitosis (MIT). Telencephalon, 9-day-old embryo. G = Golgi apparatus in the apical processes of matrix cells, and ependymoblasts. N = nucleus (30,000 ×).

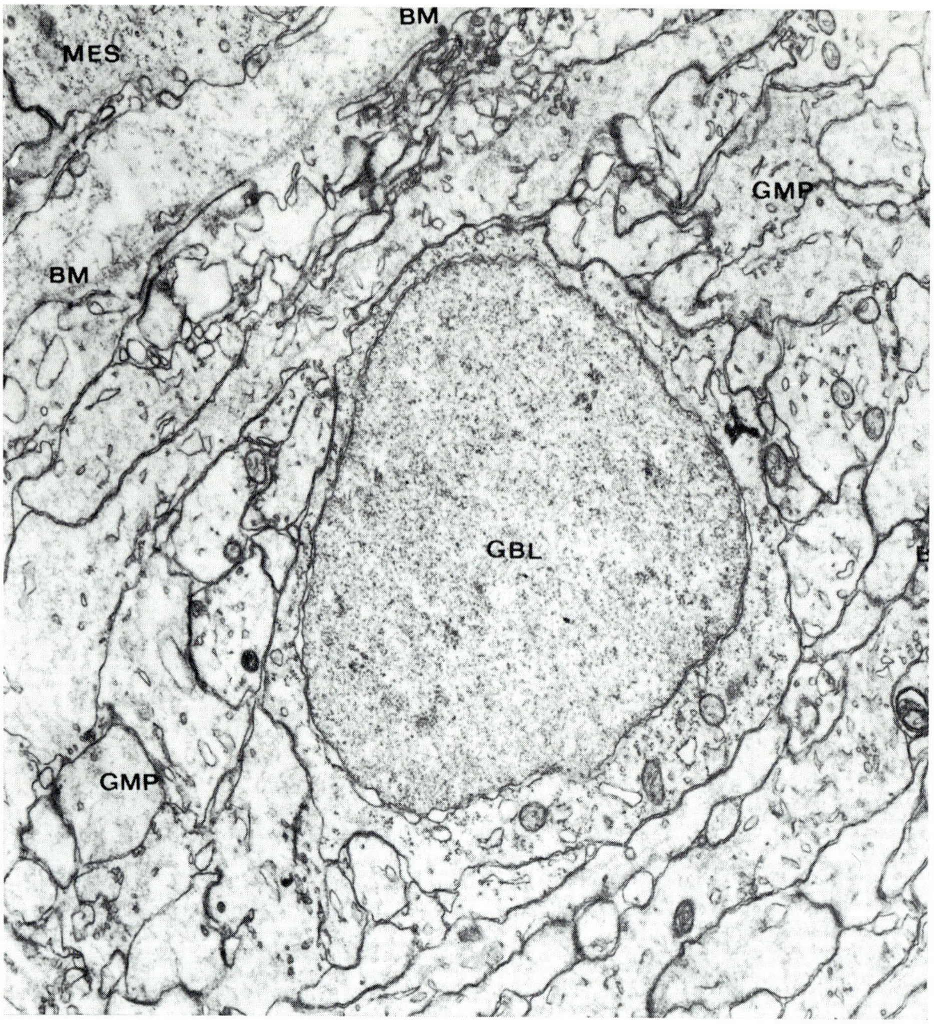

Fig. 11. Nature of the outer surface of the telencephalon, 7.5-day-old embryo. BM = superficial basement membrane; GMP = zone of the primitive marginal glia; GBL = glioblast; MES = mesenchymal cells of the meninx primitiva (25,000 ×).

but this bipolarity is not genetically fixed in a particular direction (Wechsler, 1966a). The cells of the spinal matrix of chick embryos exhibit an identical ultrastructure (Wechsler, 1963, 1965b, 1966a). The same has also been found in the matrix of the optic vesicle (Meller, 1964).

V. THE DIFFERENTIATION OF NEURONS

Neuronal development passes through stages which are characteristic for this type of cell. One of these features is the organization of a highly specialized endoplasmic reticulum (Bellairs, 1959; Fujita and Fujita, 1963; Glees and Meller, 1964; Meller *et al.*, 1966a; Pappas and Purpura, 1964; Tennyson, 1962; Wechsler, 1963, 1965b,

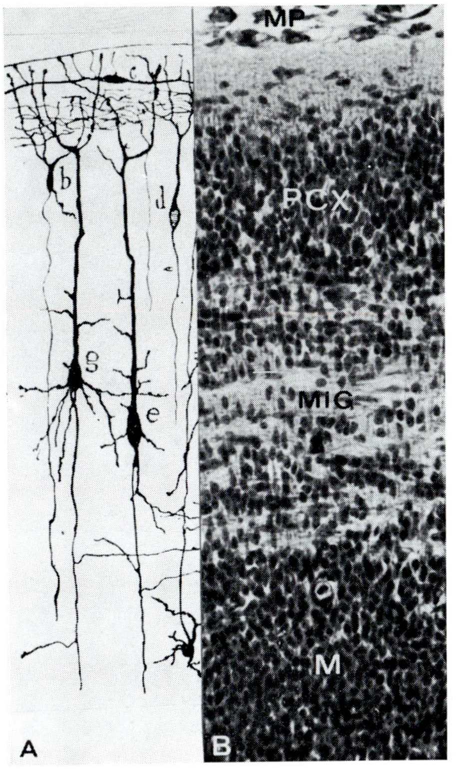

Fig. 12. A diagrammatic representation of the general development and differentiation of the nerve cells. A, Differentiation of the cortical nerve cells; note the progressive proliferation of the dendritic processes and the formation of the axon collaterals (Cajal, 1952); B, Beginning of the cytoarchitectural differentiation in optic tectum, 6.5-day-old embryo. M = matrix; MIG = migratory zone; PCX = primary cortex; MP = primitive meninges.

1966c, f). We assume from our observations that multipolar nerve cells of the CNS take their origin from bi- and multipolar precursor cell types and that perikaryon, axon, dendrites and synapses follow a special pattern of cytoplasmic differentiation. It follows from this that the development of nerve cells must be related to growth of the cell body, the elaboration of axonal and dendritic processes, and the heteropolar differentiation of cytoplasmic structures (Wechsler, 1965b, 1966c, f).

First we shall consider the cells migrating from the matrix, *e.g.* the neuroblasts of the transitional or migratory zone (Wechsler and Meller, 1963b); we will then continue our investigations by studying the ultrastructure of the unipolar neuroblasts of the primary cortex (Wechsler and Meller, 1963a). Finally, we would like to discuss the maturation phenomena of multipolar neurons.

The cells of the migratory zone of the telencephalon and mesencephalon are difficult to classify, but we believe that 3 types occur: neuroblasts, glioblasts and undifferentiated cells. The neuroblasts of the migratory zone are, on the basis of their ultrastructure, still very immature neurocytes (Fig. 13). More mature cells, or cells easier to classify, can be found in the walls of the telencephalic hemispheres and the highly differentiated

References p. 141–144

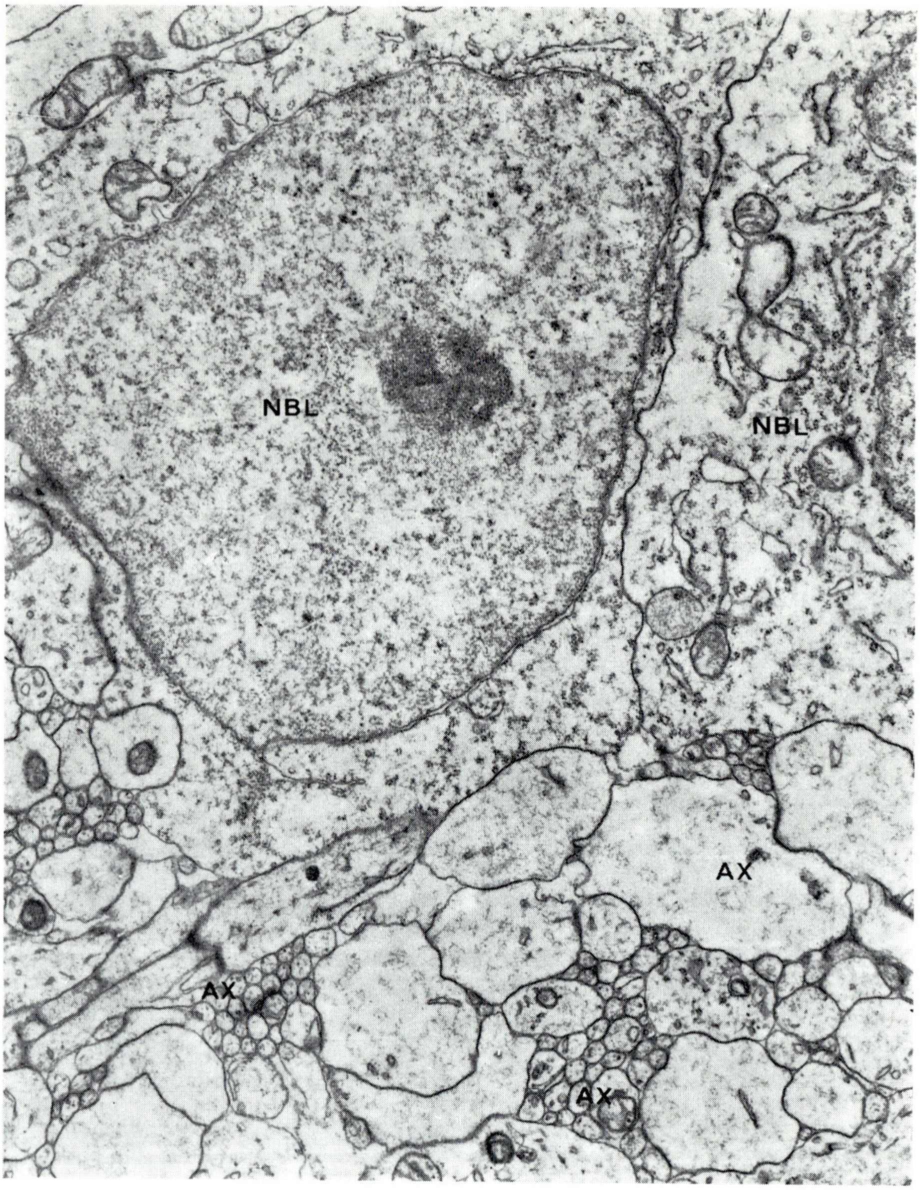

Fig. 13. Migrating neuroblast from the migratory zone, optic tectum, 7-day-old embryo. NBL = Neuroblast; AX = embryonic axon (18,000 ×).

tectum opticum: groups of unipolar neuroblasts are present, which are separated by very few processes (Fig. 14). These neuroblasts have an ovoid nucleus and a larger nucleolus, while numerous ribosomes are detectable in the perinuclear cytoplasm. The endoplasmic reticulum is relatively well developed and of the granular type, but Nissl complexes are missing. Mitochondria are present in large numbers and the Golgi apparatus is localized on both sides of the nuclei (s. Fig. 3A). The axons and dendrites of these unipolar neuroblasts are between 0.2 and 2 μ thick in diameter. Obviously most of them would escape observation under the light microscope. Even in electron microscopy they are often not identifiable by morphological features; but ribosomes are only present in dendrites in contrast to the axons (Figs. 14 and 20).

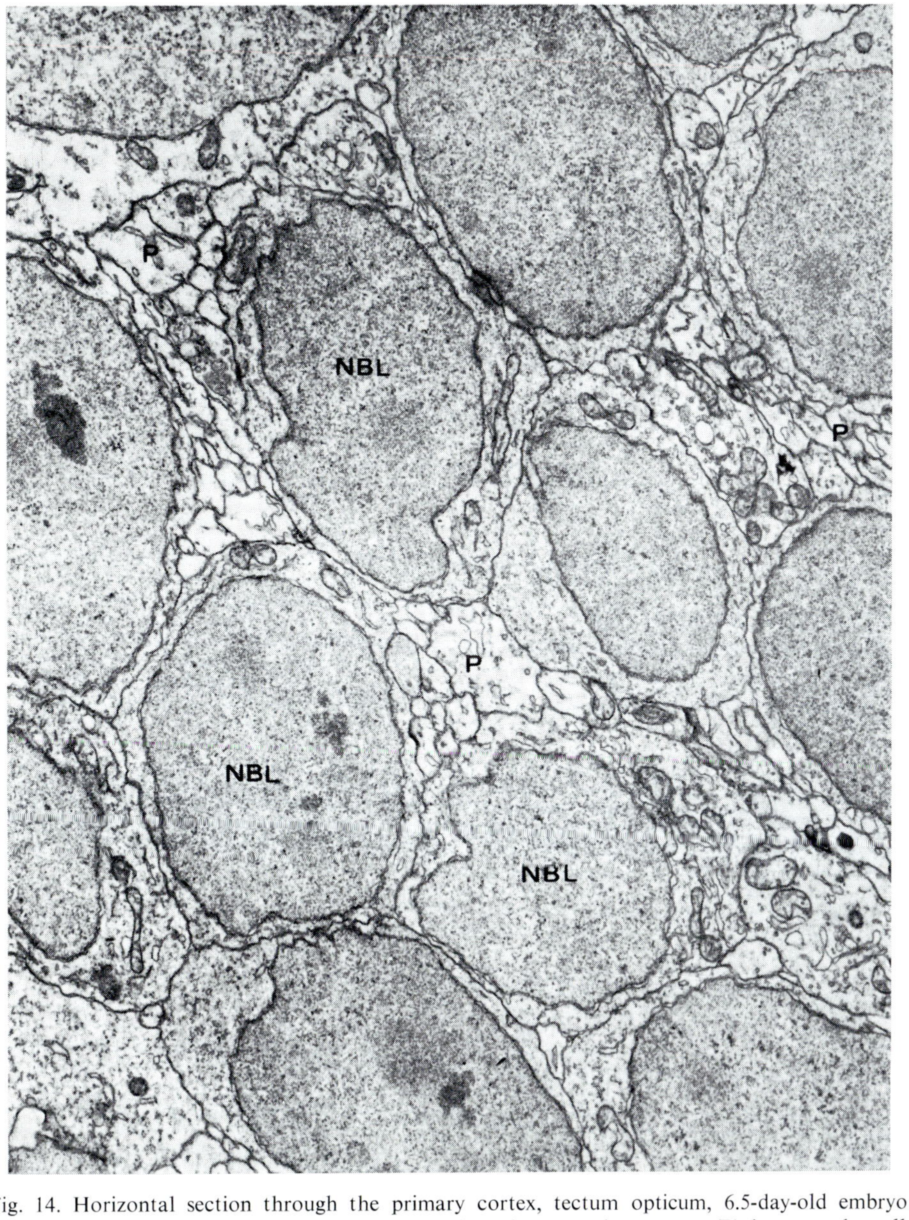

Fig. 14. Horizontal section through the primary cortex, tectum opticum, 6.5-day-old embryo. Densely packed unipolar neuroblasts (NBL), only a few neural processes (P) between the cells (12,000 ×).

References p. 141–144

Final differentiation and maturation of the neuronal cell body

In the final stage of cytological maturation the cytoplasmic differentiation of multipolar neuroblasts and maturing neurons becomes more and more obvious. The cell body enlarges, its nucleus becomes round and its internal structure less electrondense, while the nucleolus appears even prominent (Fig. 15). The differentiation of cytoplasmic organelles parallels this. The Golgi complex becomes more extensive and can now be found in all portions of the perikaryon. The number and shape of mitochondria increases. Secondary structures, such as lysosomes, appear and increase in multipolar neuroblasts, but lipofuscin is still lacking. Neurofilaments and microtubuli are relatively scarce. The most characteristic sign of maturation of the perikaryon is the development and organization of the endoplasmic reticulum, which reaches its peak with the development of Nissl bodies. Initially loosely orientated profiles of granular endoplasmic reticulum proliferate and become arranged in the typical parallel fashion of ergastoplasm (Figs. 15–17). Using high power magnification it can be established that the endoplasmic reticulum is densely covered by ribosomes, but a considerable number of free ribosomes in the form of rosettes can be seen as well (Fig. 17).

The different stages of neuronal development exhibit distinct and measurable changes in the proportion of free and membrane-bound ribosomes. This progression towards membrane-bound ribosomes can be found in all neurons of the chick and has also been described with reference to spinal neurons (Bellairs, 1959; Eschner and Glees, 1963; Glees and Meller, 1964; Meller *et al.*, 1966a; Wechsler, 1963, 1965b), telencephalic and mesencephalic neurons (Fujita and Fujita, 1963; Wechsler and Meller, 1963), spinal ganglia (Wechsler and Schmekel, 1967), sympathetic ganglia (Wechsler and Schmekel, 1966a, b, 1967) and the retina (Meller, 1964). Similar findings have been reported for other species, including man (Pappas and Purpura, 1964; Tennyson, 1962, 1965).

Development and differentiation of neuronal processes

The development of axons is characterized by growth in length and thickness and by multiplication of branches, including the formation of collaterals. The ultrastructure of embryonic axons shows no special features apart from neurofilaments, microtubuli, vesicles, tubules and small mitochondria. They do not contain ribosomes. The adult axons have the same cytoplasmic structures but the proportions are different. Axoplasmic differentiation runs parallel with an increase in diameter. The number of filaments and microtubuli increases regularly, while the other structures decrease relatively. We have gained the impression that thick axons contain more neurofilaments while thin ones contain a relatively greater number of microtubuli (Fig. 18A–C). We would like to make some general comments regarding the *development of central nerve fibres*. After cyto- and myeloarchitectonic differentiation has ceased, the migratory zones of the hemispheres and of the tectum opticum supply the fibres and cells of the white matter. In addition to migratory cells, the migratory zones contain relatively large areas of neuronal processes, with many embryonic axons aggre-

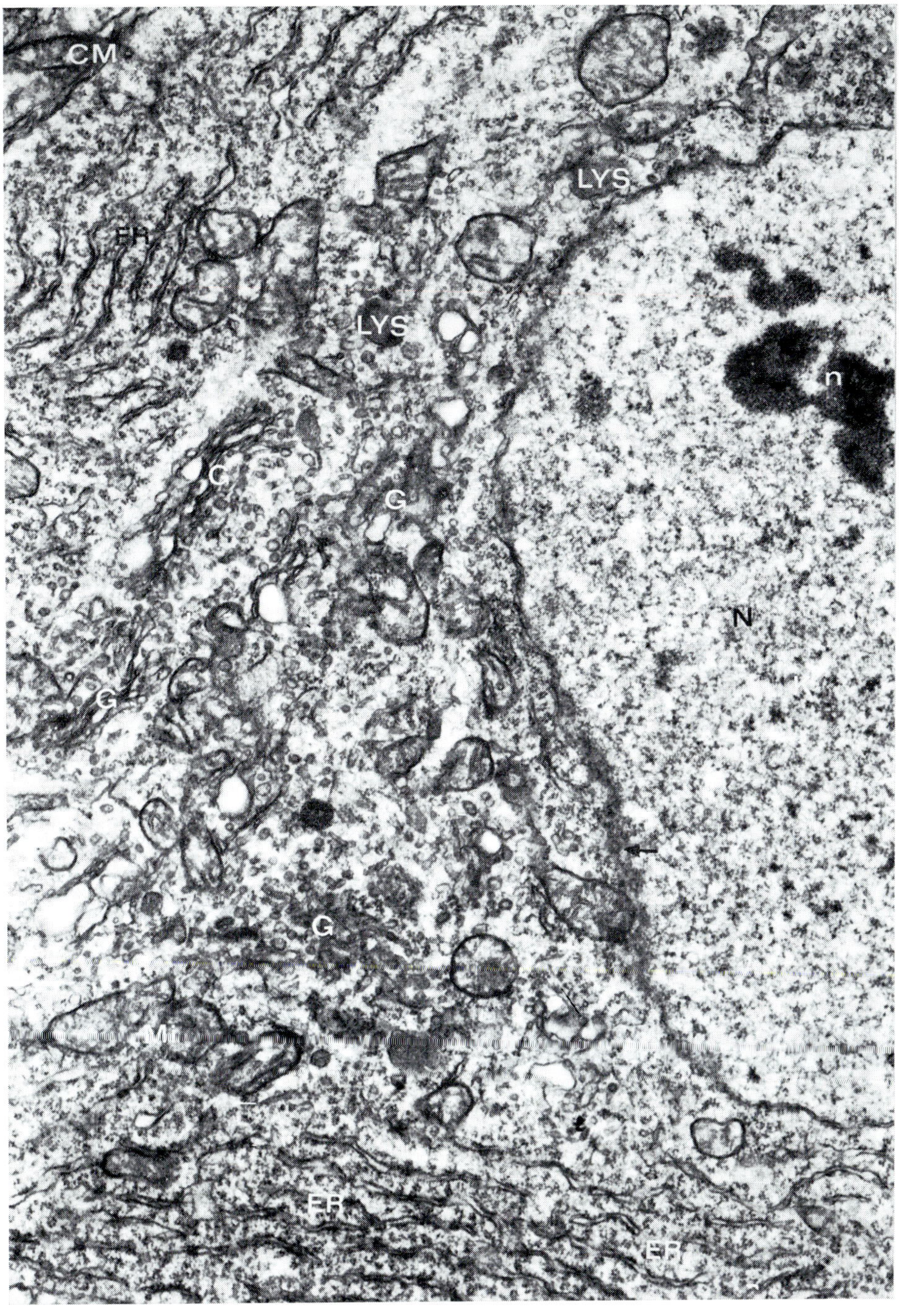

Fig. 15. Final differentiation of a pyramidal cell from the striatum of a 16-day-old embryo, a section of the perikaryon. Note the proliferation of the endoplasmic reticulum, the enlargement of the Golgi apparatus (G) and the first appearance of the lysosomes (LYS). ER = granular endoplasmic reticulum in the phase of Nissl-aggregate formation; Mi = mitochondria; CM = cell membrane; N = nucleus; n = nucleolus (35,000 ×).

References p. 141–144

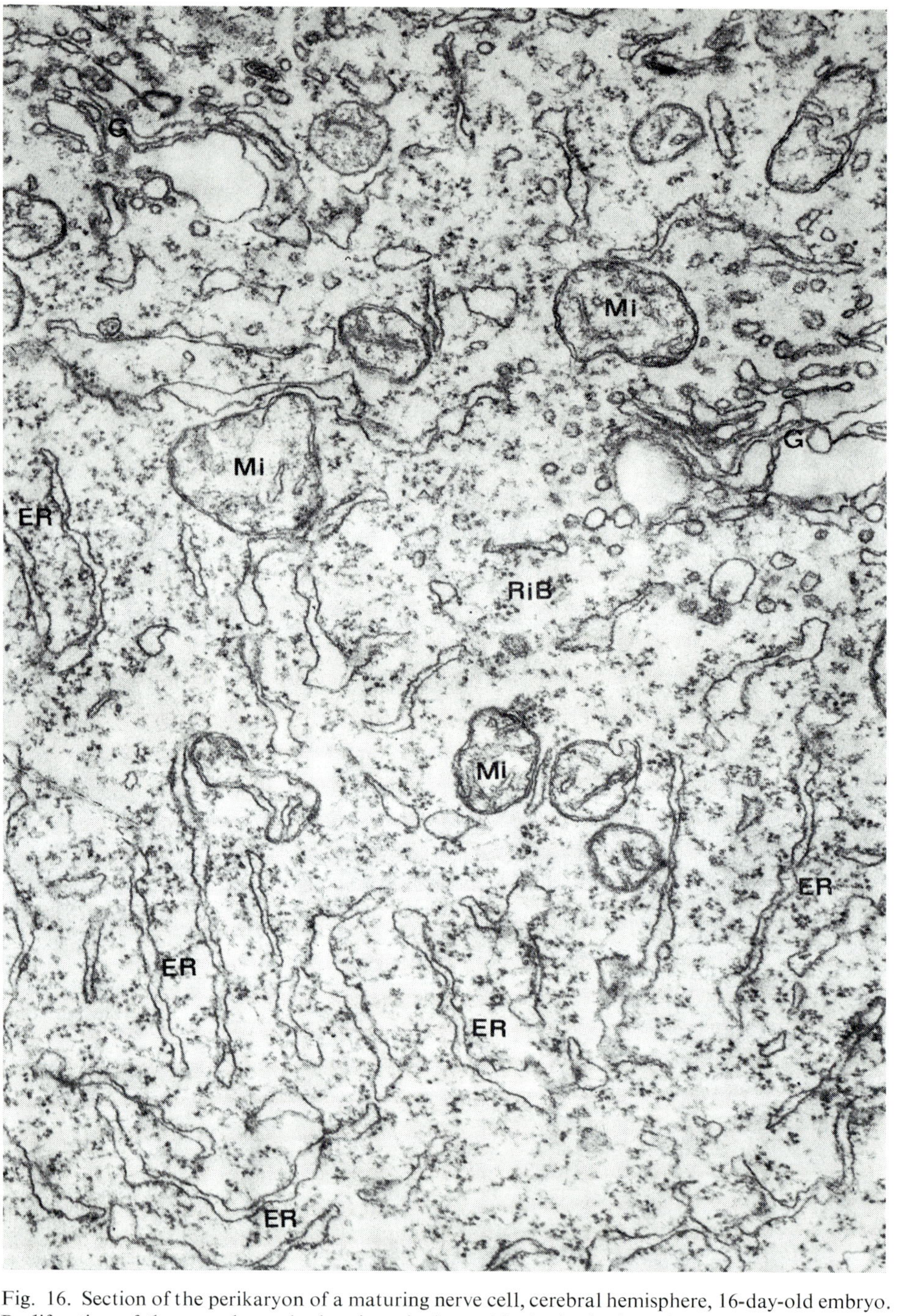

Fig. 16. Section of the perikaryon of a maturing nerve cell, cerebral hemisphere, 16-day-old embryo. Proliferation of the granular endoplasmic reticulum with the beginning of ergastoplasm formation (ER). In the cytoplasm are many free ribosomes (RiB). Mi = mitochondria; G = Golgi apparatus (50,000 ×).

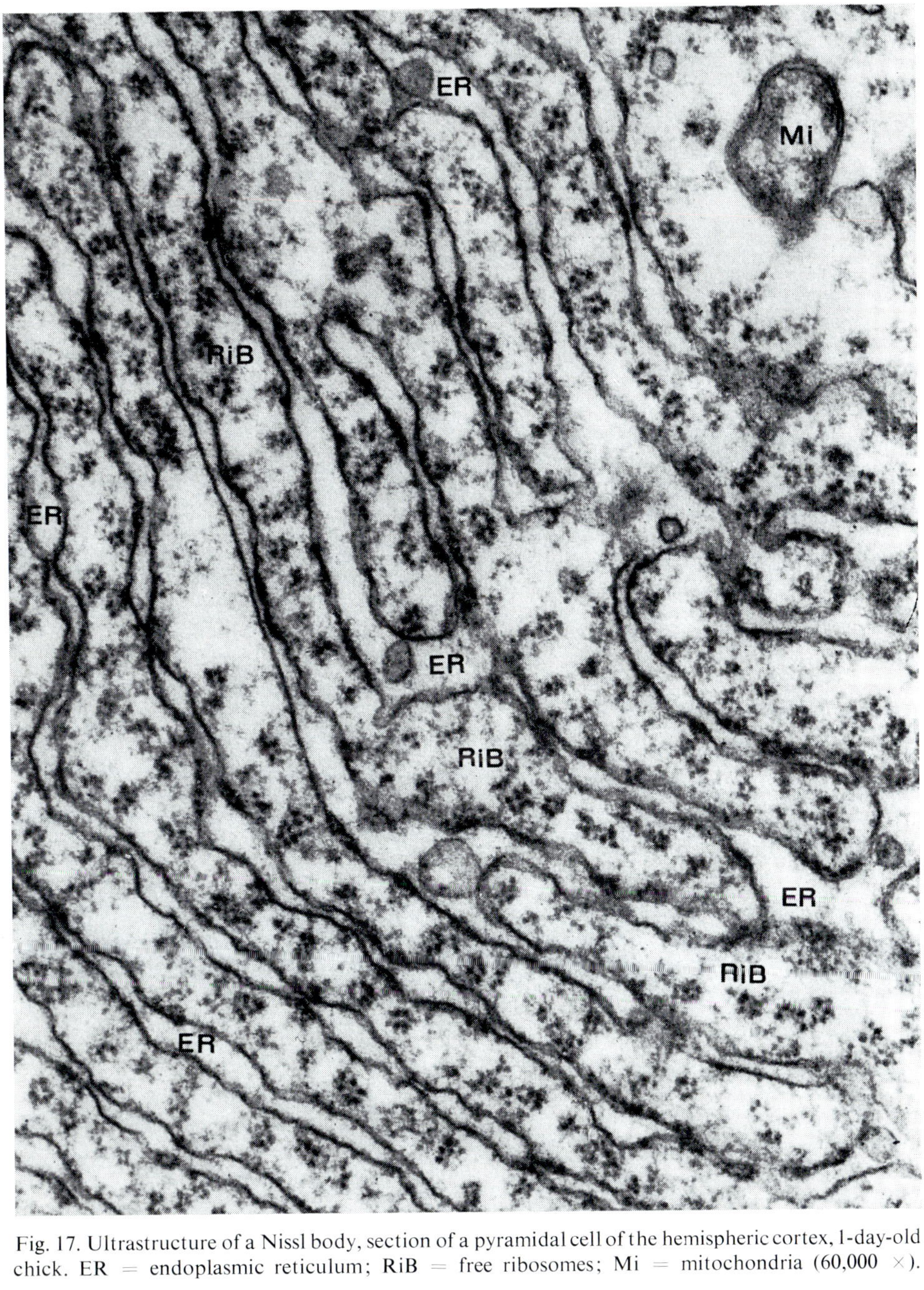

Fig. 17. Ultrastructure of a Nissl body, section of a pyramidal cell of the hemispheric cortex, 1-day-old chick. ER = endoplasmic reticulum; RiB = free ribosomes; Mi = mitochondria (60,000 ×).

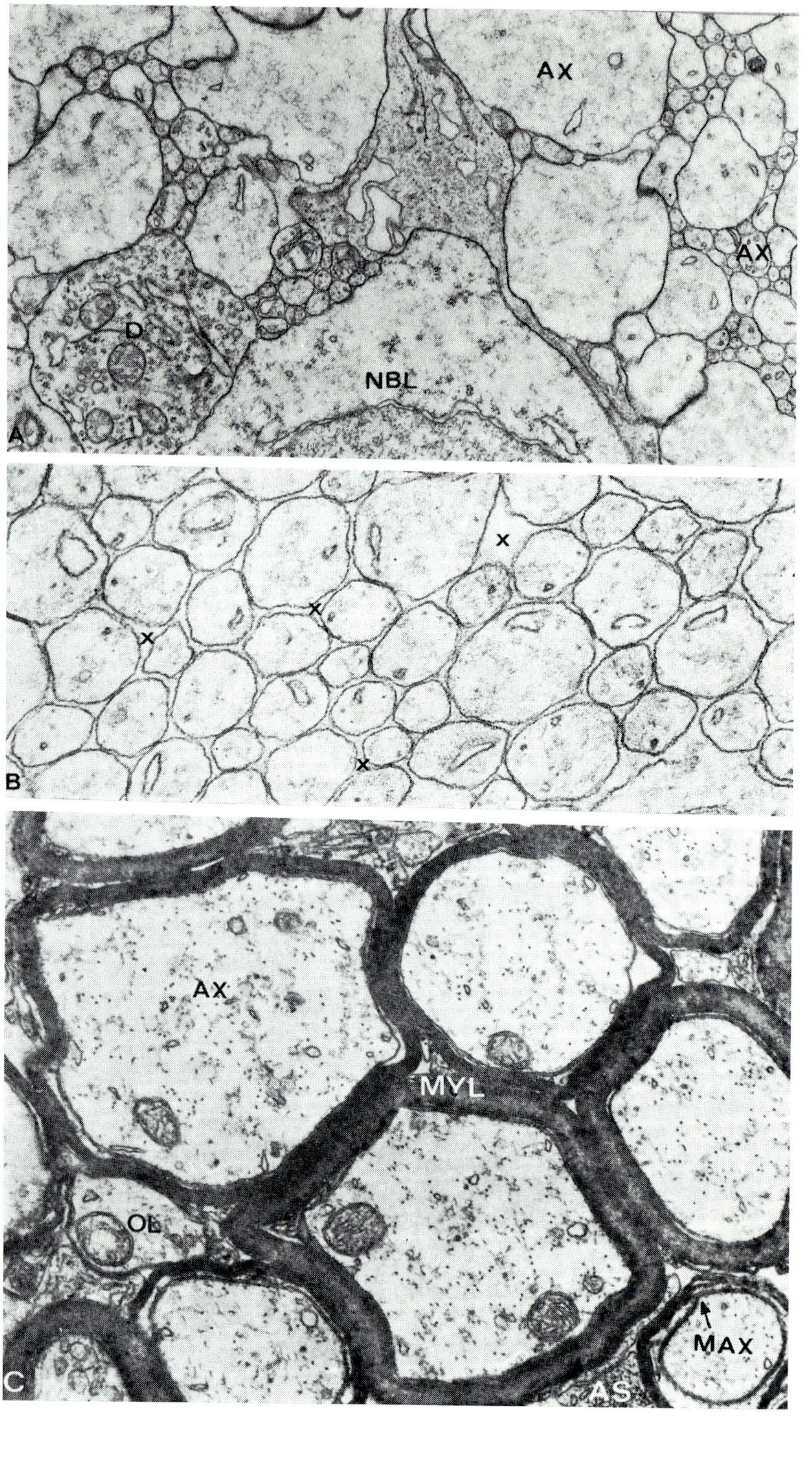
AX
AX
D
NBL
A
x
x
x
x
B
AX
MYL
OL
MAX
AS
C

gated into large bundle complexes (Figs. 13, 18a, 24, 25). In the early phases of the development of the white matter the axo-axonal relationship dominates. The first architectonic arrangement of the axon bundles is determined by the polar glioblasts and their processes. Nerve fibre formation begins only after glial differentiation has started. In this stage glioblasts differentiate into astrocytes and oligodendrocytes. The oligodendrocytes are responsible for the individual ensheathing of embryonic axons.

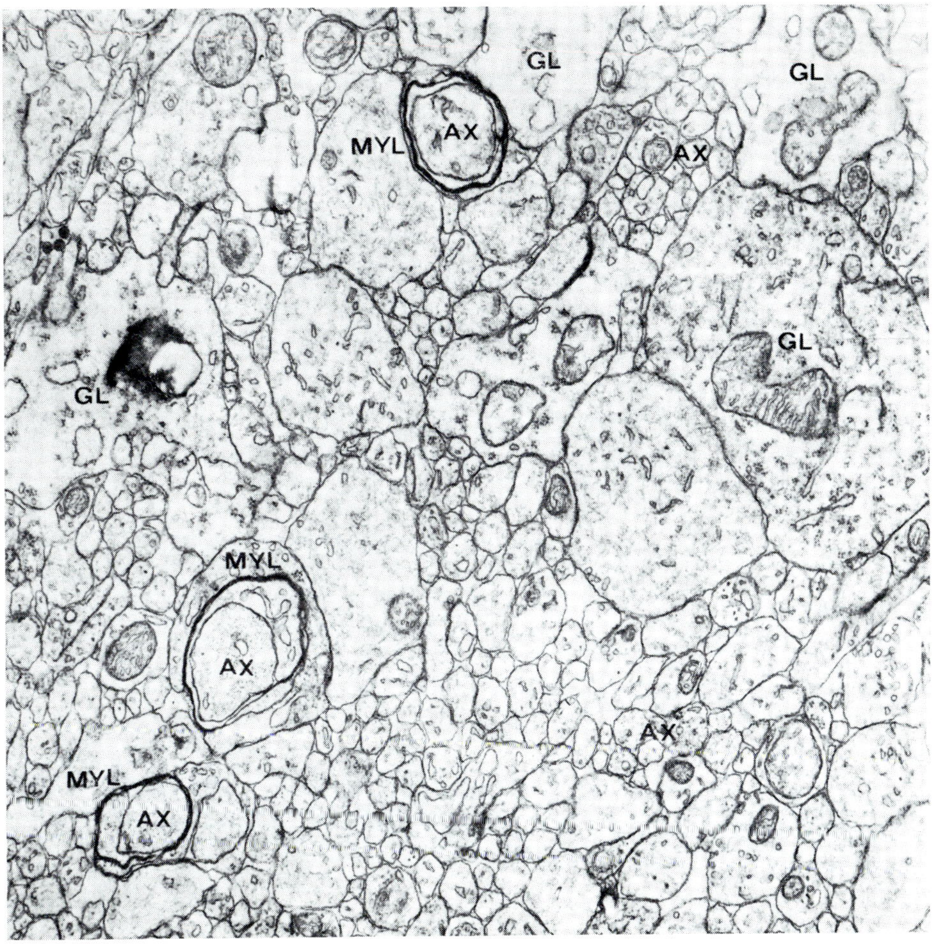

Fig. 19. Early phases of myelination, transverse section of the white matter of spinal cord, 13-day-old embryo. AX = axon bundles; GL = processes from glioblasts; MYL = first myelin spirals (18,000 ×).

Fig. 18. Ultrastructure of the embryonic and mature axons. A, The embryonic axons from th migratory zone of the telencephalon, 7.5-day-old embryo (18,000 ×); B, Migratory zone of th telencephalon, 7.5-day-old embryo (65,000 ×); C, Thin myelinated nerve fibre from the white matter 7-week-old chick (33,000 ×). NBL = neuroblast; D = dendrite; AX = axon; x = extracellular space; MYL = myelin sheath; OL = oligodendrocytic process; AS = fibrillary astrocytic process; MAX = internal mesaxon.

References p. 141–144

Similar findings have been reported from the study of the development of the white substance in the spinal cord (Wechsler, 1965b). In contrast to the cells of Schwann of the peripheral nervous system, each oligodendrocyte is capable of forming myelin around several axons. With the onset of myelogenesis the interstitial glia are pushed more and more into the background, allowing the myelin sheaths of different nerve fibres to come into contact with each other (Fig. 18C). Because the myelinating glial process retracts to a small 'glial tongue' (Peters, 1960, 1962), neighbouring myelin membranes can come into direct contact. In the areas of contact the extracellular space is obliterated and an intermediate line will be formed. These findings are valid both for the white matter of the brain and for the spinal cord in chick embryos (Fig. 19). The observations of central myelin formation reported for *Xenopus* and anura by Peters (1960, 1962), Maturana (1960), Gaze and Peters (1961) agree well with our findings in the CNS of the chick. This means that myelinization in both the central and peripheral nervous system is associated with the growth of the mesaxon, which appears to wind itself round the axon. Older views are no longer valid (Luse, 1956; De Robertis *et al.*, 1958).

In order to estimate the degree of differentiation of neurons, the dendritic proliferation is of the utmost significance. But the differentiation of dendrites can be observed electron-microscopically in a limited way only. After silver impregnation embryonic dendrites are seen to be relatively thick and to show few branches. It is possible to distinguish them from embryonic axons by means of discrete ultrastructural features, the presence of free ribosomes and poorly developed granular

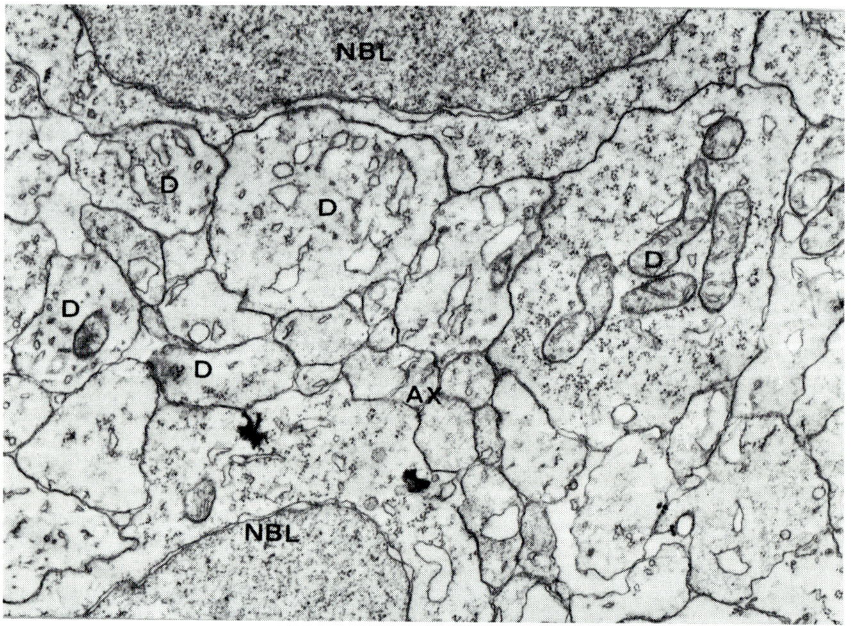

Fig. 20. Ultrastructure of the dendrites of uni- and multipolar neuroblasts. Section from the primary cortex, tectum opticum, 9-day-old embryo. NBL = neuroblast; D = dendrite; AX = axon (24,000 ×).

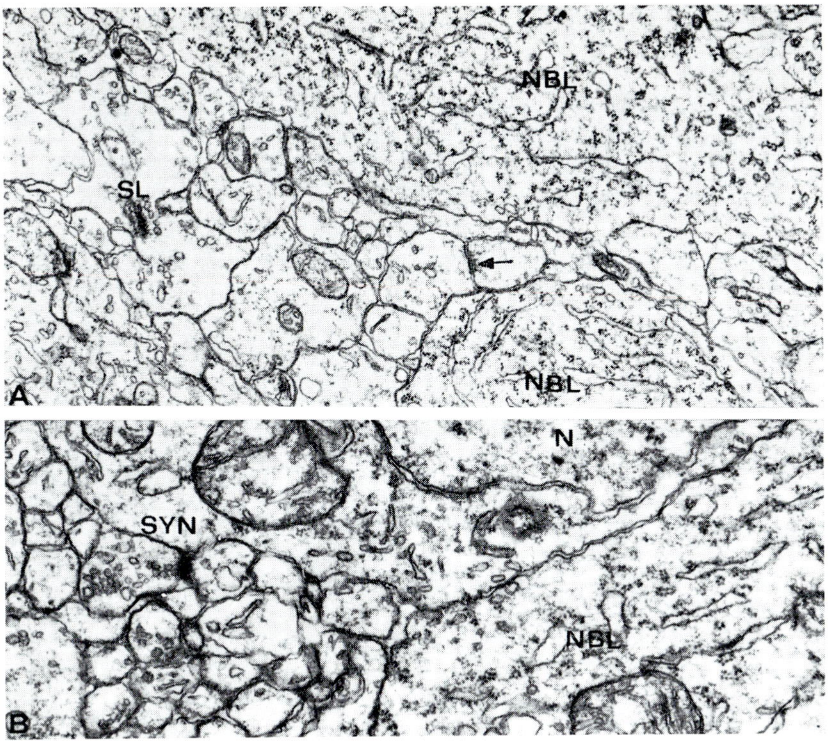

Fig. 21. Development of synapses. A, Early phases of the development of synapses, gray matter of the spinal cord, 10-day-old embryo. NBL = neuroblasts with some proliferation of the endoplasmic reticulum (ER); arrow shows the first thickening of the pre- and postsynaptic membranes, still without synaptic vesicles, SL = synaptic lamellae (21,000 ×). B, Second phase of synaptic development with the thickening of membranes on both sides of the synaptic cleft and appearance of the first synaptic vesicles (SYN). NBL = neuroblasts from the gray matter of the spinal cord, 10-day-old embryo (26,000 ×).

endoplasmic reticulum (Fig. 20). The number of microtubuli increases in relation to the growth of the dendritic tree, but electron microscopy can supply only indirect evidence of the extent to which dendrites branch and proliferate (see the development of neuropil; Figs. 38 and 39).

Synaptic development is characterized by quantitative and qualitative changes of the axoplasm (Figs. 21 and 22). New structures appear which could not be recognized before in the axoplasm. One has to discriminate between pre- and postsynaptic membrane thickenings, the appearance and accumulation of synaptic vesicles, the increase in mitochondria and the formation of special structures such as synaptic lamellae (Fig. 21B). The development of synapses has so far been mainly examined in the spinal cord of chick embryos (Glees and Meller, 1964; Glees and Sheppard, 1964; Wechsler, 1965b), but the same principles of synaptic development are also valid for brain tissue (Wechsler, 1966f). The retinal synapses have to be mentioned in this connection, for here a precise localization and recognition of synaptic contacts is possible (Meller, 1964). It should be possible to relate synaptic development to the different

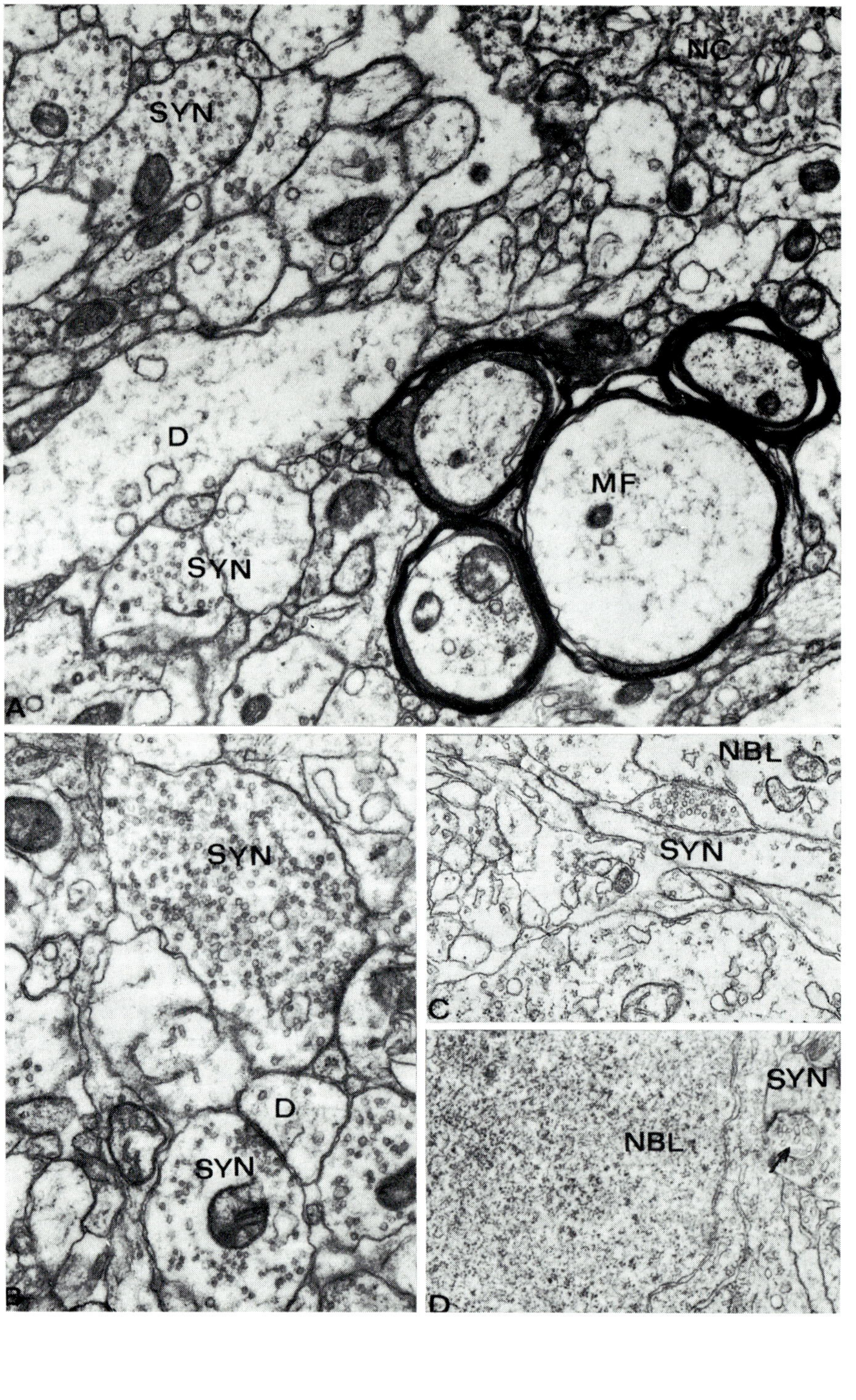

NC
SYN
D
MF
SYN
A
SYN
D
SYN
B
NBL
SYN
C
SYN
NBL
D

types of synapses described for the adult nervous system (Gray, 1964; Gray and Guillery, 1966).

VI. THE DIFFERENTIATION OF NEUROGLIA

The results of the research of neuroglia viewed under the electron microscope are available in a number of reviews (Gray, 1964; Hager, 1964; Mugnaini and Wahlberg, 1964; De Robertis, 1965; Sjöstrand, 1964).

Studies devoted to the problem of neuroglia differentiation are few. One reason is certainly the great difficulty in identifying embryonic glial cells. These difficulties are particularly great in regions containing both neurons and glia (Bellairs, 1959; Fujita and Fujita, 1963; Wechsler and Meller, 1963b). For this reason we have examined first the glial differentiation in the white matter of the spinal cord (Wechsler, 1963). Ramsey (1962) has examined this problem in newborn and young rats, studying especially the differentiation of oligodendrocytes from migrating spongioblasts in the corpus callosum. Lately, a number of criteria have been elaborated to help in the discrimination of neuroblasts from glioblasts (Meller *et al.*, 1966a). A futher contribution to the problem of gliogenesis can be found in papers dealing with the development and myelinization of central nerve fibres (Bunge *et al.*, 1962; Gaze and Peters, 1961; Luse, 1956; Maturana, 1960; Peters, 1960, 1962).

The stages of glial differentiation are diagrammatically summarized in scheme 1. Glioblasts develop from pluripotential matrix cells and are capable of forming astrocytes and oligodendrocytes. The polar ependymoglioblasts or glioblasts (formerly called polar spongioblasts) have an even wider range of differentiation potentialities. If these cells remain close to the ventricular surface they turn into glial-epithelial ependymal cells, but if they detach themselves from the inner surface, they turn into typical migrating glioblasts. We prefer the term 'glioblasts' in contrast to 'spongioblasts' as our observations show that all embryonic glial cells are individual units, and are not syncytially connected so as to deserve the name 'myelospongium' used in the classical literature.

Primitive glioblasts and neuroblasts have a similar ultrastructure. For this reason it is impossible to discriminate primitive and polar glioblasts in the matrix zones, although they have been reported after the use of silver impregnation methods (Figs. 4B and 23). The same difficulties of cellular interpretation exist in the migratory zones. However, to a limited extent it is possible to identify *polar glioblasts and migrating glioblasts* by means of their shape and localization (Figs. 24 and 25). These glioblasts have a small, spindle shaped cell body and an ovoid or moderately lobulated nucleus. The cytoplasm contains relatively few free ribosomes and the endoplasmic reticulum

Fig. 22. Development of some synapses in the brain of chick embryos. NC = nerve cell; SYN = synapsis; D = dendrite; MF = myelinated nerve fibre; NBL = neuroblast. A, Molecular layer of the hemispheric cortex, 1-day-old chick (18,000 ×); B, Mature synapses, molecular layer of the hemispheric cortex, 1-day-old chick (25,000 ×); C, Cortex of the hemispheres, 16-day-old embryo: small axosomatic type of synapsis (20,000 ×); D, Axosomatic type of synapse with spine apparatus, striatum, 16-day-old embryo.

References p. 141–144

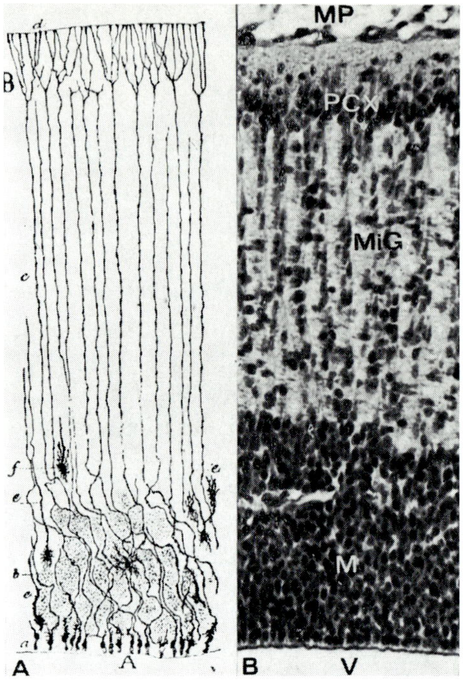

Fig. 23. A diagrammatic representation of glial differentiation. A, Differentiation of the neuroglia in the cortex (Cajal, 1952). B, Corresponding region from the brain of a 6.5-day-old chick embryo. V = ventricle; M = matrix; MiG = migratory zone; PCX = primary cortex; MP = meninx primitiva.

is little developed. Mitochondria are found in varying numbers and sizes in the cytoplasm while glial filaments are lacking. Occasionally lipid inclusions and lysosomes can be found. The following points may be helpful to discriminate glioblasts from neuroblasts: (1) the nucleus and cytoplasm of glioblasts have a greater electron density, (2) the number of ribosomes and profiles of endoplasmic reticulum is less in glioblasts than in neuroblasts, (3) the nuclear bag is more irregular in glioblasts. Similar findings have been reported for the cells in the migratory zone of the cerebral hemispheres of mice, and have contributed to the understanding of glial differentiation (Meller *et al.*, 1966b). It can be shown in the spinal cord of chick embryos that the ventral and dorsal polar glioblasts show a distinct glial-epithelial polarization in rather early stages of development (Glees and Le Vay, 1964; Wechsler, 1966e).

With progressing cytoarchitectural differentiation of the optic tectum, the striatum and the cerebral hemispheres, it becomes easier to separate small glioblasts from large neurons (Fig. 38A). The nucleus of such glioblasts is ovoid, of uniform density and shows an evenly precipitated karyoplasm (Fig. 26). The nucleoli are not so much in evidence. The perinuclear cytoplasm is narrow and contains numerous ribosomes, while only a few mitochondria are present. The amount of endoplasmic reticulum is small and glial filaments are absent. With progressive differentiation of astrocytes and oligodendrocytes the well known ultrastructural features of these glial cells become obvious. The astrocytes then show a round nucleus of medium electron-density and nucleoli-like inclusions. The cytoplasm differs slightly from that of migrating glioblasts (Figs. 26 and 27). In the case of protoplasmic and fibrillary astrocytes, processes of low density penetrate the neuropil and come into close relation with neurons and blood vessels (Figs. 27, 38 and 41). It is of interest to note that the primitive glial vascular end feet contain small glycogen granules (Meller *et al.*, 1966a). The sequence of fibrillary differentiation in astrocytes in the area of the marginal and supermarginal

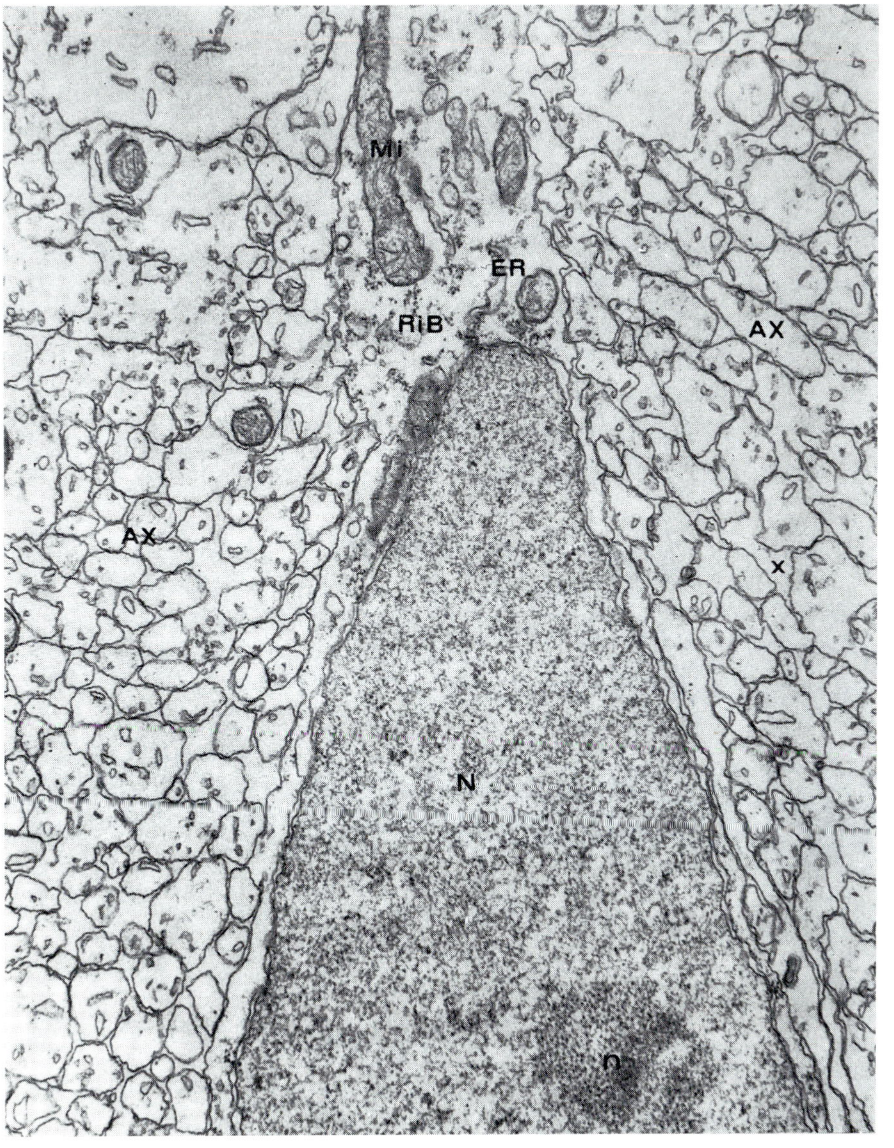

Fig. 24. Spindle-shaped glioblast from the migratory zone, telencephalon, 9-day-old embryo. N = nucleus of a longitudinally sectioned glioblast; n = nucleolus; RiB = free ribosomes; ER = endoplasmic reticulum; Mi = mitochondria; AX = embryonal axon; x = artificial slightly expanded extracellular space (30,000 ×).

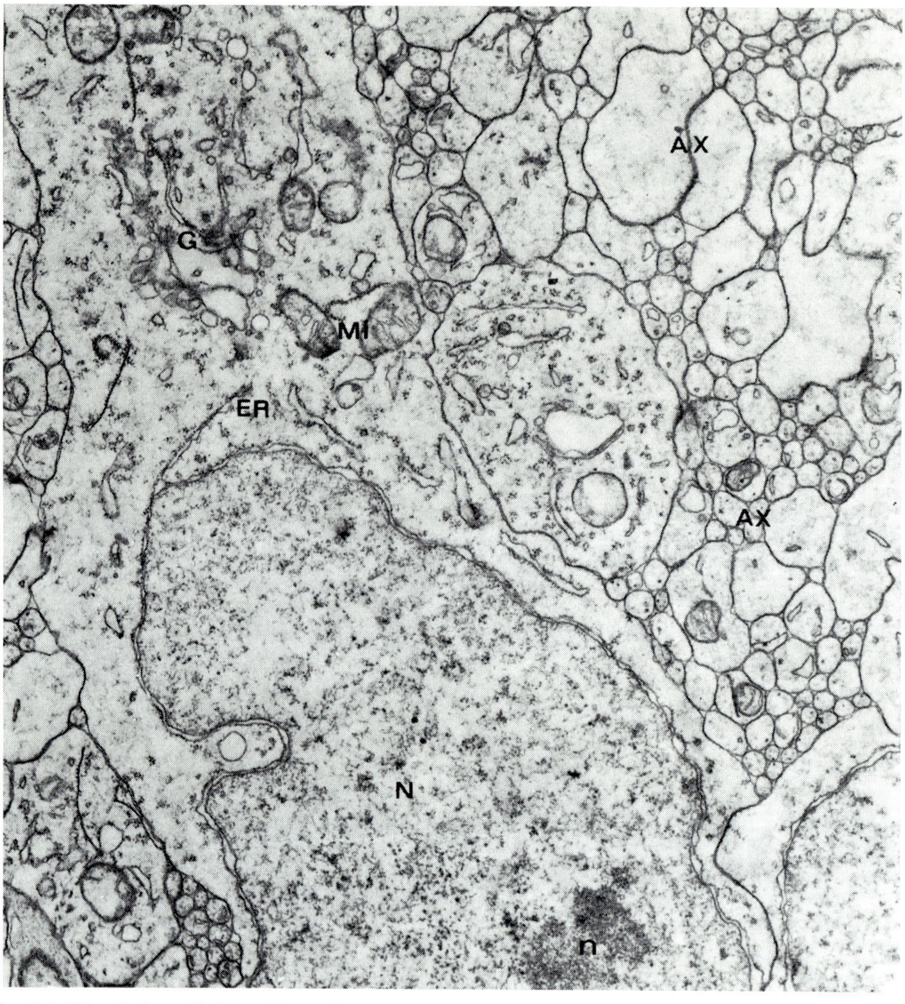

Fig. 25. Wandering glioblast from the migratory zone, telencephalon, 10-day-old embryo. N = nucleus; n = nucleolus; ER = endoplasmic reticulum; G = Golgi apparatus; Mi = mitochondria; AX = axon bundle formation (25,000 ×).

glia has been studied in particular (Fig. 39). In the second phase of embryonic development this zone consists of primitive cells and processes (Figs. 11 and 28).

Oligodendrocytes are glial cells possessing a dense nucleus, many ribosomes and a fairly well developed granular endoplasmic reticulum. The number of ribosomes and mitochondria appears to be greater than in astrocytes. Intracytoplasmic filaments are extremely rare.

VII. THE DIFFERENTIATION OF EPENDYMOBLASTS

Those matrix cells which remain attached to the inner surface of the brain produce ependymoblasts, which are the precursor cells of ependymal and chorioida epithelial

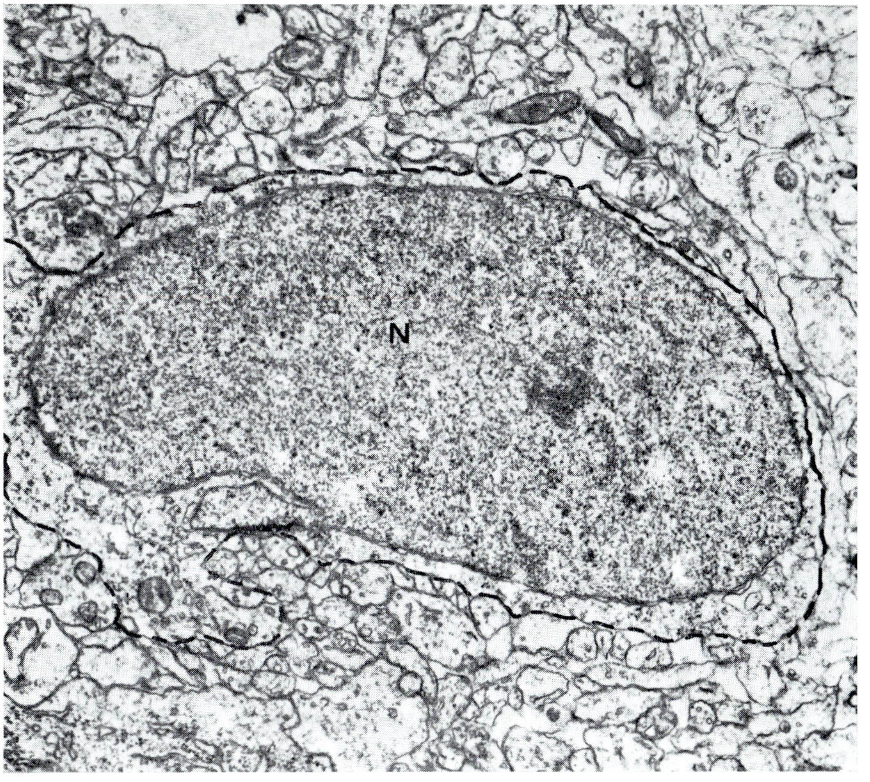

Fig. 26. Glioblast in the neuropil of the striatum, 16-day-old embryo. Cell body marked by hatched lines. N = nucleus (18,000 ×).

cells (diagram 1, p. 94). We have referred already to the significance of polar ependymoglioblasts or glioblasts for ependymal differentiation. Electron microscopical studies of the development of the ependyma and the telencephalic chorioidal plexus have been carried out, in the cerebral aqueduct of the rabbit (Tennyson and Pappas, 1962), the ventricular ependyma and plexus of the telencephalon of chick embryos (Meller and Wechsler, 1965; Wechsler, 1966b), the central canal of the spinal cord of the chick (Fujita and Fujita, 1964; Glees and Le Vay, 1964; Wechsler, 1963, 1965e), and the telencephalic plexus of the rabbit's brain (Tennyson and Pappas, 1961). It can be shown that embryonic and mature ependymal and chorioid cells differ in shape and ultrastructure.

(A) Ependyma. Matrix cells, ependymoblasts and polar glioblasts are characterized by bipolar shape and a bipolar differentiation of cytoplasmic structure. This bipolarity increases in the course of ependymal development and is terminated by a glial-epithelial type of cell. We have referred to primordial polarization of the brain surfaces and the ultrastructure of the ependymoblasts in Fig. 29. The following general rules govern ependymal differentiation.

The differentiation of apical processes is the earliest morphological sign observable and is characterized by a proliferation of microvilli and cilia. Furthermore, we see a

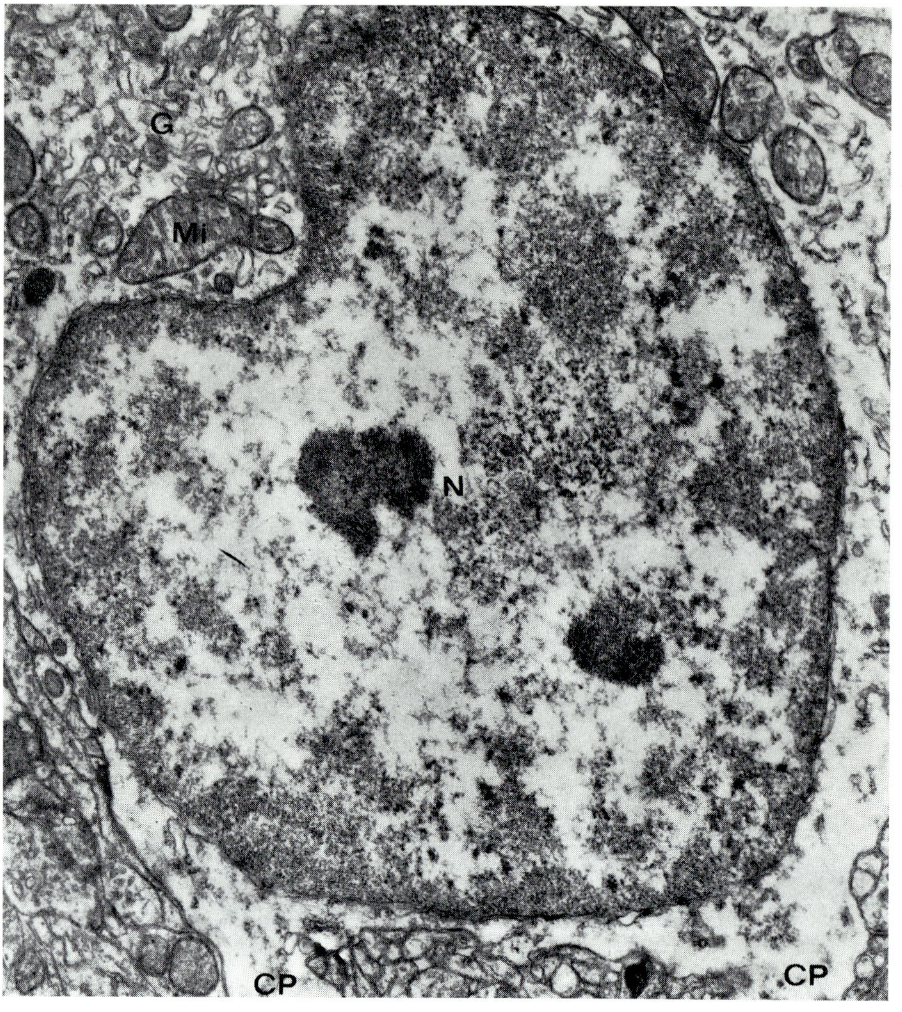

Fig. 27. Protoplasmic astrocyte, hemispheric cortex, 4-week-old chick. N = nucleus; G = Golgi apparatus; Mi = mitochondria; CP = cell processes (20,000 ×).

shift of the Golgi apparatus to the cellular apex and its enlargement. At the same time an augmentation of mitochondria, together with the appearance of more smooth cytoplasmic vesicles and tubules occurs, favouring pinocytotic activity (Figs. 30 and 31). The endoplasmic reticulum in the apical portion of ependymal cells is of both the smooth and the granular types, and is probably a combination of vesicular and tubular structures. The shape of the nucleus and its position also change during differentiation. Differentiation of basal processes, however, takes longer. Only after the reduction of the matrix zones does final differentiation of the basal portion of the ependyma and the formation of subependymal neuroglia take place. At the same time the basal ependymal processes — resembling protoplasmic astrocytic processes — make contact with glia cells, neurons and subependymal vessels. The ventricular wall is continuous

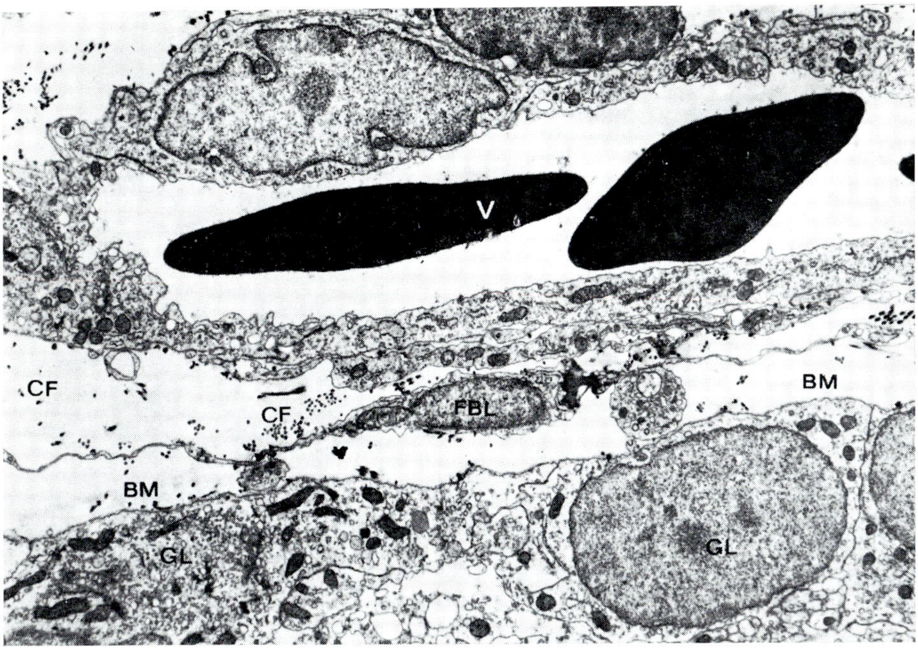

Fig. 28. Meninges and primitive marginal glia in the region of hemispherical cortex, 13-day-old embryo. GL = closed layer of protoplasmic glia cells; BM = superficial basement membrane; V = immature medium sized meningeal blood vessel; FBL = fibroblast; CF = collagen fibrils (10,000 ×).

in all stages of development and the apical indentation and desmosomal thickenings strengthen the inner lining.

(B) Plexus epithelium. The primordial cells have an elongated columnar shape, which changes during maturation into a more cubical form. The immature pseudo-stratified epithelium is polarized. The differentiation of the plexus stroma follows that of the epithelium. We distinguish three cytogenetic phases in the development of the plexus epithelium (Meller and Wechsler, 1965; Wechsler, 1966b).

Phase I: In the early stages of embryonic development of the telencephalic choroid plexus (7–10 days of incubation) the basal cytoplasm of the cells contains numerous free ribosomes, but only very few profiles of endoplasmic reticulum (Fig. 32). The number of mitochondria is relatively small. The apical parts of these columnar cells are inter-connected by desmosomes and a few microvilli and cilia protrude. The Golgi apparatus tends to be situated in the apical region. The nucleus is oval, electron-dense and contains large nucleoli (Fig. 32). It is usually situated in the centre of the cell and is only occasionally displaced towards the base or apex.

Phase II: Further progress in polar differentiation of plexus cells is observed in 13–15-day-old chick embryos. In the basal portion of the columnar epithelium the cells develop a well differentiated granular endoplasmic reticulum of a type usually associated with ergastoplasm (Figs. 33–35). In this phase the proliferation of the endoplasmic reticulum may be even more pronounced than in mature choroid cells.

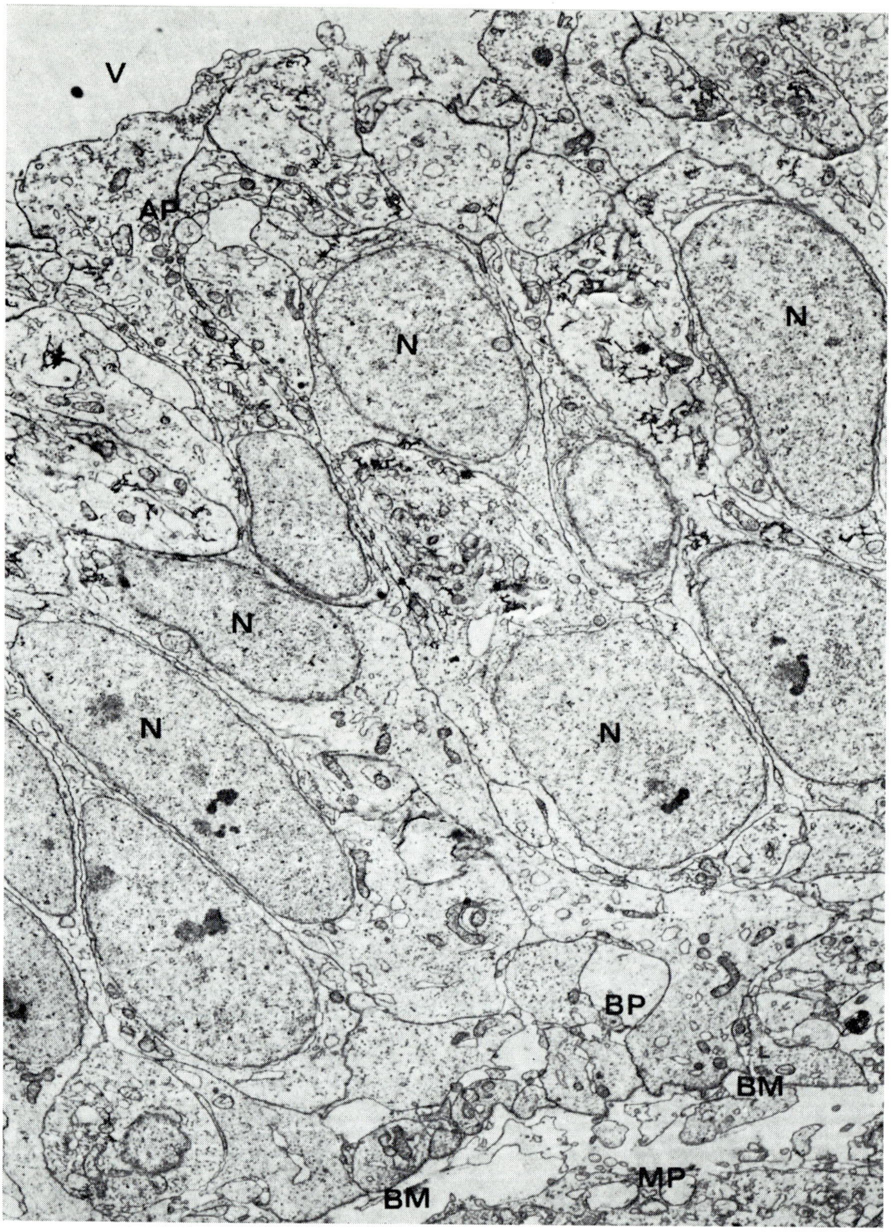

Fig. 29. Surface polarization of the wall of brain vesicle (for explanation see text). V = ventricle; AP = apical or central process of the matrix cells and of the polar ependymo-glioblasts; N = nucleus; BP = basal or peripheral processes; BM = basement membrane; MP = cells of the meninx primitiva (6000 ×).

The number of mitochondria increases and there are changes in structure in both the apical and basal portions of the cells. In the apical portion, the Golgi apparatus enlarges, the endoplasmic reticulum changes to the smooth type (Fig. 36) and a marked proliferation of microvilli and cilia takes place. A basal labyrinth is not yet present and the nuclei are found in the middle of the cells.

Phase III: The maturation of plexus epithelium begins in the last third of embryonic development. The columnar or cubically shaped cells show further apical differentiation with a considerable increase of microvilli, which now far exceed the number of cilia. Increase in the number of apical mitochondria continues as well. The rounder nuclei now occupy a more basal position and, as a result, they reduce the space avail-

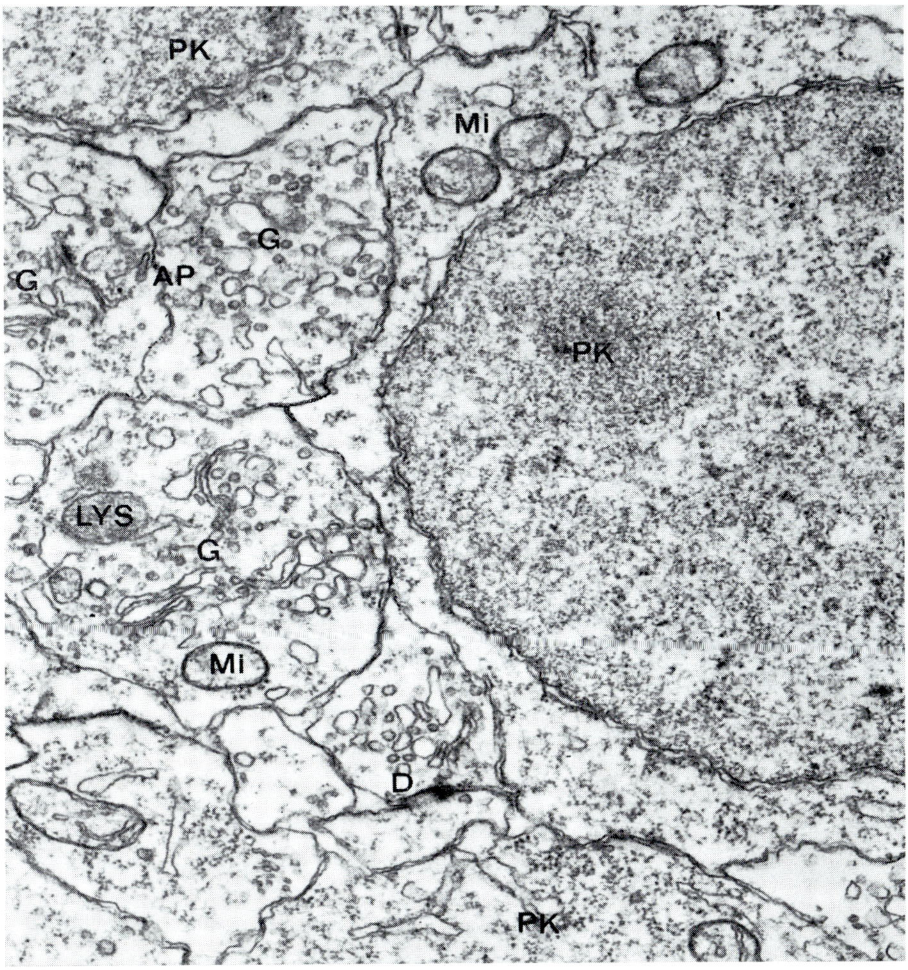

Fig. 30. Horizontal section through the ventricle wall, ependymal matrix, telencephalon, 9-day-old embryo. PK = perikaryon of an ependymoblasts; AP = apical process of ependymoblast with large Golgi apparatus (G); Mi = mitochondria; ER = endoplasmic reticulum; LYS = lysosomes; D = desmosomes (33,000 ×).

References p. 141–144

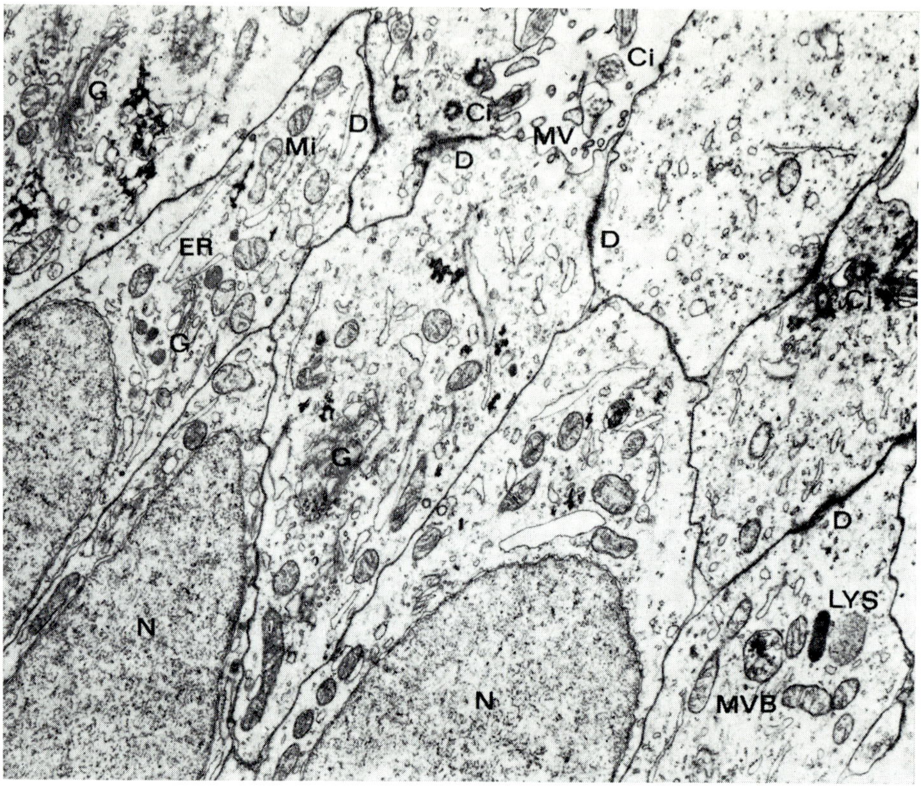

Fig. 31. Advanced differentiation of the ventricular surface with reduction of the matrix layer, telencephalon, 13-day-old embryo. N = nucleus; G = Golgi apparatus; ER = endoplasmic reticulum; Mi = mitochondria; D = desmosomes; Ci = cilia; MV = microvilli; LYS = Lysosomes; MVB = multivesicular bodies (15,000 ×).

able for ergastoplasm. An infolding of the basal plasmalemma can be observed at this stage.

We have already described the ultrastructure of the plexus stroma with respect to problems of the blood-barrier (Meller and Wechsler, 1965; Wechsler, 1966b). Maturation changes take place at both levels of the blood–cerebrospinal fluid barrier, *i.e.* in the epithelial cells and the vascular stroma. The plexus stroma consists primarly of undifferentiated mesenchymal cells and immature capillaries (Figs. 32, 33 and 37). Intercellular substances can be recognized only by the presence of fine granular or filamentous precipitation. While the basement membrane of the plexus epithelium is present from the very beginning of plexus formation, no external basement membrane can be found around embryonic vessels (Fig. 37). Differentiation of capillaries leads to a flattening of the endothelium and sometimes to the formation of pores (Fig. 37). The laying down of the basement membrane is the last step in maturation and continues after hatching. The same is also true for the synthesis of a large amount of collagen fibrils in the stroma.

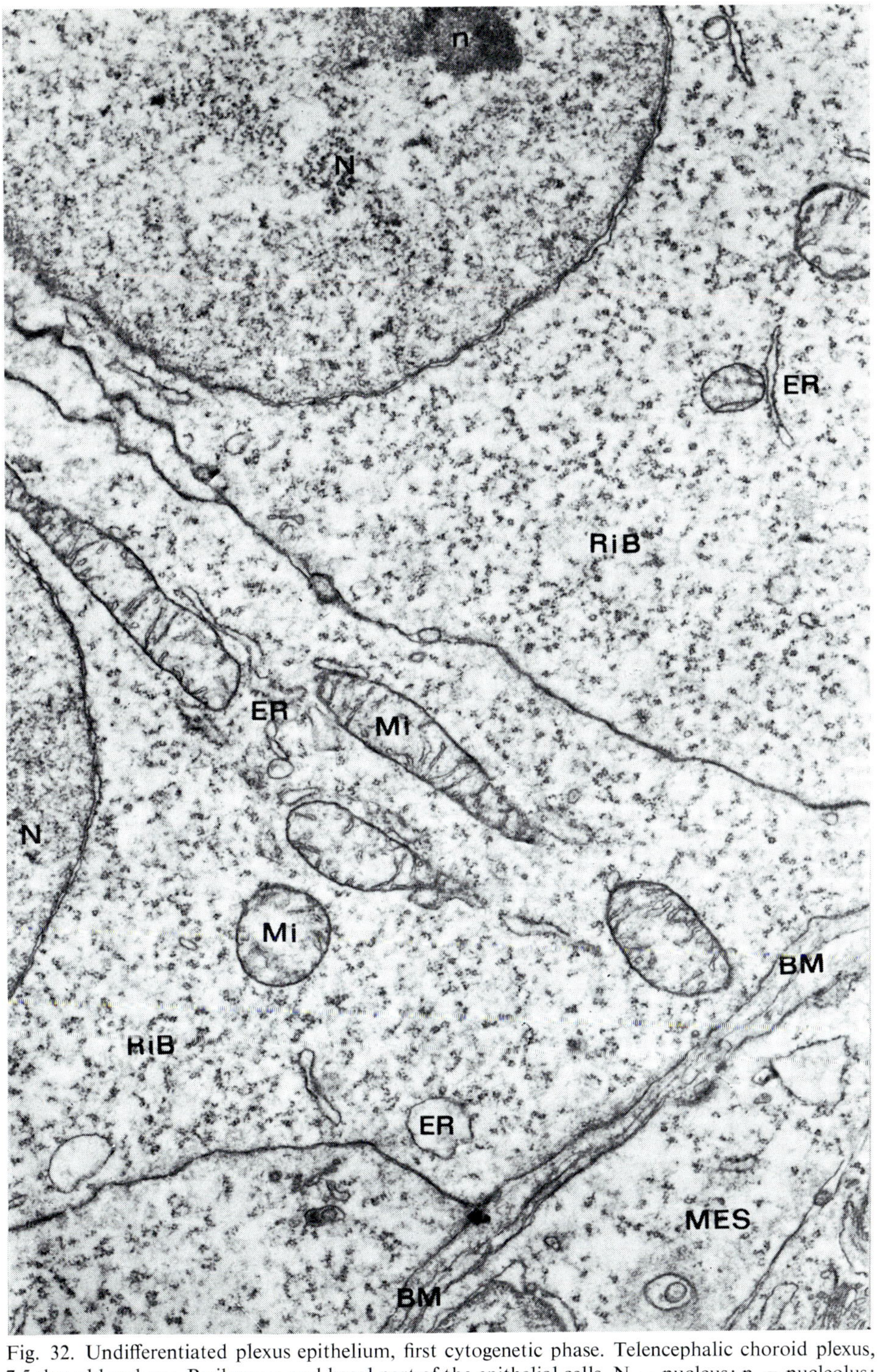

Fig. 32. Undifferentiated plexus epithelium, first cytogenetic phase. Telencephalic choroid plexus, 7.5-day-old embryo. Perikaryon and basal part of the epithelial cells. N = nucleus; n = nucleolus; RiB = free ribosomes; ER = endoplasmic reticulum; Mi = mitochondria; BM = basement membrane; MES = undifferentiated cells of the plexus stroma (25,000 ×).

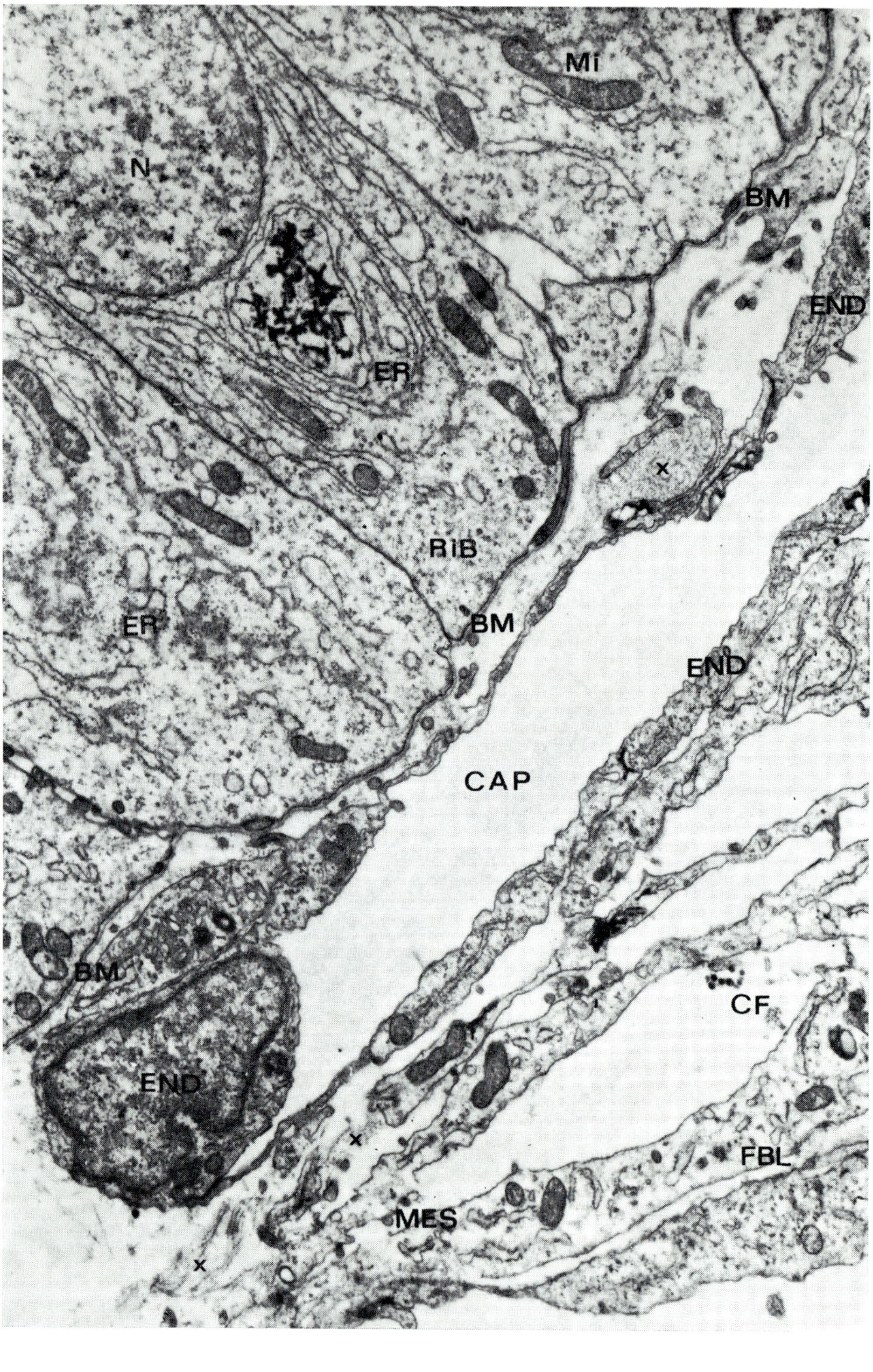
Mi
N
BM
END
ER
x
RiB
BM
ER
END
CAP
BM
CF
END
x
FBL
MES
x

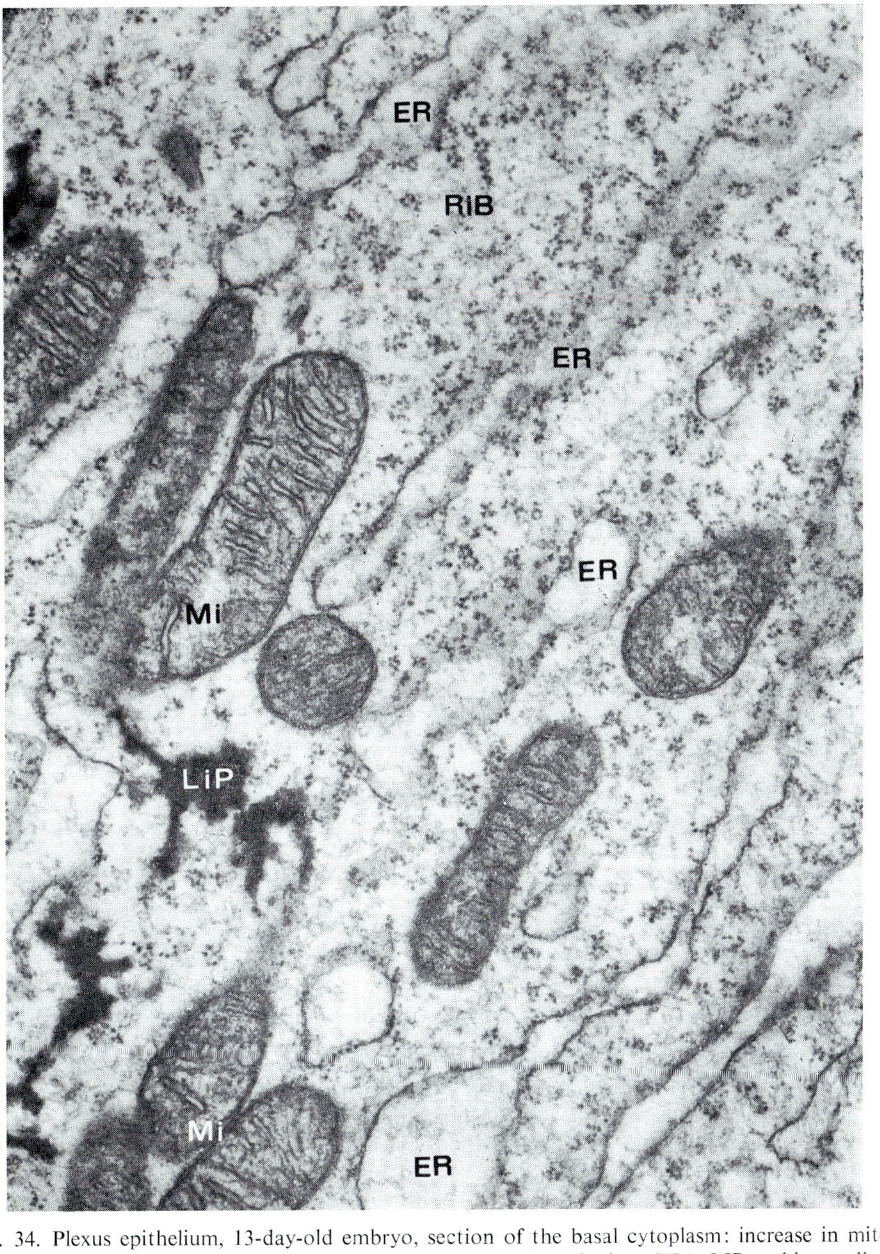

Fig. 34. Plexus epithelium, 13-day-old embryo, section of the basal cytoplasm: increase in mitochondria (Mi) and proliferation of the granular endoplasmic reticulum (ER). LIP = bizarre lipid plaques; RiB = free ribosomes (45,000 ×).

Fig. 33. Second cytogenetic phase of the differentiation of plexus epithelium, 13-day-old embryo. BM = basement membrane; N = nucleus; ER = endoplasmic reticulum; Mi = mitochondria; RiB = free ribosomes; CAP = incompletely developed stroma capillary without basement membrane; END = endothelium; MES = processes of undifferentiated mesenchyme cells and fibroblasts (FBL); CF = mature collagen fibrils; x = precursor of collagen fibrils (10,000 ×).

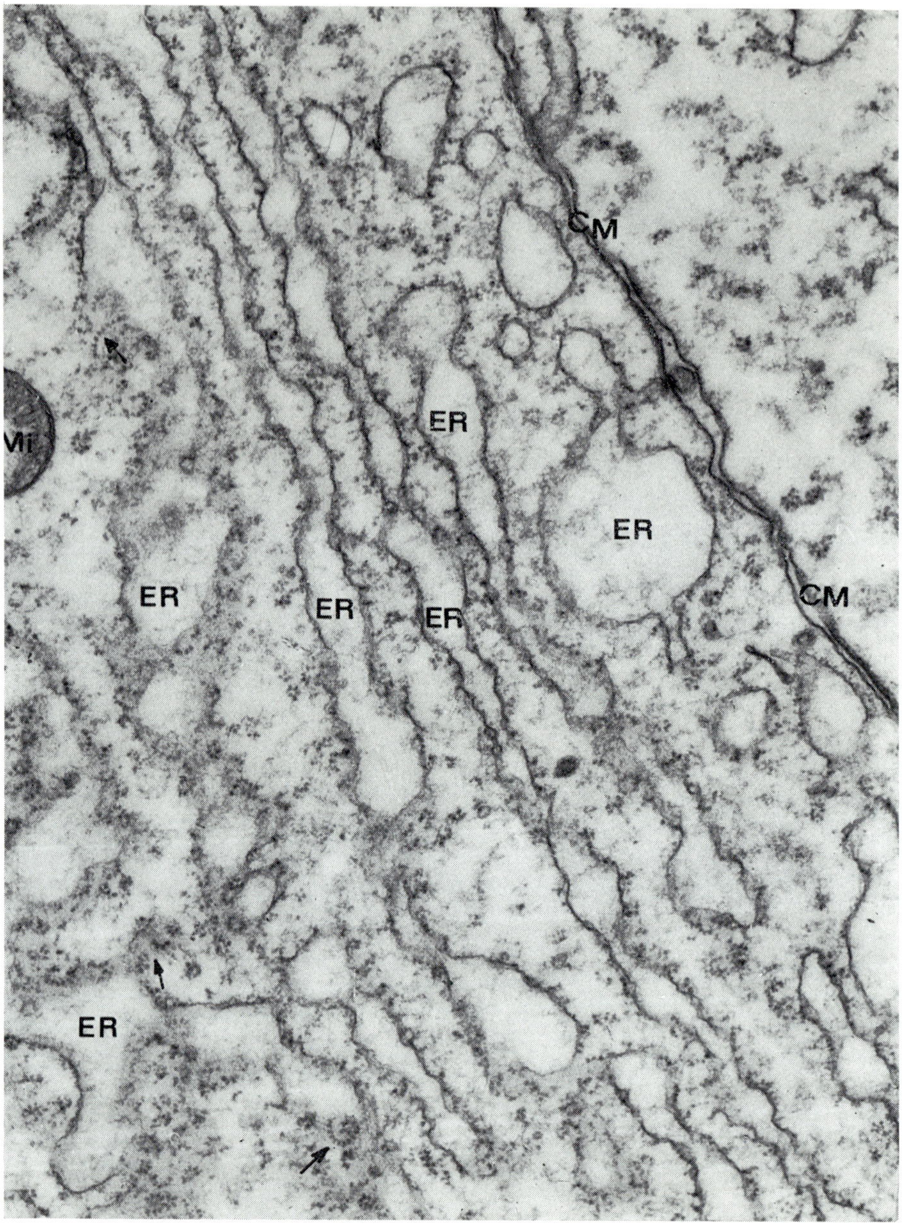

Fig. 35. Section of basal ergastoplasm in the second cytogenetic phase of the plexus development, 13-day-old embryo. CM = cell membrane; Mi = mitochondria; ER = cisterns of the basal ergastoplasm, the membrane-bound ribosomes arrange themselves on the surface of the endoplasmic membranes in the form of rosettes or circles (arrows) (45,000 ×).

Fig. 36. A and B. Different stages of the apical plexus epithelium differentiation, 13-day-old embryo. MV = microvilli; Ci = cilia; Mi = mitochondria; ER = endoplasmic reticulum; D = desmosomes; G = Golgi apparatus (33,000 ×).

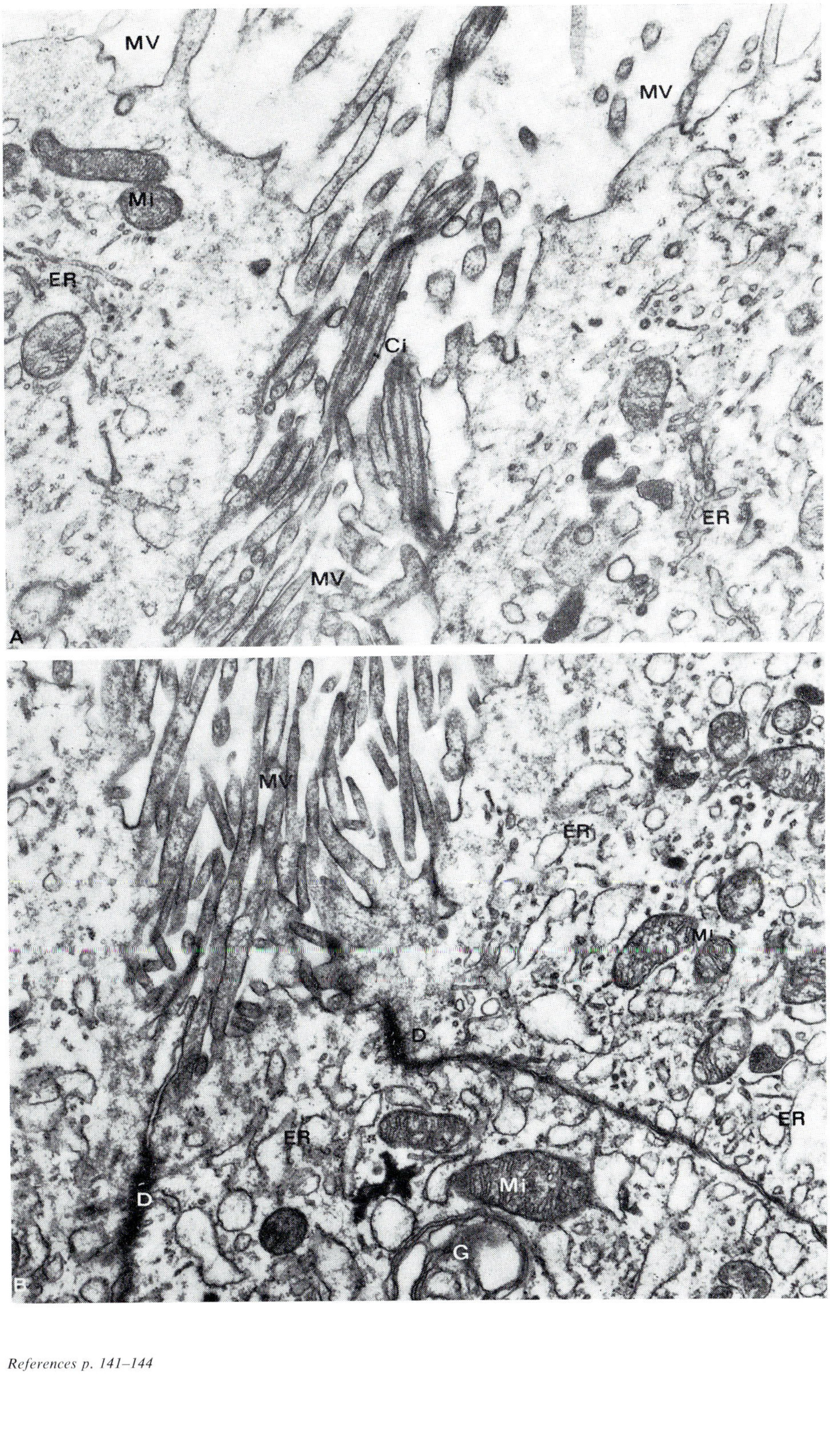
MV
MV
Mi
ER
Ci
ER
MV
A
MV
ER
Mi
D
ER
ER
D
Mi
G
B

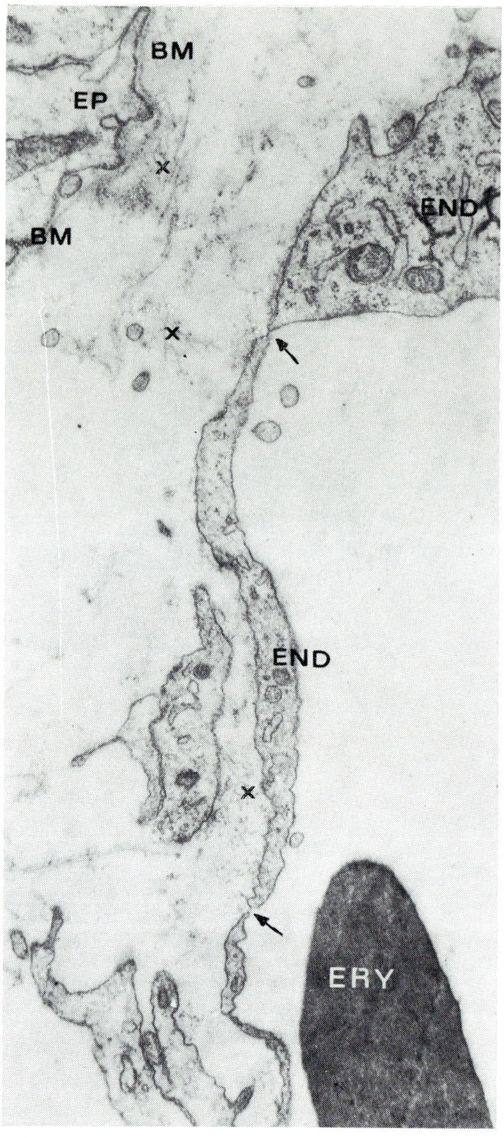

Fig. 37. Section of the plexus stroma, 13-day-old embryo. Marked degree of flattening of the capillary endothelium (END) with (arrows) pore formation; no basement membrane is visible. ERY = erythrocyte in the lumen of the vessel; BM = basement membrane of the plexus epithelium. In the interstitial ground substance no mature collagen fibrils, only some precursor material (x). EP = plexus epithelium (18,000 ×).

Fig. 38. The morphological basis of neuropil development. The decreasing neurodensity occurs due to increasing proliferation and branching of the neural and glial processes without widening of the extracellular spaces. A, Section from the striatum, 16-old-day embryo: NC = nerve cell; NBL = neuroblast;GBL = glioblast; NP = processes of the neuropil (5000 ×); B, Neuropil of the hemispheric cortex, 4-week-old chick. Increase in processes in the region of the neuropil (NP). NC = mature nerve cell (5000 ×); C, Cortex of the hemisphere, 1-day-old chick, no widening of the extracellular space. SYN = synapses (15,000 ×).

Under the electron microscope the structure of the primitive cortex is seen to be determined by individual neuroblasts and by the epithelial arrangement of the tissue

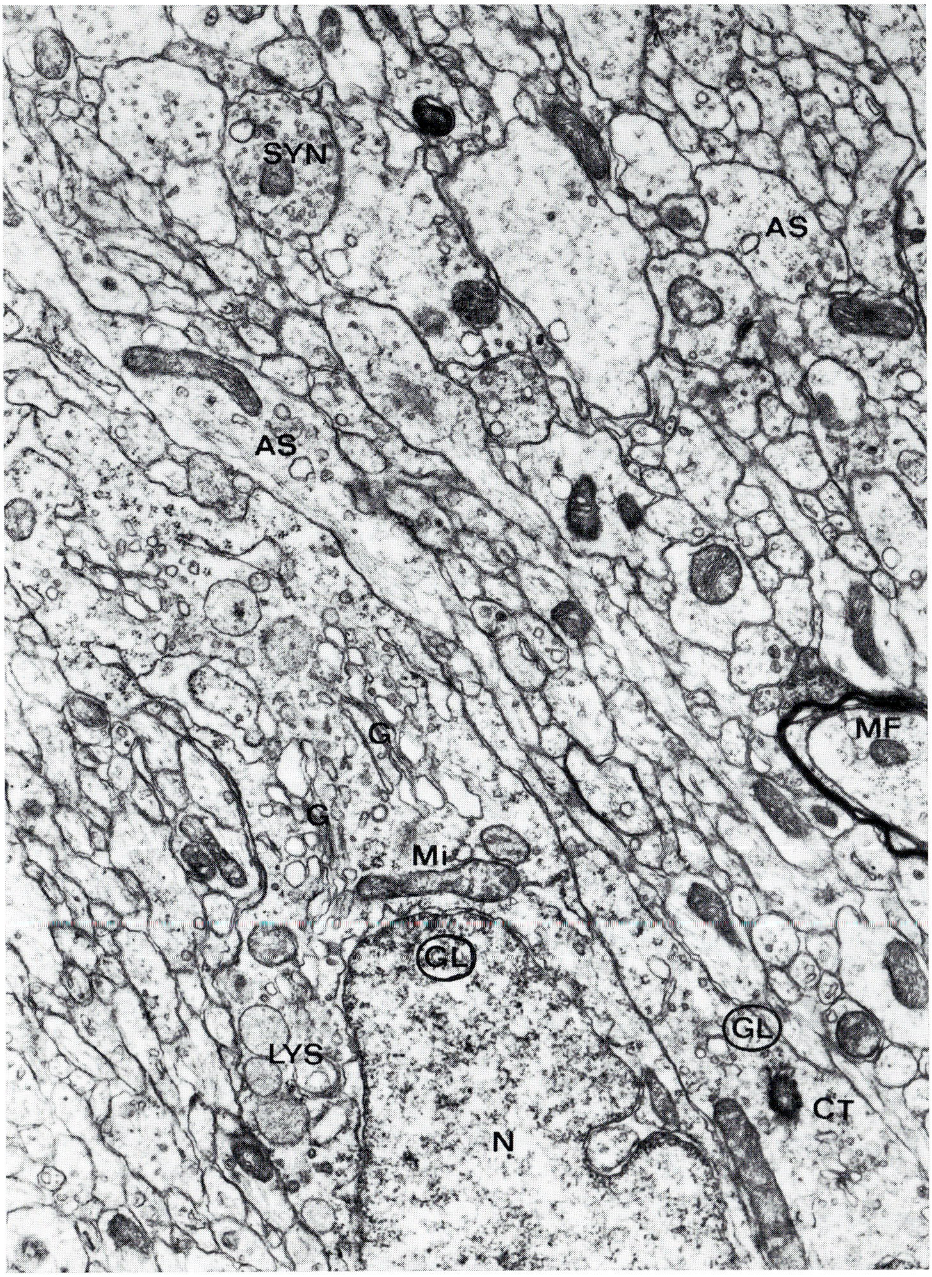

Fig. 39. Section of the molecular layer, cortex of the hemisphere, 1-day-old chick embryo. GL = glial elements of the protoplasmic type; N = nucleus; LYS = lysosomes; Mi = mitochondria; G = Golgi apparatus; CT = centriol; AS = astrocyte process; SYN = synapses; MF = small myelinated fibre (18,000 ×).

(Pappas and Purpura, 1964; Wechsler and Meller, 1963a). 'One of the chief postnatal developmental changes in feline neocortex may be viewed as a transition from appositional relationships between large elements to smaller elements of the neuropil. Cell body-to-cell body, and cell body-to-large dendrite appositions are characteristically observed in antenatal and neonatal preparations. Elaboration of fine dendritic processes from large dendrites as well as the development of small glial and axonal elements is a postnatal event. Thus the interposition of fine processes between cell bodies and cell body dendrite appositions results in the basic architectural characteristics of the adult cortical neuropil' (Pappas and Purpura, 1964).

Our own investigations show the following. The extracellular space presents no dilatation in whatever stage of development studied. In the beginning of neuropil formation, relatively thick processes of neurons are conspicuous (Fig. 14). Participation of glia is negligible and limited to the processes of polar glioblasts. In later stages of development (*e.g.* striatum, cortex of the hemispheres, tectum opticum) glial processes intermingle between neuronal processes and become more abundant. Proliferation and branching of these processes continue. Owing to this proliferation of neuronal and glial processes, nerve cells are pushed apart without any dilatation of extracellular spaces (Figs. 38 and 39). Decreasing neurodensity, therefore, does not mean an increase in ground substance such as Nissl (1903) assumed. The epithelial arrangement and the proliferation and branching of neural and glial processes are the general histogenetic principles which in turn determine the individual cytoarchitectural behaviour of various regions of the grey matter of the brain. In spite of the constant distance between adjacent cellular elements, the extracellular space increases progressively both in total volume and total surface. This increase is caused by cell proliferation together with the elaboration of a huge number of very fine terminal branches. In this way single neurons gain an extreme surface area and the increased possibility of versatile mutual contact formation.

IX. VASCULAR DEVELOPMENT

The EM findings also permit some evaluation of the problem of glial-vascular contacts, especially with respect to the development of the blood–brain barrier (Wechsler, 1965a). Attention has therefore been given to the histotopographical relations between embryonic capillaries and brain tissue, as well as to the differentiation of vessels and perivascular tissue. It has previously been shown that primitive capillaries of the CNS are not surrounded by a pericapillary free diffusion space. Capillaries in early stages of brain development do not have a continuous basement membrane. The thickening of the basement membrane is a prominent feature of maturing capillaries (Dahl, 1963; Donahue, 1964; Donahue and Pappas, 1962; Pappas and Purpura, 1964; Tani and Ishii, 1963; Wechsler, 1965a).

In all phases of brain development, embryonic blood vessels are in immediate contact with the matrix cells and with the neural and glial elements. Free perivascular spaces can be observed only after the histological differentiation of small arteries and veins, but not in the capillary bed. Fig. 40 illustrates the vessels in the matrix zones.

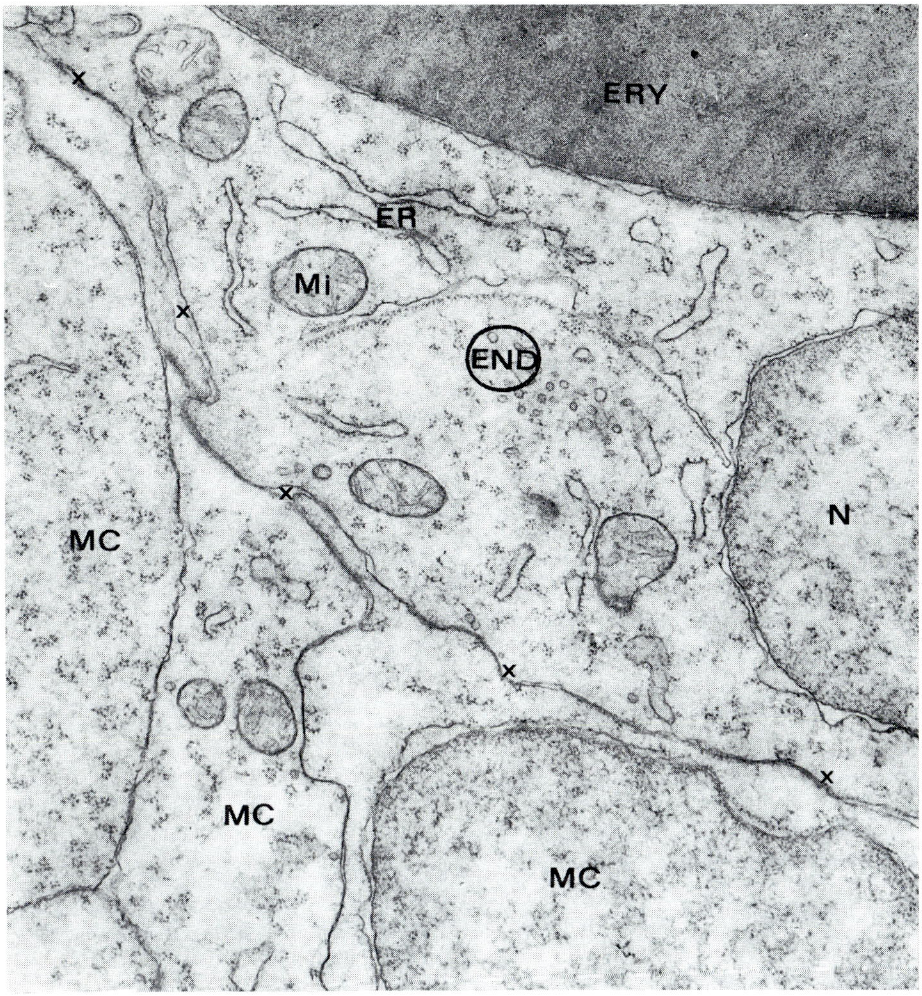

Fig. 40. Vascularization of the matrix zone, telencephalon, 7-day-old embryo. The large capillaries have no basement membrane and no widened perivascular space. ERY = erythrocyte; END = endothelium; MC = matrix cells; x = perivascular space; ER = endoplasmic reticulum; Mi = mitochondria; N = nucleus (40,000 ×).

The embryonic capillaries have a conspicuous endothelial lining and no basement membrane. It is not possible to differentiate between various types of cells in the vascular wall. The perivascular space corresponds in width to the diameter of the extracellular space. In the second phase of vascular development, immature capillaries, and small arteries and veins develop. At this stage, the formation of the basement membranes is visible. A discrete dilatation of the extracellular perivascular space parallels the formation of the basement membrane (Fig. 41). Towards the end of brain development, capillaries flatten to form a small endothelial tube while the basement membrane increases in size. This process terminates a few weeks after hatching. In view of the differentiation of perivascular spaces, which vary in different

References p. 141–144

areas of the brain, it is noteworthy that glial processes do not extend to vessels at the beginning of the vascular development. Only via a primordial sheath (Fig. 41), made of processes of astrocytes, is a complete cytoplasmic perivascular glial envelope formed (Fig. 42). From these electron microcopical observations the hypothesis is derived that already at the beginning of vascularization the brain has a different blood–tissue barrier from that in other organs. During ontogenetic development the blood–brain barrier undergoes a number of structural changes which may determine the efficiency of its function (Donahue, 1964; Pappas and Purpura, 1964; Wechsler, 1965a).

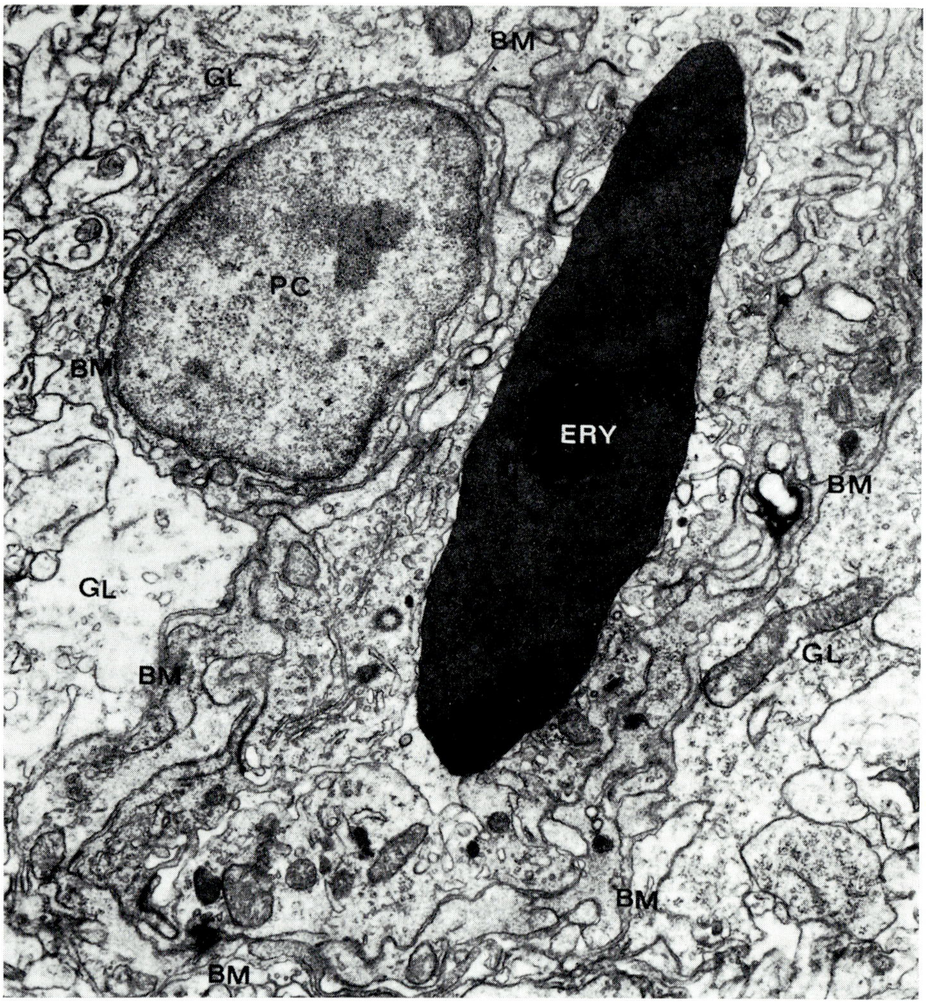

Fig. 41. Capillaries from the striatum, 16-day-old embryo. ERY = erythrocyte; PC = pericyte; GL = perivascular glial processes in various stages of differentiation; BM = basement membrane. (17,000 ×).

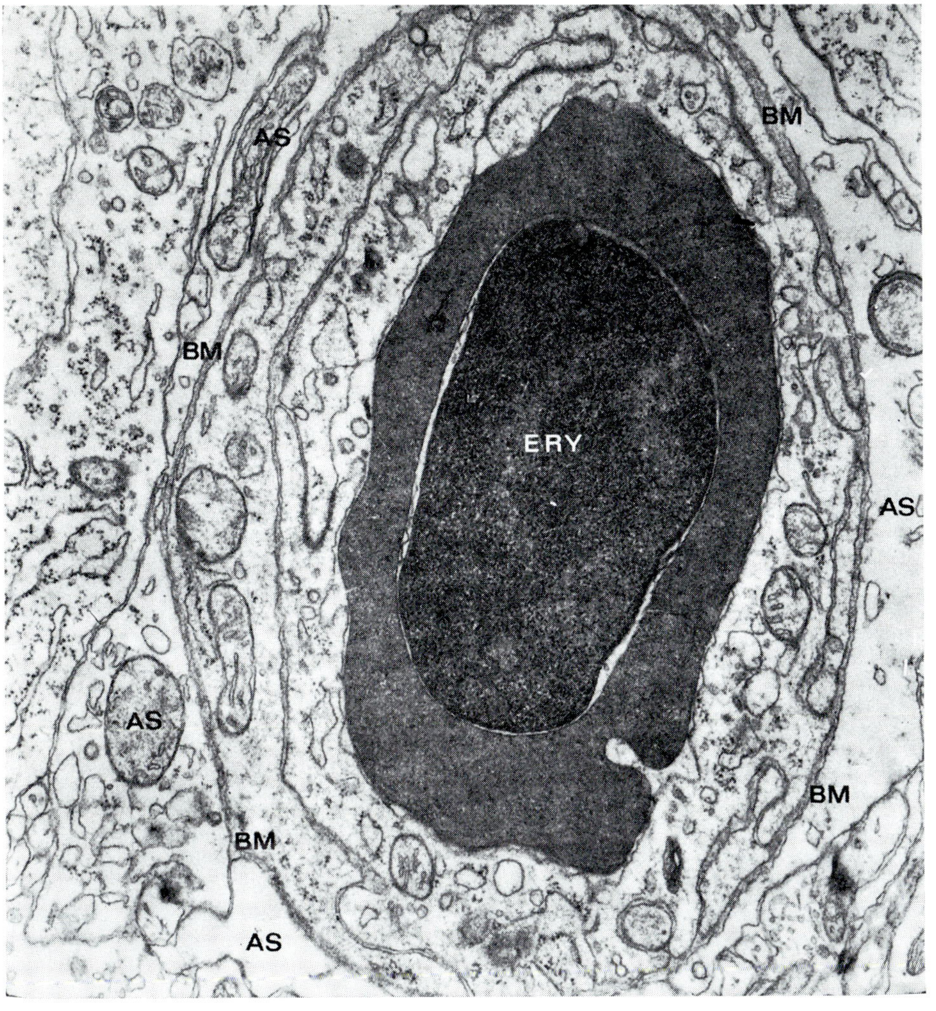

Fig. 42. Capillaries from the hemispherical cortex, 1-day-old chick. Increased thickening of the basement membrane. AS = processes of protoplasmic astrocytes; NC = perikaryon of a nerve cell; ERY = erythrocyte; BM = basement membrane (30,000 ×).

X. CONCLUSIONS

In this paragraph we would like to devote some space to the close relationship between ultrastructure and cytodifferentiation. We will, however, not discuss here the intimate relationship between cytogenesis and histogenesis, although cellular differentiation is a process governed by many factors within the framework of tissue organization and tissue differentiation.

The relationship between cytodifferentiation and ultrastructure can be traced out especially well in the CNS because the range of differentiation of the neuroectodermal matrix cells is relatively wide (see Diagram 1). These relationships are characteristic of the different phases of cellular development (Wechsler, 1966f). The pluripotential,

References p. 141–144

undifferentiated matrix cells are cells of an embryonic type and possess a primordial, bipolarity (Wechsler, 1966). In the second cytogenetic phase, the stages of primordial i.e. an unstable or early cell differentiation, it is not always possible to distinguish neuroblasts from glioblasts by means of their ultrastructure. The closest relationship between ultrastructure and differentiation exists in the third cytogenetic phase, in which the final cytological differentiation and cell maturation occur (see Fig. 3A and B).

The nucleoprotein synthesizing system, in its relationship to cell differentiation, is one of the most important points which deserves discussion (Beermann, 1963; Grobstein, 1959; Herrmann, 1960). It is thought that biochemical differentiation precedes the start of morphological differentiation. In favour of this view are the findings on transplantation of nuclei (King and Briggs, 1955). Biological specificity is achieved in embryonic cells, which possess topochemically a simple cytoplasmic structure. In contrast to the convential light microscopic image, electron micrographs reveal that the neuroectodermal matrix cells, as well as the differentiating neuro- and glioblasts, are crowded with organelles, some of which provide the machinery for cellular energetics and protein synthesis. All that these cells have to do in the course of differentiation must, therefore, be done with the same basic machinery which other embryonic cells use. Among the organelles the free ribosomes seem to be the dominant structures. They are most likely the primary cytoplasmic tools of cytological differentiation. The specific organization of endoplasmic reticulum occurs later in the course of progressive cytodifferentiation and maturation. Mitochondria, Golgi apparatus, filaments, microtubuli and numerous special surface structures of the cell membranes take part in the process of differentiation, *e.g.* Weber (1962) emphasized the significance of mitochondria, and Porter (1961) the importance of the development of the endoplasmic reticulum.

Based upon EM observations, the differentiation of neuroectodermal cells reflects 3 basic types of cytodifferentiation:

(1) cells with a *uniform* type of cytoplasmic differentiation, *viz.* astrocytes and oligodendrocytes,

(2) cells having a *bipolar* type of differentiation, *viz.* ependyma and plexus epithelium, and

(3) cells with a *hetero- or multipolar* differentiation of cytoplasmic structure, *viz.* neurons.

Although in this way electron microscopical studies contribute to our knowledge of cytodifferentiation, the problem of the mechanisms by which the genetic code anchored in the nucleus is translated into cytoplasmic structure is so far inaccessible to electron microscopical analysis. It is of particular importance that in chick embryos catecholamincontaining granules of adrenergic neurons (sympathetic ganglia) are synthesized within the pericaryon of the neuroblasts in very early stages of cellular differentiation (Wechsler und Schmekel, 1966a and b, 1967). The same principle seems to be valid for the production of neurosecretory elementary granules, according to electron microscopical and histochemical studies in the developing neurohypophysis of the chick, a study which is under investigation (Fioroni, Bock and Wechsler). These observations indicate that organels later involved in synaptic or humoral transmission mechanisms can be synthesized prior to synaptic development. In this way we have achieved new evidence for the fact, that biochemical differentiation occurs already in the phase of primordial cytodifferentiation.

ACKNOWLEDGEMENT

Wir danken Herrn Prof. Glees für die englische Übersetzung des Manuskriptes

REFERENCES

Apathy, St. von, (1897); Das leitende Element des Nervensystems und seine topographischen Beziehungen zu den Zellen. *Mitt. Zool. Stat. Neapel*, **12**, 495.

Bauer, K. F., (1953); *Organisation des Nervengewebes und Neurencytiumtheorie*. München/Berlin, Urban und Schwarzenberg.

Bauer, K. F., und Vester, G., (1965); Strukturprobleme des menschlichen Gehirns. II. Elektronenmikroskopische Beobachtungen an der foetalen Hirnrinde des Menschen. Z. *naturwiss.-med. Grundlagenforsch.*, **2**, 361–409.

Beermann, W., (1963); Cytologische Aspekte der Informationsübertragung von den Chromosomen in das Cytoplasma. *Induktion und Morphogenese*, 13. Coll. d. Ges. f. phys. Chemie, 1962, in Mosbach/Baden. Berlin, Göttingen, Heidelberg, Springer-Verlag, pp. 64–100.

Bellairs, R., (1959); The development of the nervous system in chick embryos, studied by electron microscopy. *J. Embryol. exp. Morph.*, **7**, 94–115.

Briggs, J., and King, T., (1955); Specificity of nuclear function in embryonic development. *Biological Specificity and Growth*. E. G. Butler, Editor. Princeton, Univ. Press, pp. 207–228.

Bunge, M. B., Bunge, R. P., and Pappas, G. D., (1962); Electron microscopic demonstration of connections between glia and myelin sheaths in the developing mammalian central nervous system. *J. Cell Biol.*, **12**, 448–453.

Cajal, S. Ramón y, (1929); *Etudes sur la Neurogenèse de Quelques Vertébrés*. Madrid, Instituto Ramón y Cajal.

Cajal, S. Ramón y, (1952); *Histologie du Système Nerveux de l'Homme et des Vertébrés*. Madrid, Instituto Ramón y Cajal.

Dahl, V., (1963); The ultrastructure of capillaries in cerebral tissue of human embryos. *Dan. med. Bull.*, **10**, 196–199.

De Robertis, E. D. P., (1965); Some new electron microscopical contributions to the biology of neuroglia. *Progress in Brain Research, Vol. 15, Biology of Neuroglia*, E. D. P. De Robertis and R. Carrea, Editors. Amsterdam, Elsevier, pp. 1–11.

De Robertis, E. D. P., Gerschenfeld, H. M., and Wald, F., (1958); Cellular mechanism of myelination in the central nervous system. *J. biophys. biochem. Cytol.*, **4**, 651–658.

Donahue, S., (1964); A relationship between fine structure and function of blood vessels in the central nervous system of rabbit fetuses. *Amer. J. Anat.*, **115**, 17–26.

Donahue, S., and Pappas, G. D., (1962); The fine structure of capillaries in the cerebral cortex of fetal and adult rats. *IVth Int. Congr. Neuropath., München, 1961*, Vol. 2. Stuttgart, Thieme-Verlag, pp. 77–80.

Eschner, J., and Glees, P., (1963); Free and membrane-bound ribosomes in maturing neurons of the chick and their possible functional significance. *Experientia (Basel)*, **19**, 301–303.

Fujita, S., (1963); Matrix cell and cytogenesis in the central nervous system. *J. comp. Neurol.*, **120**, 37–42.

Fujita, S., (1965); The matrix cell and histogenesis of the central nervous system. *Laval méd.*, **36**, 125–130.

Fujita, H., and Fujita, S., (1963); Electron microscopic studies on the histogenesis of the central nervous system of the domestic fowl. II. Neuroglia. *Kaibogaku Zasshi (Acta anat. Nippon)*, **38**, 107–108.

Fujita, H., and Fujita, S., (1963); Electron microscopic studies on neuroblast differentiation in the central nervous system of domestic fowl. *Z. Zellforsch.*, **60**, 463–478.

FUJITA, H., AND FUJITA, S., (1964); Electron microscopic studies on the differentiation of the ependymal cells and the glioblast in the spinal cord of domestic fowl. *Z. Zellforsch.*, **64**, 262–272.

GAZE, R. M., AND PETERS, A., (1961); The development, structure and composition of the optic nerve of *Xenopus laevis* (Dandin). *Quart. J. exp. Physiol.*, **46**, 299–309.

GLEES, P., AND MELLER, K., (1964); The finer structure of synapses and neurones. A review of recent electronmicroscopical studies. *Paraplegia*, **2**, 77–95.

GLEES, P., AND LE VAY, S., (1964); Some electron microscopical observations on the ependymal cells of the chick embryo. *J. Hirnforsch.*, **6**, 355–360.

GLEES, P., AND SHEPPARD, B. L., (1964); Electron microscopical studies of the synapse in the developing chick spinal cord. *Z. Zellforsch.*, **62**, 356–362.

GRAY, E. G., (1964); Tissue of the central nervous system. *Electron Microscopic Anatomy*, St. M. Kurtz, Editor. New York/London, Academic Press, pp. 369–427.

GRAY, E. G., AND GUILLERY, R. W., (1966); Synaptic morphology in the normal and degenerating nervous system. *Int. Rev. Cytol.*, **19**, 111–182.

GROBSTEIN, C., (1959); Differentiation of vertebrate cells. *The Cell*, Vol. 1. Jean Brachet and Alfred E. Mirsky, Editors. New York/London, Academic Press, Ch. 11, pp. 437–496.

HAGER, H., (1959); Elektronenmikroskopische Untersuchungen über die Feinstruktur der sogenannten Grundsubstanz der Gross- und Kleinhirnrinde des Säugetieres. *Arch. Psychiat.*, **198**, 574–600.

HAGER, H., (1964); Die feinere Cytologie und Cytopathologie des Nervensystems. *Veröffentl. morphol. Pathol.*, **67**.

HAMBURGER, V., AND HAMILTON, A., (1951); A series of normal stages in the development of the chick embryo. *J. Morph.*, **88**, 49–92.

HELD, H., (1909); *Die Entwicklung des Nervengewebes bei den Wirbeltieren.* Leipzig, Barth-Verlag.

HERRMANN, H., (1960); Molecular mechanism of differentiation. *Fundamental Aspects of Normal and Malignant Growth.* W. W. Nowinsky, Editor. Amsterdam, Elsevier, pp. 495–545.

HIS, W., (1889); Die Neuroblasten und deren Entstehung im embryonalen Rückenmark. *Abh. math.-phys. Klasse d. Königl. Sächs. Ges. Wissensch.*, **XV**, 331–372.

HOLTFRETER, J., AND HAMBURGER, V., (1955); Embryogenesis: progressive differentiation. I. Amphibians. *Analysis of Development.* B. H. Willier, P. Weiss and V. Hamburger, Editors. Philadelphia & London, Saunders, pp. 230–296.

HORSTMANN, E., (1957); Die Struktur der molekularen Schichten im Gehirn der Wirbeltiere. *Naturwissenschaften*, **44**, 448.

HORSTMANN, E., (1958); Über die Frage der Grundsubstanz im Zentralnervensystem. *Verh. anat. Ges. (Jena)*, **55**, 100–108.

HORSTMANN, E., AND MEVES, H., (1959); Die Feinstruktur des molekularen Rindengraus und ihre physiologische Bedeutung. *Z. Zellforsch.*, **49**, 569–589.

KÄLLÉN, B., (1962); Mitotic pattern in the central nervous system of chick embryos. *Z. Anat. Entwickl.-Gesch.*, **123**, 309–319.

KING, T. J., AND BRIGGS, R., (1955); Changes in the nuclei of differentiating gastrula cells, as demonstrated by nuclear transplantation. *Proc. nat. Acad. Sci. (Wash.)*, **41**, 321–325.

LUSE, S. A., (1956a); Electron microscopic observations of the central nervous system. *J. biophys. biochem. Cytol.*, **2**, 531–542.

LUSE, S. A., (1956b); Formation of myelin in the central nervous system of mice and rats, as studied with electron microscopy. *J. biophys. biochem. Cytol.*, **2**, 777–784.

MATURANA, H. R., (1960); The fine anatomy of the optic nerve of anurans. An electron microscope study. *J. biophys. biochem. Cytol.*, **7**, 107–119.

MELLER, K., (1964); Elektronenmikroskopische Befunde zur Differenzierung der Rezeptorzellen und Bipolarzellen der Retina und ihrer synaptischen Verbindungen. *Z. Zellforsch.*, **64**, 733–750.

MELLER, K., BREIPOHL, W., AND GLEES, P., (1966a); Early cytological differentiation in the cerebral hemisphere of mice. An electronmicroscopical study. *Z. Zellforsch.*, **72**, 525–533.

MELLER, K., ESCHNER, J., AND GLEES, P., (1966b); The differentiation of endoplasmic reticulum in developing neurons of the chick spinal cord. *Z. Zellforsch.*, **69**, 169–197.

MELLER, K., UND WECHSLER, W., (1964); Elektronenmikroskopische Befunde am Ependym des sich entwickelnden Gehirns von Hühnerembryonen. *Acta neuropathol.*, **3**, 609–626.

MELLER, K., UND WECHSLER, W., (1965); Elektronenmikroskopische Untersuchung der Entwicklung der telencephalen Plexus chorioides des Huhnes. *Z. Zellforsch.*, **65**, 420–444.

MUGNAINI, E., AND WALBERG, F., (1964); Ultrastructure of neuroglia. *Ergebn. Anat. Entwickl.-Gesch.*, **37**, 194–236.

NIESSING, K., UND VOGELL, W., (1957); Das elektronenoptische Bild der sogenannten Grundsubstanz der Hirnrinde. *Z. Naturforsch.*, **125**, 641–646.

NISSL, F., (1903); *Die Neuronenlehre und ihre Anhänger*. Jena, Gustav Fischer.

PANNESE, E., (1966); Structures possibly related to the formation of new mitochondria in spinal ganglion neuroblasts. *J. Ultrastruct. Res.*, **15**, 57–65.

PAPPAS, G. D., AND PURPURA, D. P., (1964); Electron microscopy of immature human and feline neocortex. *Progress in Brain Research*, Vol. 4, *Growth and Maturation of the Brain*. D. P. Purpura and J. P. Schadé, Editors. Amsterdam, Elsevier, pp. 176–186.

PETERS, A., (1960); The formation and structure of myelin sheaths in the central nervous system. *J. biophys. biochem. Cytol.*, **8**, 431–446.

PETERS, A., (1962); Myelination in the central nervous system. *4. Int. Kongr. Neuropathol.*, II. Stuttgart, Thieme, pp. 50–54.

PORTER, K., (1961); The ground substance; observations from electron microscope. *The Cell*, Vol. II. J. Brachet and A. Mirsky, Editors. New York, Academic Press, pp. 621–676.

RAMSEY, H., (1962); Differentiation of oligodendroglia from migratory spongioblasts. *5. Int. Congr. Electron Microsc., Philadelphia, 1962*, Vol. II, N-3. New York, Academic Press.

REISER, K. A., (1959); Die Nervenzelle. *Handbuch der mikroskopischen Anatomie des Menschen.*, Bd. IV/4. Berlin/Göttingen/Heidelberg, Springer-Verlag, pp. 185–514.

SAUER, M. E., AND WALKER, B. E., (1959); Radioautographic study of interkinetic nuclear migration in the neural tube. *Proc. Soc. exp. Biol. (N.Y.)*, **101**, 557–560.

SIDMAN, R. L., AND ANGEVINE JR., J. B., (1962); Autoradiographic analysis of time of origin of nuclear versus cortical components of mouse telencephalon. *Anat. Rec.*, **142**, 326–327.

SJÖSTRAND, F. S., (1964); The endoplasmic reticulum. *Cytology and Cell Physiology*. G. H. Bourne, Editor. New York, Academic Press, pp. 311–375.

TANI, E., AND ISHII, S., (1963); Ontogenic studies on the rat brain capillaries in relation to the human brain tumor vessels. *Acta neuropath.*, **2**, 253–270.

TENNYSON, V. M., (1962); Electron microscopic observations of the development of the neuroblast in the rabbit embryo. *5th Int. Congr. Electron Microsc, Philadelphia, 1962*, Vol. II, N-8.

TENNYSON, V. M., (1965); Electron microscopic study of the developing neuroblast of the dorsal root ganglia of the rabbit embryo. *J. comp. Neurol.*, **124**, 267–318.

TENNYSON, V. M., AND PAPPAS, G. D., (1961); Electron microscopic studies of the developing telencephalic choroid plexus in normal and hydrocephalic rabbits. *Disorders of the Developing Nervous System*. W. S. Fields and M. M. Desmond, Editors. Springfield/Ill., Thomas, pp. 267–325.

TENNYSON, V. M., AND PAPPAS, G. D., (1962); An electronmicroscopic study of ependymal cells of the fetal, early postnatal and adult rabbit. *Z. Zellforsch.*, **56**, 595–618.

TORACK, R. M., (1965); The extracellular space of rat brain following perfusion fixation with glutaraldehyde and hydroxyadipaldehyde. *Z. Zellforsch.*, **66**, 352–364.

VAN HARREVELD, A., CROWELL, J., AND MALHOTRA, S. K., (1965); A study of extracellular space in central nervous tissue by freeze-substitution. *J. Cell Biol.*, **25**, 117–137.

WATTERSON, T. L., VENEZIANO, P., AND BERTHA, A., (1956); Absence of a true germinal zone in neural tubes of young chick embryos as demonstrated by the colchicine technique. *Anat. Rec.*, **124**, 379.

WEBER, R., (1962); Electron microscopy in the study of embryonic differentiation. *The Interpretation of Ultrastructure*, Vol. I. R. J. C. Harris, Editor. New York, Academic Press, pp. 393–409.

WECHSLER, W., (1963); Elektronenmikroskopischer Beitrag zur Entwicklung und Differenzierung von Zellen am Beispiel des Nervensystems. *Verh. dtsch. Ges. Path.*, **47**, 316–322.

WECHSLER, W., (1964a); Zur Feinstruktur des peripheren Randschleiers des sich entwickelnden Rückenmarks von Hühnerembryonen. *Naturwissenschaften*, **51**, 113–114.

WECHSLER, W., (1964b); Zur Feinstruktur der Vorderhornregion des sich entwickelnden Rückenmarks von Hühnerembryonen. *Naturwissenschaften*, **51**, 114.

WECHSLER, W., (1964c); Die Differenzierung des Neurons. Elektronenmikroskopische Untersuchungen bei Hühnerembryonen. *Electron Microscopy*. 3rd Eur. Reg. Conf. Electr. Micr. Prague, Publ. House Czechoslovak Acad. Sci., pp. 279–280.

WECHSLER, W., (1965a); Die Entwicklung der Gefässe und perivaskulären Gewebsräume im Zentralnervensystem von Hühnern. Elektronenmikroskopischer Beitrag zur Kenntnis der morphologischen Grundlagen der Bluthirnschranke während der Ontogenese. *Z. Anat. Entwickl.-Gesch.*, **124**, 367–395.

WECHSLER, W., (1965b); Elektronenmikroskopische Untersuchungen der Entwicklung von Nervenzellen und Nervenfasern bei Hühnerembryonen. Verh. anat. Ges., 60. Sitz., Ergänzungsheft. *Anat. Anz.*, **115**, 287–302.

WECHSLER, W., (1966a); Die Feinstruktur des Neuralrohres und der neuroektodermalen Matrixzellen am Zentralnervensystem von Hühnerembryonen. *Z. Zellforsch.*, **70**, 240–268.

WECHSLER, W., (1966b); Zur Entwicklung der Liquorräume des Gehirns von *Gallus domesticus. Wiener Z. Nervenheilk.*, Suppl. **1**, 49–69.

WECHSLER, W., (1966c); Elektronenmikroskopischer Beitrag zur Nervenzelldifferenzierung und Histogenese der grauen Substanz des Rückenmarks von Hühnerembryonen. *Z. Zellforsch.*, **74**, 401–422.

WECHSLER, W., (1966d); Elektronenmikroskopischer Beitrag zur Histogenese der weissen Substanz des Rückenmarks von Hühnerembryonen. *Z. Zellforsch.*, **74**, 232–251.

WECHSLER, W., (1966e); Elektronenmikroskopischer Beitrag zur Differenzierung des Ependyms am Rückenmark von Hühnerembryonen. *Z. Zellforsch.*, **74**, 423–442.

WECHSLER, W., (1966f); Electron microscopy of the cytodifferentiation in the developing brain of chick embryo. *Evolution of the Forebrain.* R. Hassler and H. Stephan (Eds.), Stuttgart, Thieme-Verlag, pp. 213–224.

WECHSLER, W., UND MELLER, K., (1963a); Zur Feinstruktur des primären Cortex von Hühnerembryonen. *Naturwissenschaften*, **50**, 694–695.

WECHSLER, W., UND MELLER, K., (1963b); Zur Feinstruktur der Schwärmzone des Telencephalons von Hühnerembryonen. *Naturwissenschaften*, **50**, 714–715.

WECHSLER, W., UND SCHMEKEL, L., (1966a); Elektronenmikroskopischer Nachweis spezifischer Grana in den Sympathicoblasten der Grenzstrangganglien von Hühnerembryonen. *Experientia*, **22**, 296.

WECHSLER, W., UND SCHMEKEL, L., (1966b); Elektronenmikroskopischer Nachweis spezifischer Grana in den Sympathicoblasten des Grenzstranges von Enten- und Gänseembryonen. *Naturwissenschaften*, **53**, 409.

WECHSLER, W., UND SCHMEKEL, L., (1967); Elektronenmikroskopische Untersuchung der vegetativen (Grenzstrang) und spinalen Ganglien bei *Gallus domesticus. Acta neurovegetativa*, in press.

WEISS, P., (1955); Special vertebrate organogenesis. Nervous system (neurogenesis). *Analysis of Development.* B. J. Willier, P. A. Weiss, V. Hamburger, Editors. Philadelphia, Saunders, pp. 346–401.

WOHLFARTH-BOTTERMANN, K. E., (1957); Die Kontrastierung tierischer Zellen und Gewebe im Rahmen ihrer elektronenmikroskopischen Untersuchung an ultradünnen Schnitten. *Naturwissenschaften*, **44**, 287–288.

Developmental Patterns in the Central Nervous System of Birds

I. Electrical Activity in the Cerebral Hemisphere, Optic Lobe and Cerebellum*

M. A. CORNER, J. P. SCHADÉ, J. SEDLÁČEK, R. STOECKART AND A. P. C. BOT

Central Institute for Brain Research, Amsterdam (The Netherlands)

The chick embryo has been one of the most extensively used preparations for the study of neurogenesis. Descriptive cytological studies were already made early in this century (Ramon y Cajal, 1960) and have been carried on in recent years as well, especially with regard to cell migration and degeneration patterns (Jones and Levi-Montalcini, 1958; Levi-Montalcini, 1964). Other studies have shown histochemical aspects of neural development (Hughes, 1955; Mottet and Barron, 1954; Rogers, 1960). Experimental studies have also been carried out, demonstrating early determination of regional developmental patterns in the neural epithelium (Hara, 1961; Stefanelli, 1954) and some of the factors required for subsequent normal maturation (Hamburger, 1956, 1958; Levi-Montalcini, 1958; Peterson and Murray, 1955). The changing properties of nerve cells during maturation have been studied with respect to their response to injury (LaVelle, 1964). Still other research has demonstrated the specific affinities of growing nerve fibers, a property of great importance in the establishment of the normal pattern of innervations (Hamburger, 1961; Castro, 1963; Székely and Szentágothai, 1962; DeLong and Coulombre, 1965). Although extensive work has also been done in mammals and amphibians in certain of the areas of investigation mentioned, avian material has provided in many respects the deepest insight so far obtained into the general features of neurogenesis.

Descriptive study of the developing nervous system is again an active field, now using modern techniques of high resolution, and the chick embryo has been a frequently used material in recent ultrastructural, biochemical and electrophysiological investigations. A multi-disciplinary program has been started in this laboratory in order to establish correlations between the structural organization, functional activity and biochemical properties of the normal developing brain. We have also been interested in the relationship of these factors to behavior development. Experimental alteration of brain development then promises to be an important method for finding

* This research was supported in part by grants from the National Institute of Neurological Diseases and Blindness (NB 3048) and from the National Institute of Mental Health (MH 6825). Public Health Service, Bethesda, U.S.A.

References p. 189–192

causal relations among the various parameters which describe the central nervous system. A beginning has been made in this direction in our research program and additional techniques for analytic study of neurogenesis are planned.

A knowledge of the features of normal development is thus essential also for the interpretation of alterations brought about in brain activity by experimental interventions. A certain amount of fundamental information is now available and it is worthwhile to summarize at this time the known facts about normal central nervous development in birds (almost exclusively the chick). This will be done here in three articles: (1) electrophysiological parameters, (2) biochemical characteristics and (3) behavioral manifestations of nervous activity. Histological studies are not at the point where a review is useful, and ultra-structural changes in development are described elsewhere in this volume. A final article (4) will then, insofar as possible, interpret in terms of cellular activities the observations which have been described. This will draw both on the small amount of analytic data available for chick and on analogous mammalian observations, for which the possibilities of interpretation are much greater.

MATERIAL AND METHODS

Studies of embryos were made either in an incubator for premature infants or simply in a Faraday cage warmed by an infra-red lamp and kept humid with large dishes of water. The relative humidity was ca. 60% in the latter case and almost 80% in the former, without any noticeable differences in recorded brain activity or in motility and heartbeat. The temperature was kept between 36°–40°C, again with no difference in results seen over this range. (For precise measurement of neurophysiological constants, however, the possible significance of environmental fluctuations of this magnitude would still need to be considered.) It is of critical importance in embryos to have the head oriented so that it lies almost on a horizontal plane with the heart. Lifting the head vertically out of the shell produces signs of severe hypoxia within minutes, including the rapid loss of electrical activity from the brain. The head was immobilized by means of either moistened cotton or plaster in embryos and by a specially designed collar in post-hatching chicks.

White Leghorn embryos were incubated in a commercial chick brooder at a temperature of 38°C and humidity close to 80%. The stages were determined by measurement of the third toe according to the criteria of Hamburger and Hamilton (1951). This is extremely important since very consistent results were obtained in all parameters of functional development studied if embryos of the same stage were compared. This was not the case for chronological age even in a given brood of eggs. Moreover, the distribution of stages on successive days of incubation fluctuated slightly from one brood to another. Most *post*-hatching studies were made on male White Rock chicks obtained from a commercial hatchery at about one day of age. A few experiments involving direct brain stimulation were done with White Leghorn chicks hatched and raised in the laboratory. Post-hatching chicks were kept in a run, with a warming lamp placed so as to allow them to regulate their own body temperature.

Electrical recording of 'spontaneous' waves and evoked potentials were made in many experiments with insulated stainless steel wires (100μ diameter) inserted through small holes in the skull. In other cases the skull was partially removed and silver wires (100μ diameter) or balls up to 1 mm in diameter, chloridized at the tip, were placed on the pial surface. These variations in recording technique did not produce significant amplitude nor frequency differences among preparations of a given stage of development. Both monopolar and bipolar recordings were obtained. In addition, an electrode was placed on the skull for the purpose of monitoring both the small, almost continual movement artifacts which are prominent at the high gain used in early stages and any larger movements of the head. An electrode on the trunk registered the body movements, including respiration, and the electrocardiogram (ECG). The most satisfactory (*i.e.* isoelectric) indifferent electrode proved to be a steel plug embedded in a plaster block, in electrical contact with the embryo via a dilute salt solution. Electrode fidelity was tested prior to the experiment by recording in Ringer's solution, and afterwards by recording from the brain after death of the preparation. Slow waves lasting one second or longer were sometimes seen at some leads. They were synchronous in all parts of the brain and nearby tissues but varied greatly in amplitude from one electrode to another. Since the differences corresponded to the sensitivities of the various electrodes to movements of Ringer's solution bathing them and were electrode- rather than position-specific, these waves were assumed to reflect ionic shifts within the embryo to which well-chloridized silver wires do not react. They typically increase in amplitude after bleeding or injection of many chemical compounds but will not be further considered here. It was also found essential, especially in younger embryos, to frequently remove excess moisture from the brain surface by means of filter papers in order to avoid deceptive electrolytic artifacts (*e.g.* Sharma *et al.*, 1964). Specially constructed cables were employed in some experiments in order to record brain activity during periods of motility (Kamp *et al.*, 1965). Tektronix type 122 pre-amplifiers were used to amplify evoked potentials before displaying them on an oscilloscope (Tektronix type 502A or 565). Electroencephalograms (EEG's) were registered either with a Schwarzer electroencephalograph or with a conventional ink-writer system (Elther).

For stimulation of the brain surface in order to record the direct-evoked responses, it was found necessary to remove part of the skull and dura and to keep the exposed (stimulated) area dry. The distance between the two stimulating electrodes had to be of the order of 1 mm or more in order to evoke a detectable response and symmetrical placement of recording electrodes was essential for satisfactory reduction of the stimulus artifact. Square wave shocks were generated by a Grass model S4 stimulator. Long cathodal or anodal currents were applied from a dry cell via one of the stimulating electrodes, with the other located either a few millimeters distant or on the body surface so as to have a minimum of brain tissue lying between the poles. The sensory stimuli which have been used are: brief flashes (Philips type PR 9104 stroboscope) or sustained illumination, hand claps, and stroking various regions of the skin. Drugs were injected intra-peritoneally and stagnant anoxia was produced by severing one of the large extra-embryonic blood vessels.

References p. 189–192

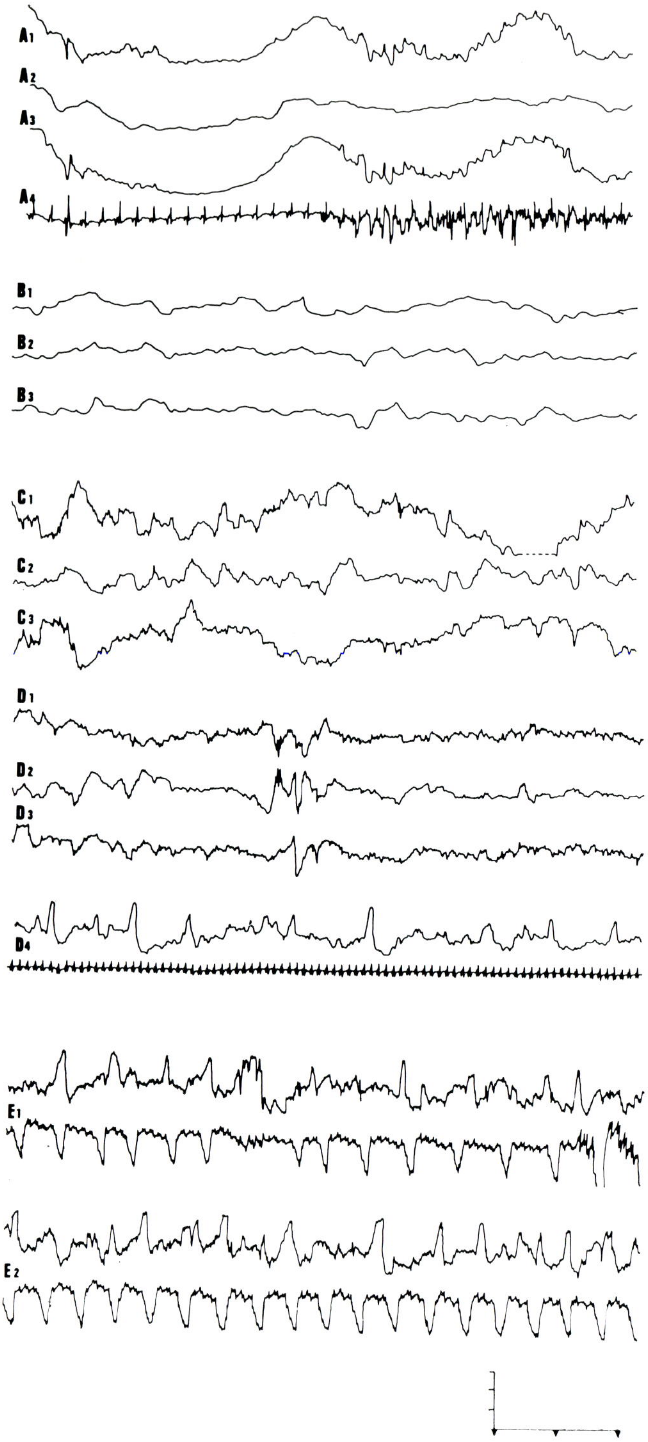
A1
A2
A3
A4
B1
B2
B3
C1
C2
C3
D1
D2
D3
D4
E1
E2

Measurements were made manually from EEG records which showed minimal or no slow fluctuations of the baseline. The isoelectric line was taken as the basis for determining wave durations and amplitudes. A 'summated amplitude' was determined for consecutive two second periods at several points in time throughout the recording. This was done by counting the number of intersections of a finely-ruled graph paper which fell between the isoelectric line and the electrical tracing. Unless otherwise indicated, an upwards deflection is *positive* in the EEG and ECG records and *negative* in the oscilloscope records.

A. Early development of spontaneous electrical activity

No activity has been recorded from either the cerebral hemisphere or the optic lobe in our experience prior to *stage 41* (the 15th day of incubation in most cases; Fig. 1A). Four of the nine youngest *stage-41* embryos studied (3rd toe length 14–15 mm) showed intermittent waves in the cerebral hemisphere. Despite slight quantitative difference from one preparation to another the general features are the same. Single waves of either polarity, and trains of waves lasting up to ca. 10 sec occur at variable intervals (Fig. 1). Their *duration* ranges from ca. 100–600 msec, which values occur in an irregular sequence. The silent *intervals* between waves may be less than one second or more than ten, with no apparent regularity in the timing of their occurrence. The *amplitude* of the waves is variable and usually not greater than 10 μV, but in one case reached 30 μV on the caudal surface of the hemisphere and 20 at the frontal pole. This description agrees fully with that of Peters *et al.* (1956) on the development of cerebral electrical activity in the chick embryo. Other reports (Garcia-Austt, 1954; Peters *et al.*, 1960; Katori, 1962) have placed the first cerebral activity as early as the 13th day of incubation, which in fact is when the first individuals attain *stage 41* of development. The descriptions given for the waves at this stage agree with the present findings.

Activity in the optic lobes and cerebellum is first recorded later than in the cerebral hemispheres (Peters *et al.*, 1960). It consists of sporadic low amplitude waves (up to 10 μV) having a frequency of 10–15 c/sec and riding upon irregular slower waves.

Fig. 1. Normal spontaneous electrical activity in the cerebral hemispheres of the chick embryo.
A. Late *stage 40*, simultaneous recordings: 1, left hemisphere; 2, bilateral differential recording; 3, right hemisphere; 4, trunk lead monitoring the movement artifacts.
B. Late *stage 41*, simultaneous monopolar recordings made during a stretch free of movements: 1, left hemisphere frontal; 2, right frontal; 3, right occipital.
C. *Stage 42*, simultaneous records in a movement-free stretch: 1, left hemisphere; 2, bilateral differential record; 3, right hemisphere.
D. Early *stage 43*, *idem* (note lower gain): 1, left hemisphere; 2, differential; 3, right hemisphere; 4, monopolar recording from a different embryo, showing the 'late rhythm' more clearly (ECG underneath).
E. *Stage 44*, monopolar stretches taken from a single embryo at an interval of several minutes (E_1 and E_2), showing a difference in the frequency of high amplitude waves; the trunk lead underlying each of the EEG curves registers respiratory movements, which apparently stop during somatic motility. *Calibrations*: horizontal, 1 sec per division except in D_4 and in E, where one division is 2 sec; vertical, 20 μV per division in A–C and 50 μV per division in D and E.

References p. 199–192

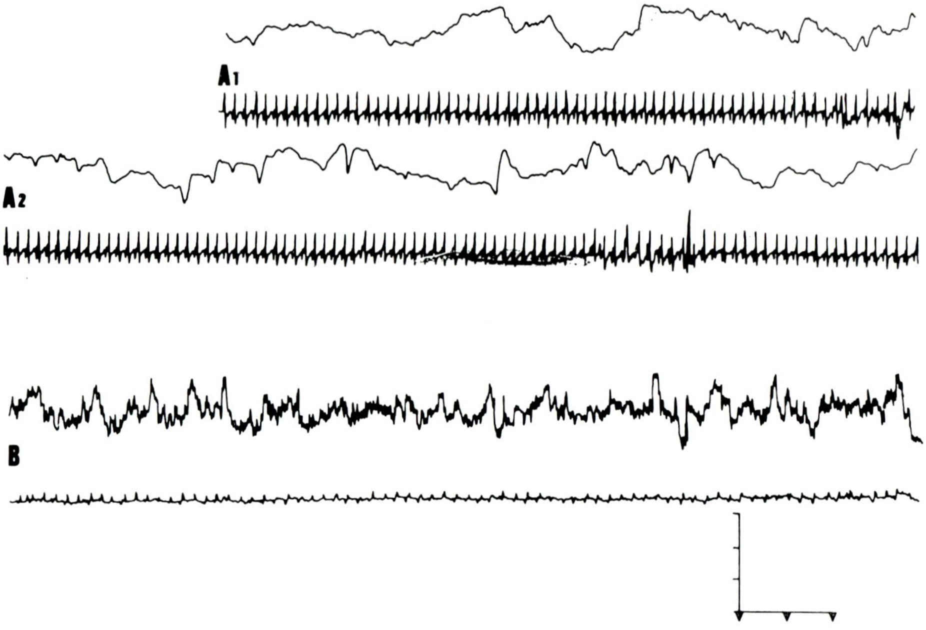

Fig. 2. Normal spontaneous electrical activity in the optic lobe of the chick embryo.
A. *Stage 42*, continuous recording (1 and 2); *upper* trace, monopolar EEG; *bottom*, ECG and body movements.
B. *stage 44*, *idem*.
Calibrations: horizontal, 1 sec per division; vertical, 20 μV per division.

Katori (1962) described similar waves in the optic lobes already on the 12th day of incubation, so that the onset of this event is not yet definitively established. Our own results for the optic lobe are in agreement with Peters, the first electric activity having

---

Fig. 3. Spatial organization of electrical activity in the embryonic chick cerebrum.
A. The cerebral EEG at early *stage 43*: 1, at a point 2 mm from the midline on the dorsal surface; 2, simultaneously at five mm from the midline; 3, trunk lead (ECG).
B. The cerebral EEG at *stage 45*: to show the typical higher amplitude waves in the lateral-most area of the dorsal surface (line 5). (The composite map below indicates all the points (black circles) at which this pattern has been encountered in *stage45* embryos; the points at which it has been found to be absent are indicated by open circles, while two points which were seen to vary from time to time are represented by half-filled circles. Lines 1–3 demonstrate both the typical *medial* pattern and the varying localization of slow waves. Lines 4, 6 show the unusually low amplitude activity which is sometimes seen at different locations in different preparations. (The numbers adjacent to the dashed lines give the distances in millimeters while those enclosed by circles refer to the electrical tracings, all recorded simultaneously.)
C. Several stretches of the cerebral record of a *stage44* preparation, showing the tendency for the occasional bilaterally synchronous waves (arrows) to be located in corresponding areas. (The last stretch also illustrates a more typical regional localization).
D. Simultaneous records from the cerebrum of a *stage45* embryo, showing the variability in the relative amplitudes of slow waves at different points and the overlapping of the spatial projections of given waves (point 3 is 1.5 mm from both 2 and 1).
Calibrations: horizontal, 1 sec per division; vertical 50 μV per division.

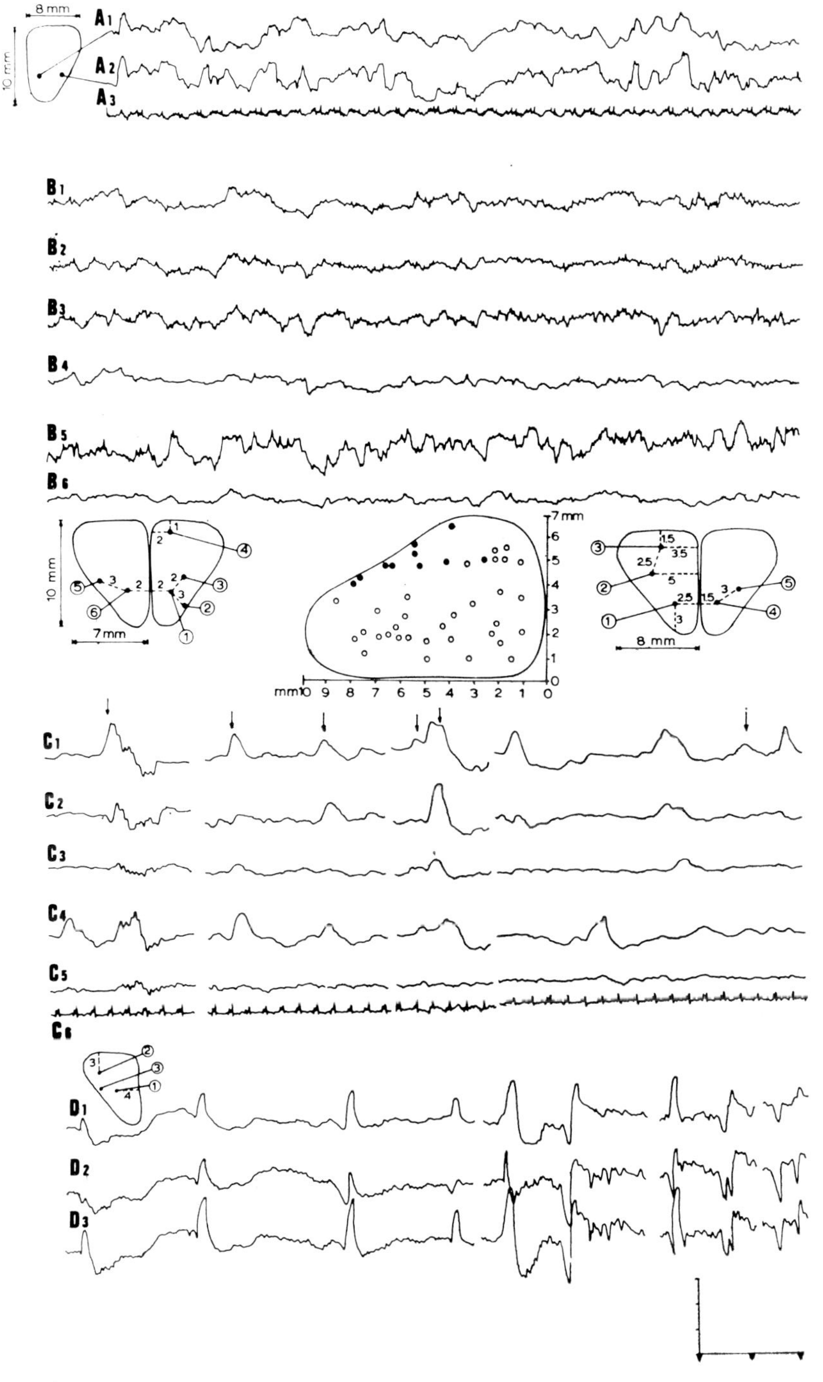
8 mm
10 mm
A1
A2
A3
B1
B2
B3
B4
B5
B6
10 mm
7 mm
7 mm
mm
8 mm
C1
C2
C3
C4
C5
C6
D1
D2
D3

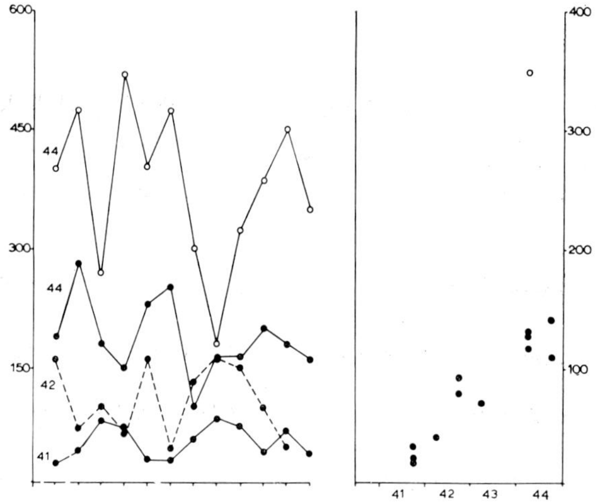

Fig. 4. *Left*, the amplitude of the cerebral EEG (in arbitrary units on the ordinate) summated over consecutive two second periods in individual embryos. Each curve is at the same time representative of the stage of development indicated by the number at the left. The uppermost curve (open circles) is taken ca. five minutes later from the same *stage-44* preparation, to show the periodic changes in amplitude.
Right, the *mean* summated amplitude (per two second stretch of EEG) as a function of development between *stages 41* and *44* (abscissa). Each point is for a different preparation except for the *open* circle, which is the mean value for one of the *stage-44* embryos during the maximum amplitude portion of its cycle. The other points for *stage 44* were all obtained during the periods of relatively low amplitude. (Increased discontinuity in the trains of slow waves causes the summated amplitude to *decline* in *stage 45*, which is not included in the graph.)

been recorded in *stage-42* embryos (Fig. 2A), but are based upon only a few cases The slow wave component is up to 30 μV in amplitude and contains waves of both polarities ranging from 100–800 msec in duration. These occur singly or in short trains at widely varying intervals.

Cerebral electrical activity in all *late stage-41* embryos (5 cases, 3rd toe 15–16 mm in length) contains in addition to slow waves an almost continuous low amplitude component having a frequency of 10–15 c/sec (Fig. 1B). In some of these embryos the slow waves (ca. 150–800 msec duration and up to 20 μV amplitude) are continuously present in an irregular sequence. In the others however, periods occur intermittently which are devoid of slow waves for as long as 3 sec. This description agrees with that given by earlier workers for the activity at about 15 days of incubation (Garcia-Austt, 1954; Peters *et al.*, 1960), and which has been called by them the 'fundamental pattern' or 'early rhythm'. Monopolar recording from several points has revealed no difference in any preparation in the type of electrical activity at different points on the surface of the hemisphere. Many waves, especially the larger ones, are synchronous over much of the hemisphere but this is not a general rule (Fig. 1B). Bilateral synchronization of waves has not been observed. The summated amplitude of the EEG fluctuates irregularly in consecutive short periods (Fig. 4) but its *mean* value varies little from one time to another or from one embryo to the next (Fig. 4).

Embryos in *early stage 42* (5 cases, 3rd toe 16–17 mm in length) show a cerebral electric pattern similar to late *stage 41* but with a slightly greater amplitude and fewer stretches devoid of slow waves. The slow waves range in duration from ca. 100 to 600 msec, with approximately a normal distribution. These values occur in an apparently random succession and are not correlated with the amplitude of the waves, which reaches a maximum ranging from 25 to 40 μV in different preparations (Fig. 1C). Successive waves may be any size relative to one another and are often of the same polarity. The fast component is in all cases steady at ca. 10 c/sec although here too the successive wave-lengths fluctuate considerably. The amplitude of this rhythm also varies but never exceeds 10 μV.

By *late stage 42* and *early stage 43* (8 cases) the overall amplitude has increased in the cerebral hemispheres and some waves now reach 70 or 80 μV, according to the preparation (Fig. 1D). The summated amplitude is comparable in all preparations (Fig. 4) and is still essentially invariant in time. The largest waves are invariably surface positive and are sometimes followed by an unusually long negative wave. In a few cases moreover, the overall amplitude/wave distribution is clearly bimodal (Fig. 5). There has thus been a second system added to the EEG at this stage, having a similar duration range to that of the earlier slow waves (ca. 100–700 msec) but with a greater amplitude. This system of waves too has a largely random character as far as the *timing* of each wave is concerned and in the *sequence* of amplitudes and of durations (Fig. 5). Garcia-Austt (1954) distinguished a 'late rhythm' appearing at

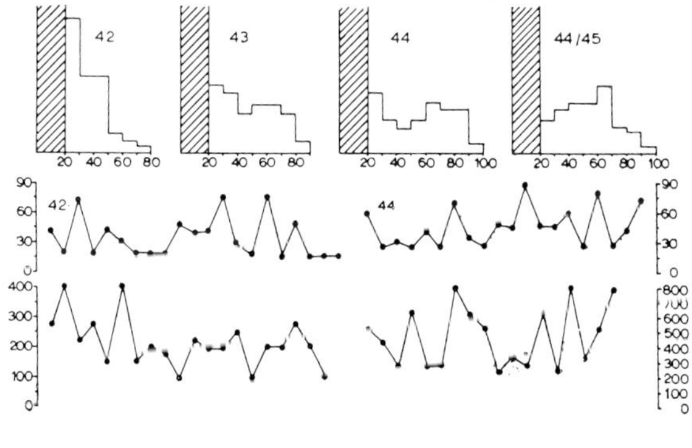

Fig. 5. *Top*, the distribution of cerebral waves according to amplitude (in microvolts on the abscissa), from single embryos at developmental *stages 42–44/45*. The ordinate gives the percentage of the total number of waves counted–which is at least 50 consecutive waves of 20 μV or larger. The plots for the two oldest embryos are from a maximum amplitude phase in order to demonstrate the development of the bimodal distribution. (During the phase of *minimal* slow wave activity the second peak is strongly reduced, causing the distribution to resemble that typical for *stage 42* or *43*.)
Middle, plots at two different stages of the amplitudes of consecutive waves equal or greater than 20 μV.
Bottom, *idem* for the duration (in msec) of consecutive waves equal or greater than 20 μV. (The absolute range and distribution of points will vary from one preparation to another but the illustrated *sequential irregularity* is always found.)

References p. 189–192

this stage but included *all* waves larger than 20 μV. We prefer to restrict the definition, however, to the predominantly surface positive, high amplitude waves which cause the bimodal distribution. The amplitude of all components of the EEG is consistently larger in the most lateral zones but otherwise the activity is similar at all points on the dorsal surface of the hemisphere (Fig. 3A). Many waves are synchronous over a wide area but with no consistent distribution, and a few of the largest waves appear simultaneously in both hemispheres. The low amplitude fast rhythm still has an essentially constant frequency in any given preparation and has increased to ca. 15 c/sec in some embryos.

The *cerebral EEG* is greatly increased in amplitude at *stage 44* over the preceding stage and contains waves of up to 150 μV in some preparations (Fig. 1E; also Sedláček, 1964). The largest waves are, as in the preceding stage, all surface positive and they are often followed by a longer negative potential of a magnitude and duration rarely seen otherwise. Changes now take place over a period of several minutes in the number of large waves and thus in the value of the *mean summated amplitude* (Fig. 4). In many cases the rapid low amplitude component of the EEG is still at ca. 10 c/sec but in other embryos it is consistently faster, up to 20 c/sec. In one preparation abrupt slowing from 10–14 c/sec to 6–8 occurred briefly at long intervals, together with a considerable increase of amplitude (Fig. 9A). The normal cerebral activity is otherwise little changed from *stage 43*. The *optic lobes* now show a continual but irregular succession of brief potentials of both polarities the amplitude of which varies up to 10 μV (Fig. 2B). Their maximum duration is about 30 msec and the frequency of their occurrence fluctuates between 15–20 c/sec. Irregular low voltage slower oscillations are also present, similar to those seen at earlier stages. The *cerebellar activity* is comparable to that of the optic lobe but lacks the fast 'spikes' (Peters *et al.*, 1960).

The activity pattern of the cerebrum at *stages 44* and *45* is basically similar at all points tested. More frequent large waves and a higher amplitude of all components of the EEG are consistently found, however, in the lateral-most areas of the hemisphere surface (Fig. 3B). Despite this distinctiveness, the lateral area frequently exhibits waves synchronous with those in more medial areas but no consistent spatial projection could be demonstrated. A point equidistant from two ipsilateral recording sites often shows a greater degree of synchronization with one than with the other, but the areas so 'linked' together differ from one preparation to the next. Bilaterally synchronous waves are seen only at infrequent intervals and tend to be regionally specific (Fig. 3C). The area covered by a given wave may be so restricted as not to be detected even 1 mm away or, on the other hand, may appear simultaneously over most of the dorsal surface. This spatial variation is not obviously correlated with the amplitude of the waves and there is a great fluctuation in the relative amplitude at any two points. The waveform often differs at different points, with topographically intermediate regions usually having an intermediate shape of potential (Fig. 3D). Depth recordings have not been made in the embryo, but in the 5 day old chick the patterns of electrical activity have been found to be similar throughout most of the cerebral hemisphere (Spooner, 1964). The ventromedial region (paleostriatum), however, shows a paucity of high amplitude waves while the ventrolateral region (ectostriatum) generates waves of greater amplitude and shorter duration, and at a higher frequency, than those anywhere else in the hemisphere. Relatively weak activity is occasionally seen at some points throughout the recording (Fig. 3B) but the location varies in different embryos. This applies equally to post-natal chicks and to full-grown chickens (Spooner, 1964; Ookawa and Gotoh, 1965).

B. Final Maturation of the Spontaneous Electrical Activity

Although the cerebral slow waves have already attained by embryonic *stage 44*

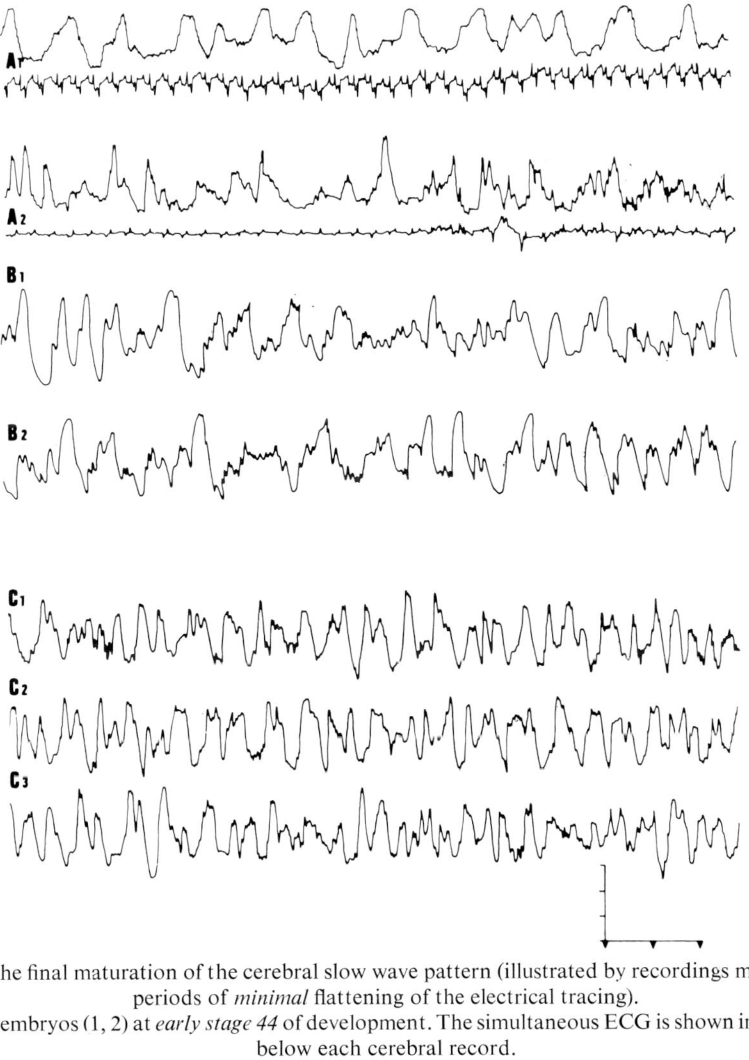

Fig. 6. The final maturation of the cerebral slow wave pattern (illustrated by recordings made during periods of *minimal* flattening of the electrical tracing).

A. Two embryos (1, 2) at *early stage 44* of development. The simultaneous ECG is shown immediately below each cerebral record.

B. A *late stage-45* embryo, showing intermittent brief periods of increased regularity of the slow rhythm (continuous monopolar recording: 1–2).

C. Characteristic cerebral activity of the *post-hatching* chick during behavioral deep sleep (continuous record: 1–3).

References p. 189–192

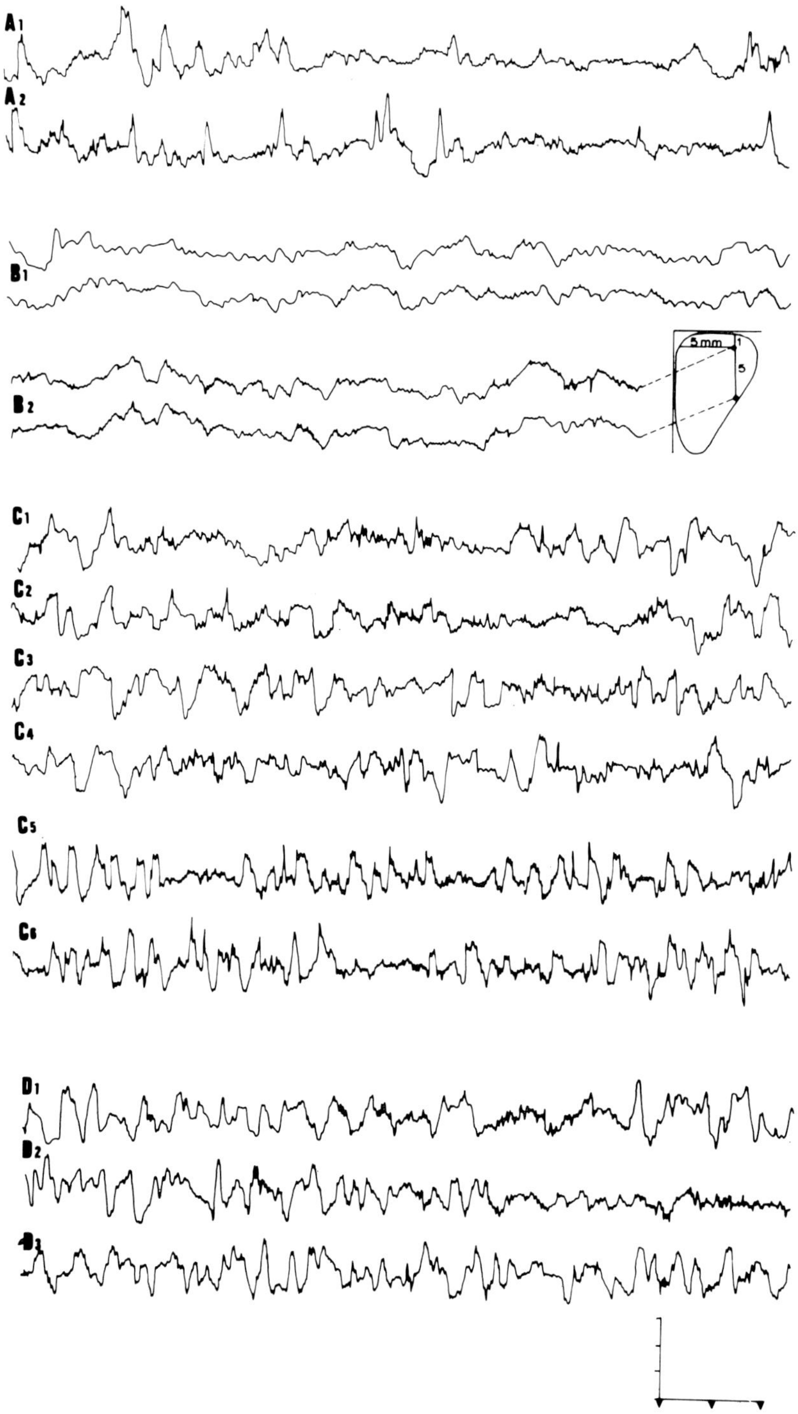
A1
A2
B1
B2
5 mm
1
5
C1
C2
C3
C4
C5
C6
D1
D2
D3

almost the amplitude reported in chicks after hatching (Key and Marley, 1962; Tuge *et al.*, 1960; Peters *et al.*, 1965; Corner *et al.*, 1966) and on the last day of incubation (Sedláček, 1964), a development of a different kind begins during or just prior to this stage. Periods in which the EEG slow waves are relatively continuous alternate with periods in which frequent brief stretches of the record are bilaterally unusually low in amplitude (Figs. 6A, 7A — and Peters *et al.*, 1965). This change occurs in a cycle

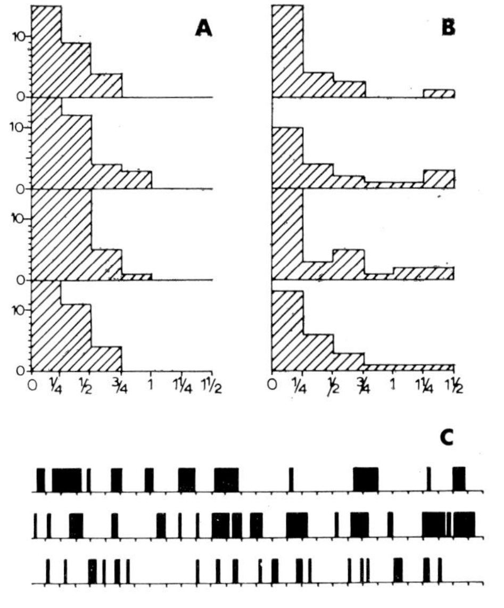

Fig. 8. The cycle of episodic flattening of the cerebral EEG at *stage 44* (the earliest that such periodicity has been seen).

Above, successive half-minute stretches selected over a period of ca. five minutes are plotted for two preparations (A, B). The *number of intervals* where the amplitude falls below 15 μV is given on the ordinate as a function of the *interval duration* (on the abscissa, in seconds).

Below, two half-minute sequences of intervals less than 15 μV in amplitude (blackened areas) in a *stage-44* embryo during the most pronounced portion of its cycle. The bottom line shows for comparison a typical stretch taken from the *least* pronounced portion. (The time scale is 1 sec per division.)

Fig 7. Development of cyclic changes in the cerebral EEG (illustrated by recordings made during periods of *maximal* flattening of the electrical tracing: compare with figure six).

A. Continuous recording (1–2) at *stage 44*: this embryo shows a more pronounced (cyclic) reduction in slow wave activity than the one illustrated in figure one (E). The simultaneously registered ECG is shown underneath the second cerebral record.

B. A typical *stage-45* embryo, showing the still more extreme reduction of slow waves at this stage during a portion of the cerebral activity cycle. Continual record (1-2) taken simultaneously at two widely separated points.

C. Continual record (1–4) from a *one-day old* chick during behavioral deep sleep: the flattened portions are less extensive than at embryonic *stage 45*, making the pattern reminiscent of *stage 44*. (C_{5-6} shows a stretch of relatively little flattening, where the episodes are very sharply delineated).

D. Continual record (1–3) from a *ten-day old* chick during sleep: the slow wave trains are more sustained than in periods of maximum flattening just following hatching (e.g. C_{1-4}) and tend to be more sharply delineated from the flattened episodes.

Calibrations: horizontal, 1 sec per division except in C_{5-6}, where it is 2 sec per division; vertical, 50 μV per division.

References p. 189–192

of several minutes in all cases and is not a consequence of an overall reduction in amplitude, since the frequency and amplitude of the electrical waves are little changed between the 'flattened' stretches. The duration and timing of the flat portions of the record are highly variable and only on occasion is a hint of rhythmicity present (Fig. 8), such as is seen in the sleeping EEG of the post-hatching chick (Klein *et al.*, 1964; Jouvet, 1965; Ookawa and Gotoh, 1964). By *stage 45* the EEG flattening has become more pronounced in all embryos (Fig. 7B), to a greater degree in some than in others, but the slow fluctuation is still present (also Peters *et al.*, 1965). This fluctuation persists after hatching as a characteristic feature of the EEG during behavioral sleep, wherein the 'paradoxical' phases (*i.e.* cerebral EEG flattening) occur chiefly within recurring periods of several minutes duration (Figs. 6C, 7C— also Jouvet, 1965; Peters *et al.*,

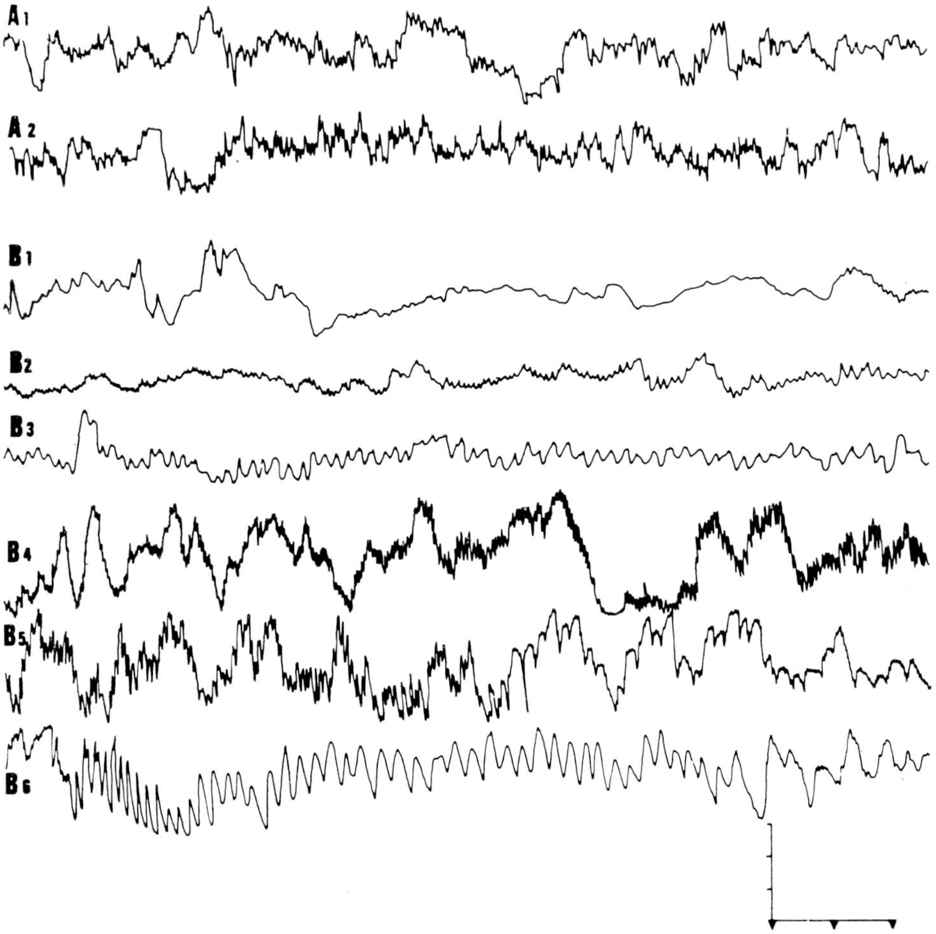

Fig. 9. Unusual electrical patterns observed 'spontaneously' in the cerebral EEG (monopolar recordings).
A. Brief episodes of high amplitude, surface positive fast waves at embryonic *stage 44* (line 1) and at ca. *one week* after hatching (line 2).
B. Build-up in a *stage-45* embryo of fast waves into large, regular slow ones (three sequences in order to show some of the large quantitative variations: 1–3, 4–5, and 6).

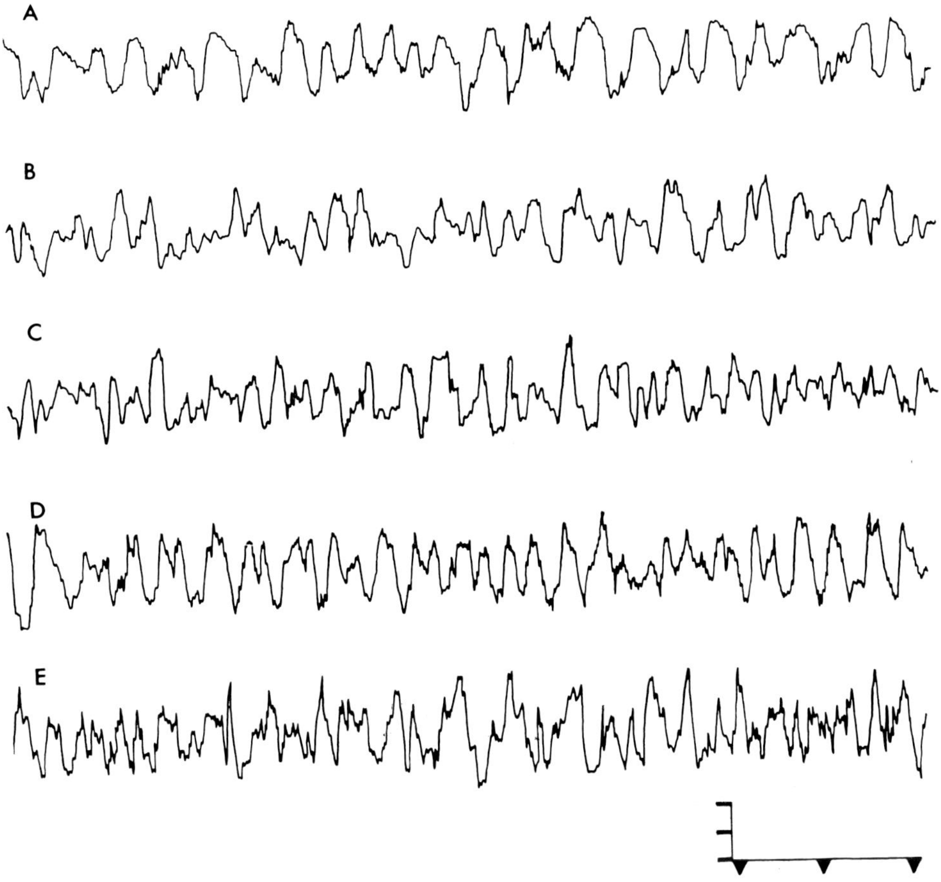

Fig. 10. Differential recordings from the cerebral hemisphere during behavioral sleep in five chicks (A–E), showing the typical individual variation which is seen from one day to at least two weeks after hatching.
Calibrations: horizontal, 1 sec per division; vertical, 50 μV per division.

1965). 'Paradoxical' EEG episodes during sleep are very variable in duration and timing, resembling *stage-44* embryonic records, but with maturation they become more clearly phasic during the periods of maximum activity (Fig. 7D — also Peters *et al.*, 1965; Corner *et al.*, 1966). The percentage of the sleep record occupied by paradoxical phases falls from ca. 0.5% in the one day old chick to half this value in the adult bird (Klein, 1963).

Regularity in the *slow wave* sequences first appears briefly in the cerebral record towards the end of *stage 45* (Fig. 6B). Comparison with the post-hatching *sleep* record shows that the cerebral EEG has with this last development essentially achieved full maturation. The electrical activity of a sleeping chick is characterized, except for the short "paradoxical" phases, by a similar sequence of large irregular slow waves which become strongly rhythmic for variable periods (also Schadé *et al.*, 1965). The frequency of this slow sleep rhythm has been reported to undergo development after hatching, from ca. 2 c/sec to 5–6 in the two to three weeks old chick (Peters *et al.*, 1965). In our experience however, this range of values represents individual variations which can be demonstrated at all ages (Fig. 10). The fast low amplitude component of the electrical activity, on the other hand, does increase in frequency during the first days after hatching, from 15–20 to ca. 25 c/sec (also Key and Marley, 1962; Tuge *et al.*, 1960). It is present in essentially constant form throughout all behavioral states and degrees of EEG slow wave activity (Corner *et al.*, 1966). The normal cerebral activity of the adult chicken is essentially the same as that already achieved by the young chick (Ookawa and Gotoh, 1965; Key and Marley, 1962; Tuge *et al.*, 1960).

An abnormally high amplitude fast cerebral rhythm has once been seen briefly in a chick of about one week of age (Fig. 9A). It is reminiscent of the unusual intermittent activity pattern described earlier for one of the *stage-44* embryos. In another young chick and in two *stage-45* embryos, a similar abnormal spontaneous pattern was seen which progressed into larger, slower waves of great regularity (Fig. 9B).

The spontaneous activity recorded from the *optic tectum* at *stage 45* (all five cases) is little changed for most of the time from the preceding stage. An irregular train of very low amplitude waves of short duration is superimposed upon sporadic small

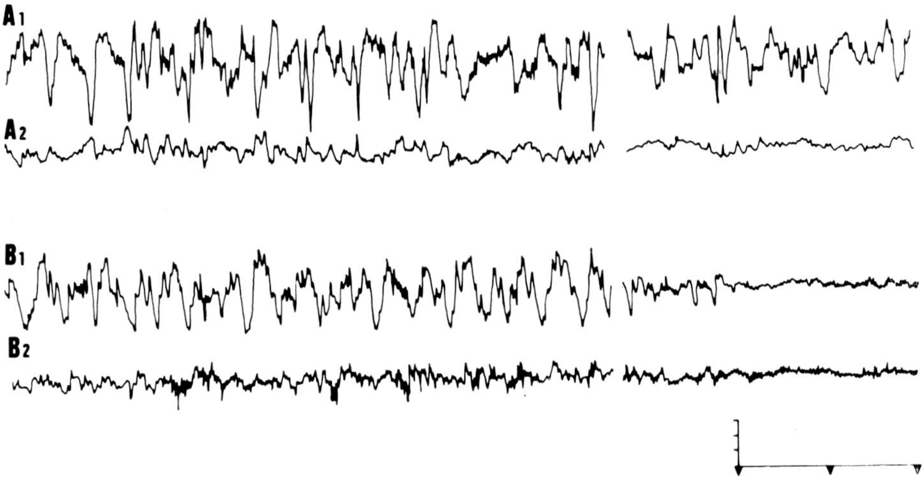

Fig. 11. A. Simultaneous recordings from the cerebral hemisphere (1) and the optic tectum (2) at embryonic *stage 45*; the first stretch shows a period of augmented tectal slow waves while the second stretch illustrates the usual tectal pattern (note the *lower gain* here than in figure two).
B. *idem*, in a *three-day old* chick: the first stretch shows the typical sleeping pattern and the second the waking one.
Calibrations: horizontal, 2 sec per division; vertical, 50 μV per division.

slow waves. In most of the preparations in addition, a period lasting several minutes has been seen at least once during the recording session in which the slow waves increase greatly in amplitude (Fig. 11A). Many of them are synchronous with ipsilaterally recorded cerebral slow waves, usually of opposite polarity and comparable duration. The lack of correlation between the amplitudes of synchronous waves in the two brain structures, plus their appearance in the optic lobe only at infrequent intervals, raises the possibility that they do not simply represent electrotonic spreading from the cerebral lobe. In *post*-hatching chicks relatively large slow waves are seen almost continually in the optic lobes during sleep (Fig. 11B). Their amplitude does not increase significantly with maturation, rarely exceeding 30 μV even in the oldest birds studied here or in adult chickens (Ookawa and Gotoh, 1965).

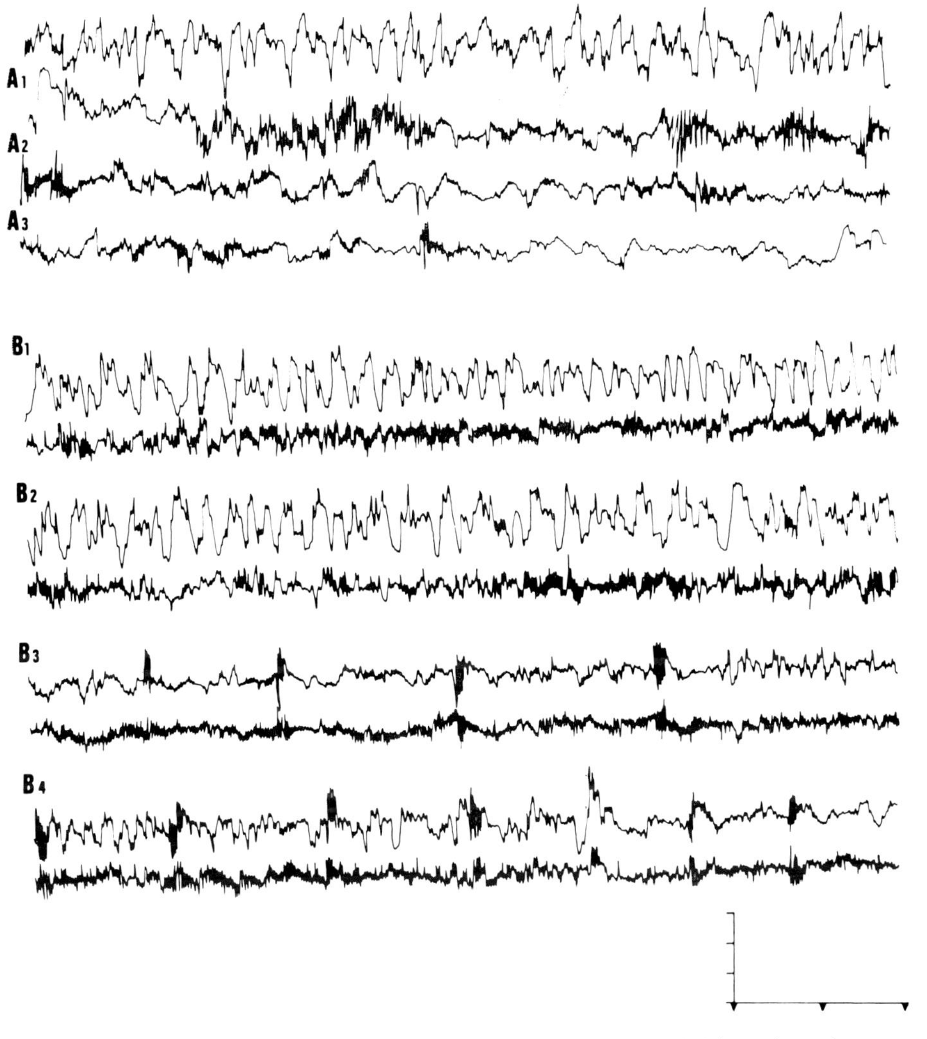

Fig. 12. Maturation of the normal 'spontaneous' electrical activity recorded from the optic tectum. A. Embryo at *stage 45* of development: continuous recording (1–3) illustrating the variability of high frequency bursts during an 'active' period. (The simultaneous cerebral EEG is included above the first portion of the tectal record.)
B. *Three days* after hatching: simultaneous activity recorded from the cerebrum (upper trace of each pair) and the optic lobe. Continuous records during sleep (1–2) and during waking (3–4), the latter showing periodic eyeball movements and reduced amplitude of the tectal spikes.
Calibrations: horizontal, 1 sec per division; vertical, 50 μV per division for the upper trace and 25 μV for the lower trace of each pair.

References p. 189–192

An additional change in the optic lobe electrical activity first appears in the last stage of embryonic development (i.e. Hamburger and Hamilton, *stage 45*). The irregular 15–20 c/sec waves increase greatly in amplitude (sometimes almost to 100 μV in either direction) in bursts of variable duration. In one case this occurred frequently throughout the record but rarely for longer than about one second per burst. In another case no such activity was seen for many minutes but when the bursts began they lasted much longer than in the first preparation, often being made up of highly regular sinusoidal waves. The wave amplitudes and the timing and duration of the bursts are highly variable in all cases however, and do not coincide with any obvious changes in the cerebral EEG (Fig. 12A). It is this type of activity which in a previous study (Peters *et al.*, 1960) is illustrated as typical for the optic lobe in the late embryo but it should be emphasized that such high amplitudes actually occur only sporadically. This is still the case in the *newly hatched* chick, as is seen by comparing the different stretches of optic lobe EEG contained both in the above-mentioned publication and in a subsequent one by the same authors (Peters *et al.*, 1964). Even one day after hatching, long periods of time can go by without seeing any increase in the amplitude of fast waves above their normal maximum of ca. 15 μV (also Scholes and Roberts, 1964).

By three days of age an almost continuous train of high amplitude 'spike'-like waves of about 25 msec duration is recorded from surface of the optic tectum (Fig.

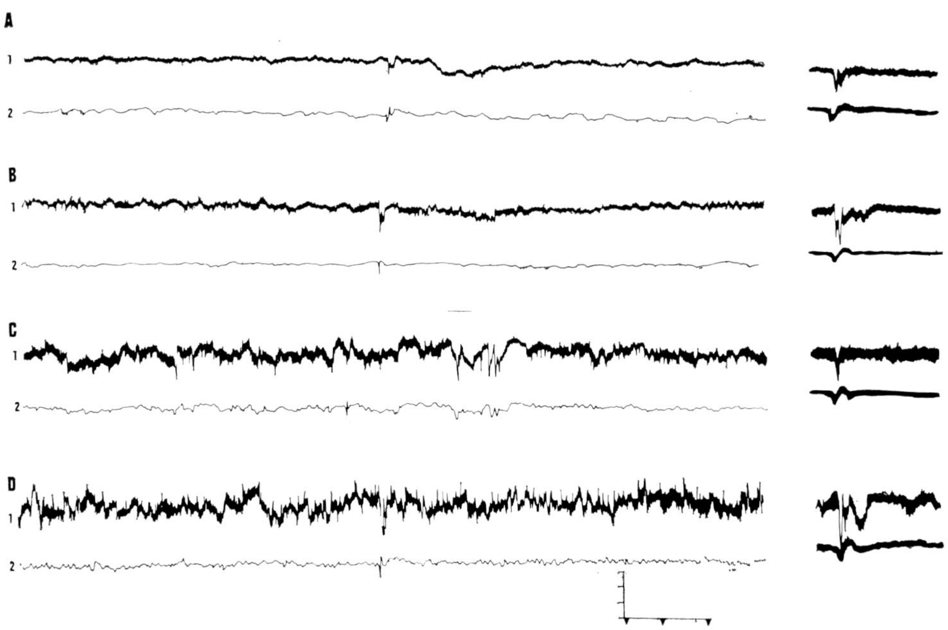

Fig. 13. Electrical activity in the optic tectum of the chick during maturation (line 1). A. 1 day after hatching, B. 5 days, C. 9 days, D. 38 days. The simultaneous electroretinogram is included (line 2) in order to mark the occurrence of a flash. The insert at the right of each paper record shows five superimposed flash-evoked responses photographed from a cathode-ray oscilloscope at six times the sweep speed indicated below.

Calibrations: horizontal, 1 sec per division; vertical, 100 μV per division. (*Courtesy of Dr. N. W. Scholes*, slightly modified.)

12B). Their frequency fluctuates rapidly in an irregular way, with short bursts of up to 35–40 spikes per second occurring as well as stretches with few or none. The spikes are usually equally of both polarities but stretches are seen where they are predominantly positive. The overall pattern just described appears invariant over long periods of time, independent of behavioral and cerebral EEG changes or the level of background illumination (also Ookawa and Gotoh, 1965). The only further striking development through two weeks after hatching is that stretches containing predominantly surface positive spikes are no longer seen in birds 7 days of age or older (three cases at each age studied, recording over several hours). Scholes and Roberts (1964; Fig. 13), working with a different breed of chick, have illustrated a progressive increase in the amplitude and frequency of the optic lobe spikes throughout the entire first week after hatching, however, and barrages of positive spikes even nine days after. The records at 5 weeks (Scholes and Roberts, 1964) and in the adult chicken (Ookawa and Gotoh, 1965) are identical to the pattern described in our experiments at one week of age and older.

The *cerebellar EEG* undergoes a slight increase in amplitude from *stage 44* to *45* both in the slow waves, which may now reach 50 μV, and in the irregular fast rhythm of ca. 15 c/sec (Peters *et al.*, 1960). In contrast to the optic lobes, the only further development evident through at least two weeks after hatching is a slight increase in the frequency of the fast rhythm (Fig. 14). Except for the absence in the cerebellum

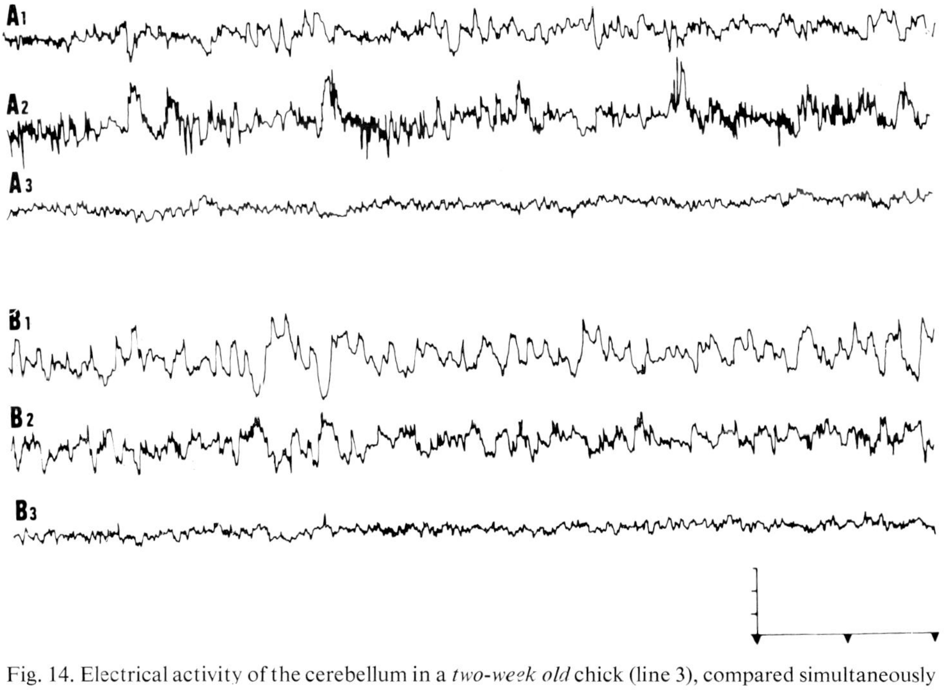

Fig. 14. Electrical activity of the cerebellum in a *two-week old* chick (line 3), compared simultaneously with the cerebral hemisphere (1) and the optic tectum (2). A is recorded during behavioral waking, B during sleep.
Calibrations: horizontal, 1 sec per division; vertical, 50 μV per division in lines 1 and 3, 25 μV in line 2.

of high amplitude spiking, the gross electrical activity pattern is thus similar in the two structures. The largest slow waves in both occur for the most part during sleep and are sometimes synchronous.

C. Responses of the brain to sensory input

The earliest electrical response to sensory stimulation which has so far been recorded is a *transient potential change* evoked in the optic tectum by illumination of the contralateral retina. This occurs clearly at the beginning of *stage 45* simultaneously with or slightly later than the earliest observed response in the eye itself (Peters *et al.*, 1958; Garcia–Austt and Patetta–Queirolo, 1961). A few embryos thus show a response to single and repetitive flashes on the 19th day of incubation (Pisareva, 1965) while most of them reach this stage on the following day (Peters *et al.*, 1958). An optic-evoked tectal potential can be revealed more than a day earlier, however, by superimposing several successive responses (Sedláček, unpublished). The evoked response appears to consist of an initial surface positive wave, ca. 150 msec in duration and up to 50 μV in amplitude, followed by a smaller negative wave lasting several hundred msec; *ON* and *OFF* responses to sustained retinal illumination have the same waveform except for the addition of a prolonged low amplitude positive after-potential (Peters *et al.*, 1958). The amplitude of the evoked potential then increases throughout *stage 45*, with no significant alteration of the waveform, and attains values up to 150 μV shortly before the time of hatching (Fig. 15 — also Pisareva, 1965).

Throughout the late embryonic period, and also in the newly hatched chick (Peters *et al.*, 1958) and adult pigeon (Hambdi and Whitteridge, 1954) the optic lobe can usually *follow* flashes only up to 4–5 per second before there is a reduction in amplitude after the initial response. The eye is not the limiting factor, being already able in the late embryo to follow rates of more than 10 per second (Peters *et al.*, 1958). The response disappears completely from the tectum at ca. 10 flashes per second in early *stage-45* embryos, at ca. 20 per second one day later, and above 40 per second in the newly hatched chick (Peters *et al.*, 1958; Pisareva, 1965; the present study). An irregular fluctuation in 'excitability' (*i.e.* response amplitude) has been observed in all three of the above-mentioned studies (Fig. 15).

The *waveform* of the evoked response at the tectal surface following a flash differs in the newly hatched chick from that in the late embryo by an initial negativity which usually precedes the positive wave and by a shorter after-negativity (Peters *et al.*, 1958). The overall duration declines to the mature range of 100–200 msec during the first day after hatching. This basic waveform is then preserved throughout post-hatching life but remains extremely variable in its fine details (Rougeul, 1957; Scholes, 1966). With computer averaging however, both the positive and the early negative wave can be resolved into two peaks (Scholes, 1966), suggesting a complex consistent response mechanism despite the great variability. The complexity of the neural mechanisms in the chick tectum is further emphasized by the varied waveforms which appear upon administration of certain drugs (Scholes, 1966) and by large changes when the electrode penetrates even slightly below the surface (Paulson, 1965). Depth

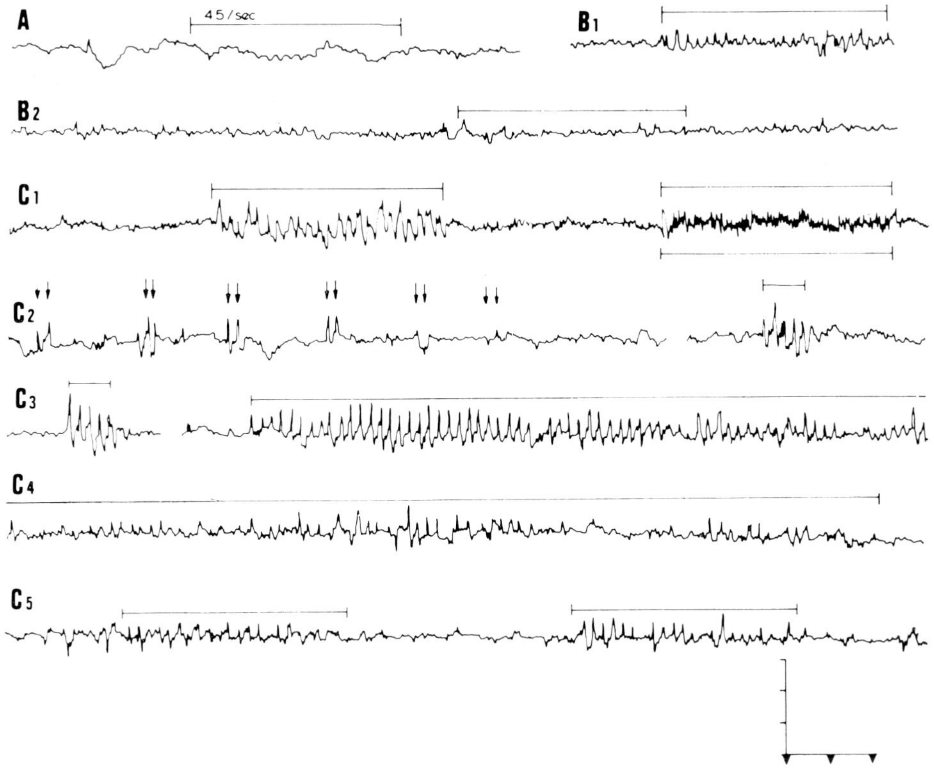

Fig. 15. Electrical responses in the optic tectum to illumination of the contralateral eye by trains of flashes (the frequency and the duration of the stimulation is indicated above the corresponding tracing).
A. *Stage-44* embryo, showing no response.
B. Continuous record (1–2) at *early stage 45*: despite a large irregular variation in response amplitude, the tectum follows the low frequency but vanishes rapidly at the higher one.
C. At *late stage 45* the response is diminished but still present throughout high frequency stimulation (line 1). Several different durations of *low* frequency stimulation are presented from a different preparation (2–5) in order to demonstrate the changes in excitability.
Calibrations: horizontal, 1 sec per division; vertical, 50 μV per division.

analysis in four different species of adult birds has in fact distinguished several populations of neurons by means of differences in the latency of the response to a flash and the differing location of the electric field and action potentials (O'Leary and Bishop, 1943; Cragg *et al.*, 1954; Hambdi and Whitteridge, 1954). Furthermore, the retinal projection upon the tectum is such that each surface evoked response bears a point-to-point relationship to the area illuminated. The deeper responses have a much wider receptive field and fatigue more readily than those near the surface (Hambdi and Whitteridge, 1954). The existence has also been demonstrated of a direct projection from the retina to the *ipsi*lateral tectum, evoking electrical responses almost identical to those in the contralateral one (Rougeul, 1957). If the optic nerve is stimulated directly by a brief shock the tectal response is considerably shorter than that evoked by a flash (only 10–20 msec) but is similarly polyphasic and variable with depth under the surface (O'Leary and Bishop, 1943; Cragg *et al.*, 1954).

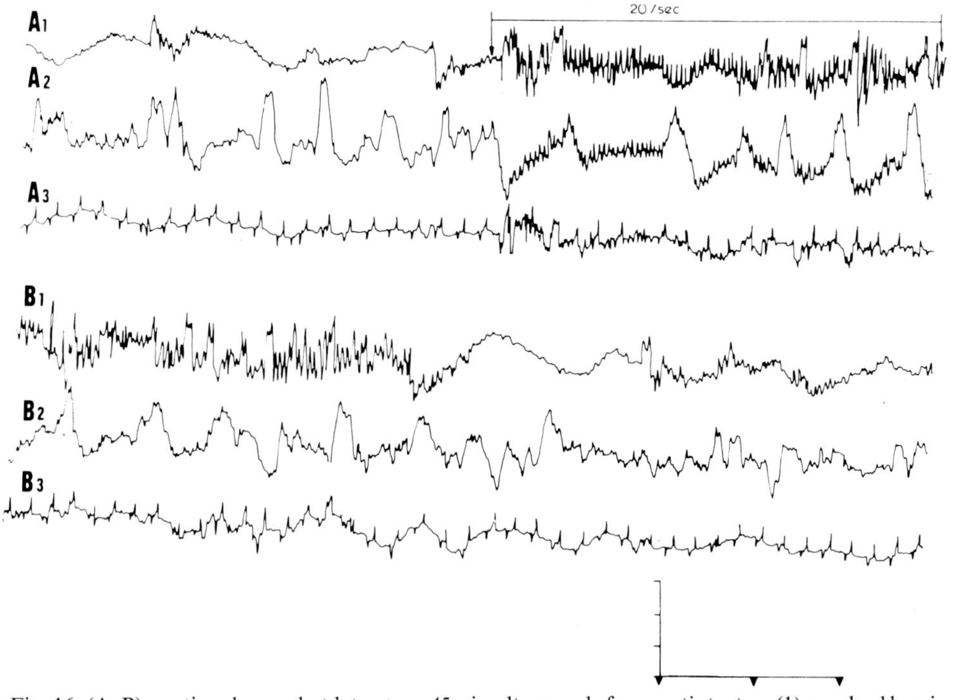

Fig. 16. (A–B) continual record at late *stage 45*, simultaneously from optic tectum (1), cerebral hemisphere (2), and trunk (3).
Calibrations: horizontal, 1 sec per division; vertical, 50 μV per division in line 1, 100 μV in line 2, and 200 μV in line 3.

Afterdischarges have been observed in the tectum following single flashes, for the first in late *stage-45* embryos (Pisareva, 1965). They consist of irregular 'spikes' occurring at 5–10 per second and lasting up to two seconds. They are much more susceptible to repeated presentation of the stimulation than are the primary evoked responses, and even after hatching can be elicited only during certain periods in a recording session (Peters *et al.*, 1958; Scholes and Roberts, 1964). We have sometimes seen irregular oscillatory afterdischarges at late *stage 45* following high frequency flash stimulation (Fig. 16), solely during periods when similar discharges also occurred spontaneously. This kind of response would no longer be conspicuous at the age when continual spike discharges occur spontaneously. The presence of a barrage of spikes following each flash has been revealed, however, by average response computation and by the use of drugs which suppress the background electrical activity (Fig. 17).

Light-evoked potentials can be recorded from the surface of the cerebral hemisphere as well as from the optic tectum. In the duckling they have been reported from the time the retina first responds to light and are almost identical in latency, duration and waveform to those seen simultaneously in the tectum (Paulson, 1965). In the chick the first cerebral response appears late in *stage 45* (observed in all cases where the third toe was longer than 24 mm and in none earlier), thus later than the tectal response. A surface positive wave begins 75–100 msec after illumination and is usually

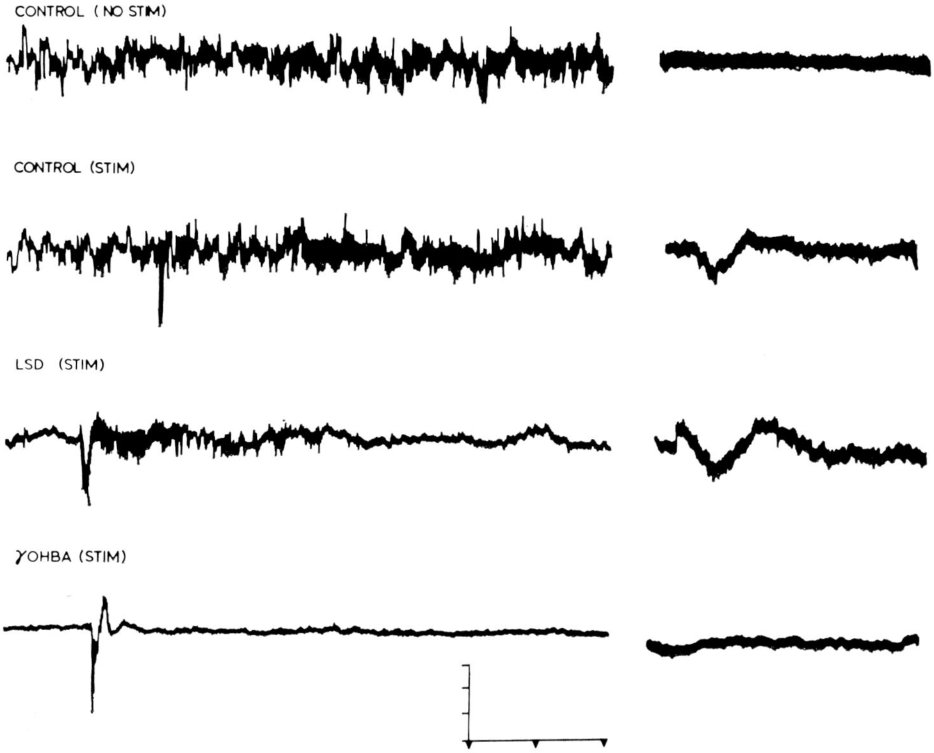

Fig. 17. Spike barrages following flash-evoked potentials in the optic tectum of the chick. These are normally masked by the background activity (A) but their presence is indicated by the computed *average response* (B). Drugs such as *d*-lysergic acid diethylamide (LSD) reveal the evoked barrage by suppressing the background spikes (note, however, the similar averaged response). γ-Hydroxybutyric acid (GOHBA) suppresses evoked as well as background spikes. (*Courtesy of Dr. N. W. Scholes*, slightly modified.)
Calibrations: horizontal, 1 sec per division; vertical, 100 μV per division.

followed by a longer negative wave (Fig. 18A). The *ON* response to steady illumination is similar but much longer, while the *OFF* response is of the opposite polarity (Fig. 18B). In the newly hatched chick the cerebral response to a flash is shorter than in the embryo (but longer than the corresponding *tectal* potential) and a negative spike often precedes the positive wave (Fig. 18C). These electrical events are restricted to the medial (dorsal) surface of the contralateral hemisphere and, in the one case extensively mapped, strongest anteriorly (Fig. 18A). The light-evoked response in the adult bird is also found in the anterior-medial region of the hemisphere (Rougeul and Buser, 1953; Rougeul, 1957). Each retina now projects to both hemispheres however, evoking an almost identical, usually biphasic response in each. It is strongest several millimeters below the surface and gradually disappears with still greater depth, the two component waves having different spatial distributions (Rougeul, 1957). The latency is of the same order as that of the tectal response, ca. 10 msec for a shock to the optic nerve and 30 msec for retinal illumination. The same authors have also re-

References p. 189–192

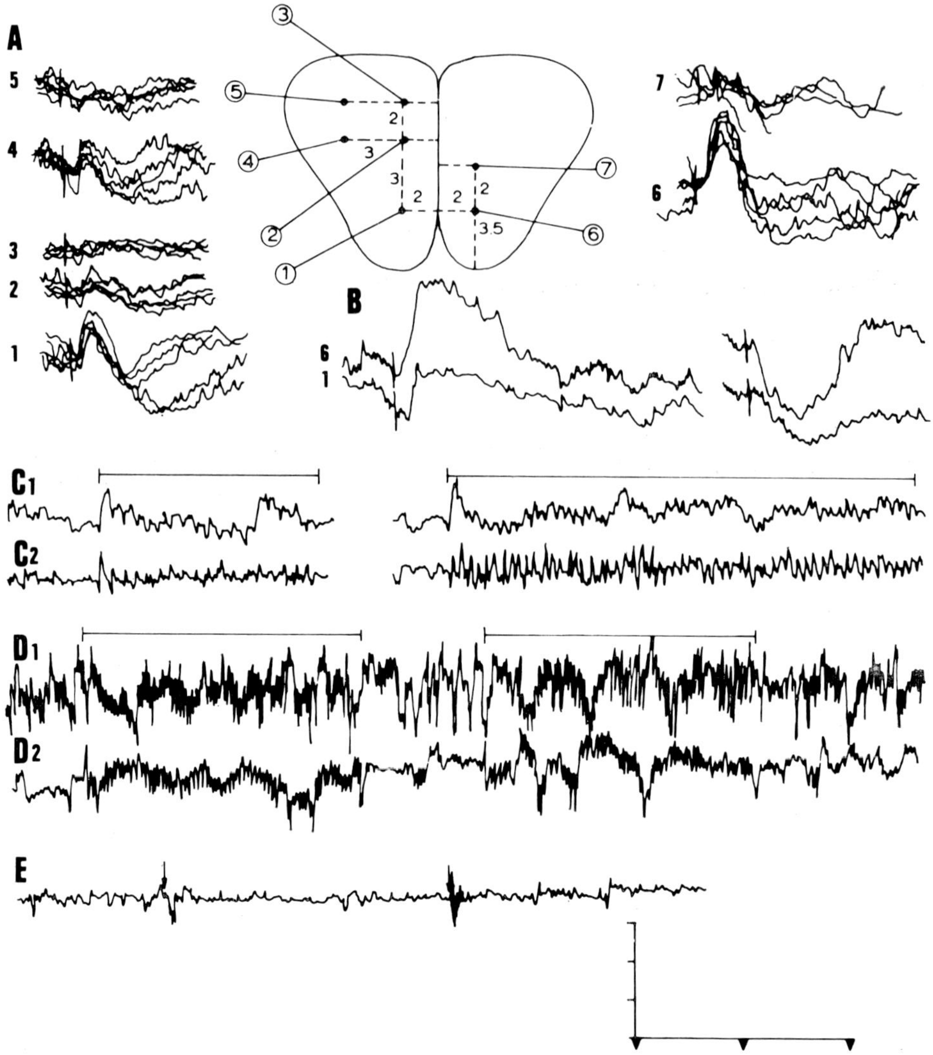

Fig. 18. Visual-evoked potentials in the cerebral hemisphere of the chick.
A. Simultaneous recordings at *stage 45* from seven points (1–7) on both hemispheres, five consecutive responses superimposed (traced from the paper record). Electrode positions are indicated on the sketch by the corresponding numbers; distances are given in millimeters next to the dashed lines. (Anterior is *downwards* on the sketch of the dorsal surface of the hemispheres.) The right eye was more strongly illuminated, resulting in larger responses from the left cerebrum.
B. An *ON*- and an *OFF*-response recorded bilaterally from the anterior-medial electrode sites (1 and 6) with a time constant of 0.3 sec.
C. The cerebral response to five/sec flashes (line 1) in a *newly hatched* chick, recorded simultaneously with the ipsilateral optic tectum (line 2).
D. The cerebral response to 20/sec flashes (line 1) in a *stage-45* embryo, recorded simultaneously with the ipsilateral optic tectum (line 2) and illustrating the failure of the hemisphere (first sequence) to always follow the stimuli.
E. Potentials evoked in the cerebrum of a *stage-45* embryo by single claps (arrows), recorded 5 mm below the dorsal surface.
Calibrations: horizontal, 1 sec per division in A and B, 2 sec in C–E; vertical, 100 μV per division.

ported short and long latency responses in the *cerebellum* following stimulation of the optic nerve, the former already appearing at about 10 msec after a shock and the latter up to 50 msec later (Buser and Rougeul, 1954; Rougeul, 1957). Short latency responses (up to 20 msec following a flash) have also been found in a part of the *thalamus* (n. rotundum) and in the *archistriatum* of the adult chicken (Phillips, 1966).

Fluctuations occur in the 'excitability' of the hemisphere which need not be simultaneous with the similar changes in the optic lobe (Fig. 18C). These affect both the amplitude of the initial and subsequent responses and the ability to follow rapid flashes, which is less in the cerebrum than in the tectum (Fig. 18D). Sheff and Tureen (1962) report that in chicks two weeks after hatching the cerebral hemisphere can follow flashes up to 14 per second before a reduction occurs in the amplitude of the responses. We have seen occasions, however, when no reduction occurred even at 20 per second, while at other times in the same bird a stimulus rate of only 5 per second produced a large decline in amplitude.

Auditory and tactile stimuli fail to evoke potential waves in any of the forebrain structures so far discussed (Erulkar, 1955; Phillips, 1966). Such responses have been reported however, bilaterally within small overlapping portions of the neostriatum in the adult pigeon (Erulkar, 1955). We have encountered an auditory evoked response already at embryonic *stage 45* but, similarly, only deep under the surface of the cerebrum (Fig. 18E). Average response computation, however (Spooner, 1964), has revealed the presence after a click of a small potential in a superficial cerebral structure as well (accessory hyperstriatum) — in addition to the expected short latency wave complex in the medulla. Single neurons, on the other hand, have been encountered throughout the hemisphere which discharge in response to several modalities of stimulation: visual, auditory and tactile (Gogan, 1963).

The cerebral electrical activity shows no obvious response to sensory input throughout the embryonic period other than the evoked potentials described (also Sedláček, 1963). Transient flattening of the EEG occasionally follows a visual, auditory or tactile stimulus but, since such episodes also frequently occur spontaneously, no causal relationship to the sensory input can be indicated. This apparently unresponsive state of the cerebrum persists for several hours after hatching (also Peters *et al.*, 1965). The EEG pattern then changes gradually to one of greatly reduced slow wave activity and begins to respond to stimulation by a transient further diminution of the slow waves (Fig. 19A). This transition is conceivably stimulated by the increased sensory input to the brain after hatching, possibly by proprioceptive stimulation as the bird slowly achieves a standing posture. In the pigeon (Tuge *et al.*, 1960) the cerebral EEG at the time of hatching resembles that of a chick embryo one week earlier. Its subsequent development is similar and there is no response to stimulation nor transition to the state of prolonged reduction of slow waves until late in the second week after hatching.

The cerebral activity in the newly-hatched chick thus changes with 'waking' to a pattern of *continuous low amplitude waves* of ca. 20 c/sec with intermittent slower waves superimposed (fig. 19B). This change occurs simultaneously throughout the entire hemisphere (Spooner, 1964). Frequent shifts occur in the number and amplitude

References p. 189–192

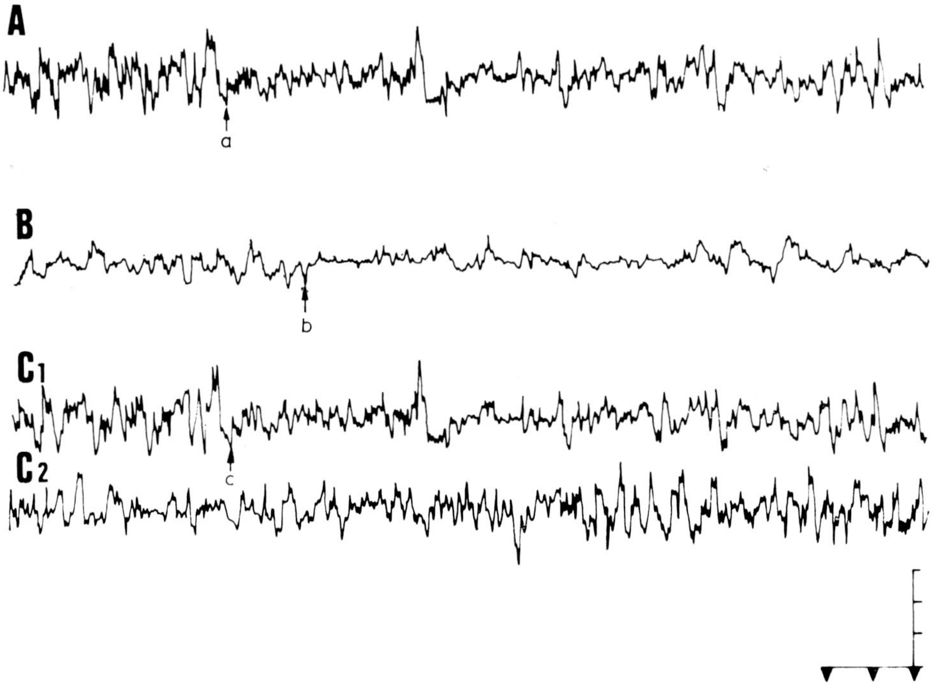

Fig. 19. The cerebral EEG on the first day after hatching.
A. During the *transitional period* to behavioral alertness. The slow waves have become smaller, and sensory stimulation produces a transient further reduction in amplitude (*a*).
B. After the attainment of *waking* behavior. Small slow waves are present which largely disappear after a sensory stimulus (*b*).
C. During the transition to *sleeping* behavior. The increasing amplitude of the slow waves is frequently reversed temporarily (as at *c*) before a stable level of large waves is reached.
Calibrations: horizontal, 1 sec per division; vertical, 50 μV per division.

of the slow waves (which are correlated with the motor activity of the chick in a way described in the third paper of this series). Any brief adequate stimulus then produces a reduction in slow wave activity, the degree and duration of which tend to reflect the intensity of the stimulus. The continual slight fluctuations in slow wave activity appear to reflect an endogenous process as well as the intensity and variety of environmental stimuli. With maturation the fast component of the EEG increases up to 30 c/sec (also Key and Marley, 1962; Tuge *et al.*, 1960), and possibly a reduction in small slow wave activity during *waking* occurs as well (Corner *et al.*, 1966; Peters *et al.*, 1965).

The fluctuating electrical pattern just described gives way after a time to a progressive *increase in slow wave activity*, simultaneously throughout the cerebral hemisphere (Spooner, 1964), ultimately returning to the large amplitude waves described in the previous section of this paper or stabilizing at an intermediate level. This transition could be due partly to decreasing proprioceptive input as the body relaxes at the same time. It is a gradual process of variable speed, usually with large fluctuations and frequent brief returns of the low amplitude wave pattern (Fig. 19C). Adequate stimulation during the slow wave state or the transition to it also produces a reduction or disappearance of the slow waves, which may be *uni*lateral (Spooner, 1964; Peters *et al.*, 1965). The effect may be transient or prolonged, depending both upon the intensity of stimulation and upon an endogenous fluctuation in responsiveness (Corner *et al.*, 1966). The same phenomenon often occurs without any evident sensory stimulation and may similarly be either brief or prolonged, in the latter case accompanied by an abrupt return of muscle tone which could play a causal role. In a long-immobilized chick the cerebral responsiveness falls to the point where it is almost insensitive to stimulation and 'spontaneous' disappearance of the slow waves is always very brief (Corner *et al.*, 1966). This condition is quickly reversed upon release of the bird.

The cerebrum of the chick is in the state of prolonged *absence of large slow waves* for only brief periods at first. These periods increase rapidly in duration in a given environment throughout the first day of post-hatching life (also Klein, 1963). The duration of low amplitude cerebral electrical activity can be prolonged by cold or by background noise and shortened by moderate warmth. In birds over one week of age there is a rapid transition to the large amplitude wave pattern upon being placed in a dark container (Corner *et al.*, 1966). This has little effect upon younger chicks unless the experience has been repeated several times. Intermittent return to the low amplitude state of cerebral activity occurs in the dark at all ages, lasting for variable

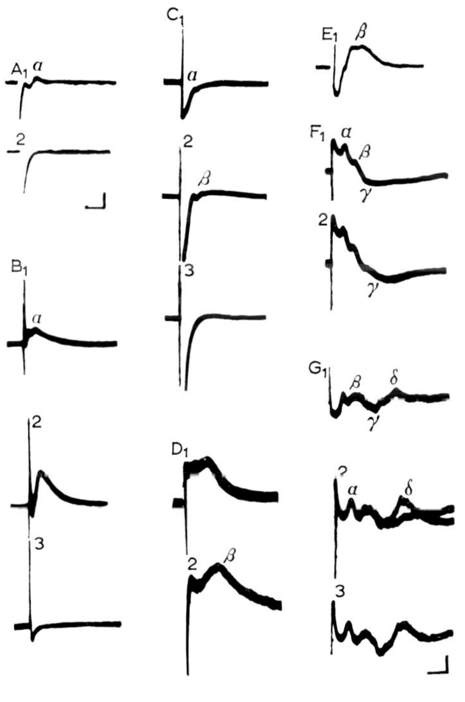

Fig. 20. The cerebral electrical response evoked at the site of stimulation by a brief shock, at increasing intensity (B–F: 1–2; G: 1–3). Lines A_2, B_3, and C_3 show the stimulus artifact (after disappearance of the active response) at the strongest shock intensity used.
A, embryonic *stage 38*; B, *stages 39* to *41*; C, *stage 42*; D, *late stage 43*; E, *stage 44*; F, *early stage 45*; G, *stage 45/46* (just prior to hatching).
Calibrations: 10 msec and 100 μV.

periods of time. *Social* factors also influence the changes in cerebral electrical activity, such that the individual organisms' cycles have a strong tendency to synchronize with one another (also Key and Marley, 1962).

D. Electrical stimulation of the cerebral hemisphere

A response is evoked by a brief shock to the dorsal surface of the cerebrum which is characteristic for the stage of development (Fig. 20). Similar waveforms have been obtained from at least five preparations at each stage and from widely separated points on the hemisphere. The earliest response is at embryonic *stage 38* (the 12th day of incubation in most cases) and consists of a surface negative wave ('α') lasting ca. 5 msec (A^1). It is never larger than 50 μV and often seems to be preceded by a smaller negative wave (also B^1). At *stages 39* to *41* this wave complex can attain a much larger amplitude and the duration seems longer, due to the exponential falling phase (B^2). The rise-time is ca. 7 msec and the time constant is 7–8 msec for a *one-half* reduction in amplitude. A very low amplitude, longer duration surface negative wave ('β') appears in *stage 42*, at a higher threshold than the initial waves ($C^{1,2}$). It is still small early in *stage 43* but develops rapidly, so that towards the end of this stage of development the amplitude often exceeds 100 μV (D^2). The rise-time is estimated at 10 msec or slightly longer, followed by a slower, exponential decay. The response is little changed at *stage 44* and sometimes shows a partial resolution of the β-wave into more than one peak (E^1). Only *on site* responses have been recorded throughout this entire period of development. The evoked potentials were usually undetectable further than one mm from the stimulating electrodes, but in a few cases the identical waveform was present up to 2–3 mm distant.

At *stage 45* all cases show, up to a certain stimulus intensity, the same response as in the preceding stage. The picture shown in Fig. 20$F_{1,2}$ then appeared in two preparations after relatively strong shocks. A surface positive wave ('γ') of 40–50 msec duration immediately follows the α-wave (s), and upon which the β-complex is superimposed. *Propagation* of the response is found in all embryos at this stage. In the four cases successfully studied, a negative wave lasting about 5 msec appeared at points up to at least 4 mm distance from the stimulus center (Fig. 21A). The threshold was higher than for the *on site* α-wave and the latencies measured at the various distances indicated a propagation velocity of between 400 and 600 mm/sec. In two of these preparations, also longer-lasting potentials were evoked at some points (Fig. 21B, C).

One chick was studied shortly before hatching and gave an *on site* response as shown in Fig. 20G. The β-wave is more prominent now relative to the longer duration (positive) γ-wave, and a late, high threshold surface negative wave ('δ') has appeared. It begins ca. 30 msec after the shock and lasts 15–20 msec, sometimes failing to appear when the stimulus intensity is only slightly above threshold (G2). This waveform has also been recorded one week after hatching, so that it may represent essentially the mature type of superficial cerebral response in the chick. *Repetitive* stimulation has not yet been studied systematically but some observations are worth mentioning.

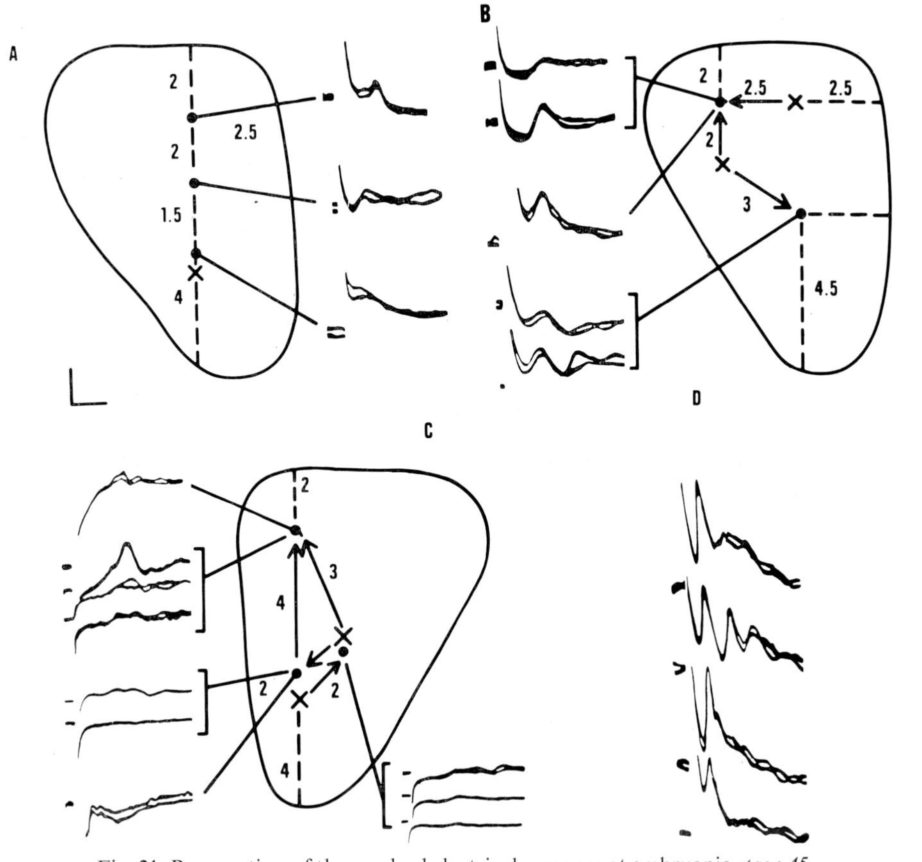

Fig. 21. Propagation of the cerebral electrical response at embryonic *stage 45*.
A. Two superimposed, ca. threshold responses at each of three distances (●) from the site of stimulation (×).
B. Longer latency waves evoked at two points in the same preparation (●) in response to stimulation 2–3 mm distant (×). *Maximal* responses are illustrated, and in two of the situations the *liminal* responses as well (upper traces).
C. A different *stage-45* embryo, showing various *on site* and *distance* responses. Each curve is made up of two superimposed consecutive responses; they are arranged at each point from bottom to top in the order of increasing stimulus intensity.
D. Effect of steady low frequency stimulation (ca. 1/sec) on the response recorded near the stimulus site (at *stage 45*). *Top*, after about 1 min the late wave (β) becomes inconsistent; thereafter (top to bottom) it breaks up into three peaks which disappear gradually within 1 min. The initial wave (α), on the contrary, is hardly affected. Two consecutive responses are superimposed in each trace.
The numbers on the sketches of the hemisphere give distances in millimeters; arrows indicate the stimulation sites which evoke the indicated responses.
Calibrations: 10 msec and 400 μV except in D, where the sweep speed is reduced to one-half.

At *stage 43* the β-wave is stable up to ca. 3 shocks per second but vanishes rapidly at 10 per second, becoming first inconsistent in shape and then progressively smaller. The α-wave, on the other hand, is not affected even at higher frequencies. In one of the older embryos the β-wave broke up into a number of regularly spaced peaks (Fig. 21D) shortly after showing waveform inconstancy during steady low frequency stimulation over a long period.

References p. 189–192

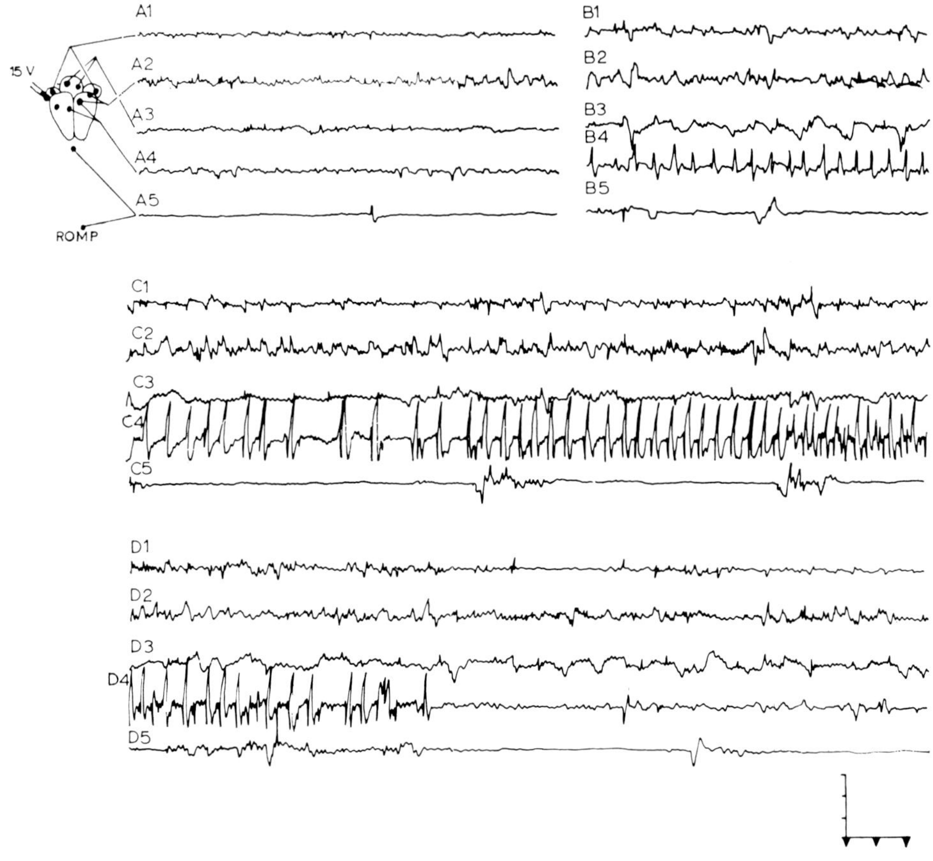

Fig. 22. Irregular spike-wave train evoked in a *stage-45* embryo by a long D.C. stimulus (5 sec, 15 V) at the dorsal surface of the right hemisphere. The stimulus electrodes were 1–2 mm apart and the ipsilateral recording site is 5 mm deep (line 4). The other brain leads are on the surface in the positions indicated. A is the activity prior to stimulation, B shows the change at 40 sec and C–D (continuous record) at 70 sec after the stimulus.
Calibrations: horizontal, 1 sec per division; vertical, 50 μV per division except line 5, which is one-half the gain.

Short pulses, even in high frequency trains or over long periods of time, have not been observed to affect the spontaneous electrical activity. Long pulses of the same intensity (up to 15 V) delivered directly to the cerebrum can have, on the contrary, a strong effect. Figure 22 shows the elicitation of a spike-wave train in a sub-surface region of the cerebrum of a *stage-45* embryo by stimulation of the ipsilateral surface. These waves, which resemble sensory-evoked potentials, began only one-half minute after a five second current and increased gradually, first in amplitude and then in frequency, before stopping abruptly. The variable relationship between the early negative spike, the large positive wave, and the negative afterpotential is clearly demonstrated. This activity is not reflected in the optic lobes, cerebellum or contralateral hyperstriatum (Fig. 22). A long-duration *cathodal* current applied to the hemi-

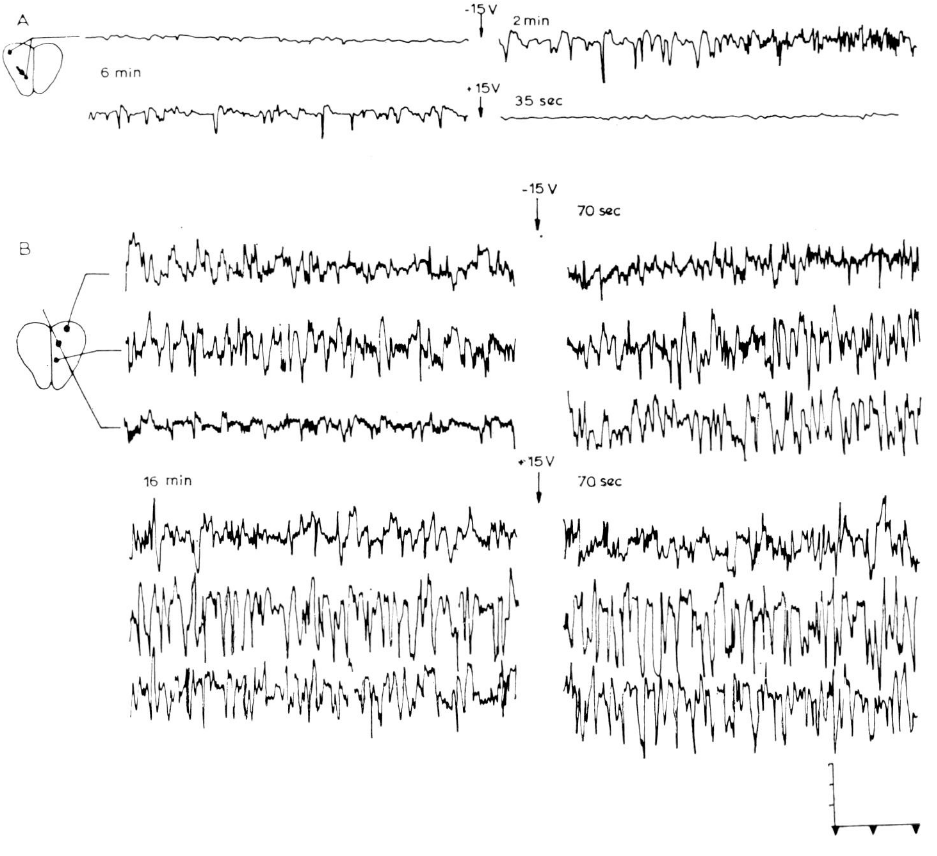

Fig. 23. Effects of surface D.C. stimulation upon the cerebral EEG in the chick one week after hatching (light nembutal anesthesia in A, heavy in B).
A. A cathodal stimulus of 15 V lasting 5 sec (arrow) results in a long-lasting amplitude increase which is then reversed by an equal anodal stimulus (bipolar recording).
B. A cathodal stimulus lasting 15 sec (15 V) at the point indicated by the arrow produces a large widespread amplitude increase over the entire hemisphere surface (simultaneous monopolar recordings). The effect continues unabated for at least one-half hour and is not affected by anodal stimulation.
Calibrations: horizontal, 1 sec per division; vertical, 100 μV per division in A, 50 μV in B.

sphere generally produces a long-lasting increase in the amplitude of the ipsilateral EEG (Fig. 23) which can sometimes be reversed by subsequent *anodal* stimulation. Local or spreading convulsion or depression, such as have been demonstrated at appropriate stages of development in the rabbit (Schadé, 1959; Schadé *et al.*, 1965), have never been seen in normal, unanesthetized chicks through at least two weeks after hatching (also Ookawa and Gotoh, 1964). In the adult pigeon however, a high amplitude cerebral surface afterdischarge can be elicited locally by an adequately intense current (Bremer *et al.*, 1939). It resembles a train of sensory-evoked potentials and lasts for only a few seconds.

No other type of electrical brain stimulation has to our knowledge been reported in

References p. 189–192

the embryonic development of any bird. The cerebral response to a wide range of stimulus parameters at various brain stem stimulation sites has been studied in the five day old chick (Spooner, 1964). Flattening of the EEG, apparently identical to that following sensory stimulation can be evoked by repetitive shocks in many regions of the thalamus, midbrain, or hindbrain. A restricted region of the thalamus evokes in addition a barrage of high amplitude, ca. six per second spikes in some parts of the ipsilateral hemisphere during the period of stimulation. They are predominantly surface positive and resemble a train of sensory-evoked potentials. No recruiting responses seem able to be elicited in the cerebrum by repetitive stimulation anywhere in the brain stem (Spooner, 1964).

Single shocks in the nucleus rotundum of the thalamus evoke strong potentials in the optic tectum (and vice-versa) but not in the archistriatum, which too is part of the direct optic projection system (Phillips, 1966). Potentials are also evoked moreover in adjacent regions of the cerebral hemisphere which are not visibly activated by flash stimulation. Direct archistriatal stimulation in turn fails to activate the n. rotundum but evokes potentials in other thalamic regions and in the tectum, and also in many parts of the hypothalamus and cerebral hemispheres (Phillips, 1966). The adjacent, non-optic regions of the hemisphere (neostriatum and paleostriatum) have in contrast much weaker projections or none at all to these structures.

E. Responses to alteration of the chemical and physical environment

The functional properties of the brain change when the temperature is either raised or lowered from its normal range of ca. 38–40°C. There is a progressive decline in the number and the amplitude of spontaneous cerebral slow waves as the temperature falls below 30°C in the late embryo and the very young chick (Peters *et al.*, 1961, 1963). Flattening of the electrical record still occurs readily following sensory stimulation however (after hatching only), and small evoked potentials are occasionally seen superimposed during repetitive flash stimulation. The EEG disappears almost completely below 25°C in *early stage-45* embryos and at a progressively lower temperature thereafter until the time of hatching. The flash-evoked potential, on the other hand, becomes much larger at these low temperature levels but now occurs only at the onset and termination of a train of stimuli. The relative amplitude of *ON* and *OFF* responses, and of the two phases in each (an initial positive wave followed by a longer negative one), varies considerably from one preparation to the next. With lowering of the temperature below 20 °C the *ON*-evoked potential vanishes earlier than the *OFF*-evoked (Peters *et al.*, 1961).

Recovery of the normal EEG occurs in almost all cases following a three hour period of hypothermia reaching ca. 15°C (Peters *et al.*, 1961) but no details of the recovery have been reported. We too have noticed that moderate hypothermia has no apparent lasting effect on cerebral activity in the chick embryo, but also that unusual electrical patterns may appear during the transition to the normal temperature level. Thus, in the case illustrated in Fig. 24 the slow waves first increase in amplitude and then form an extremely regular pattern of unusually large, long duration waves

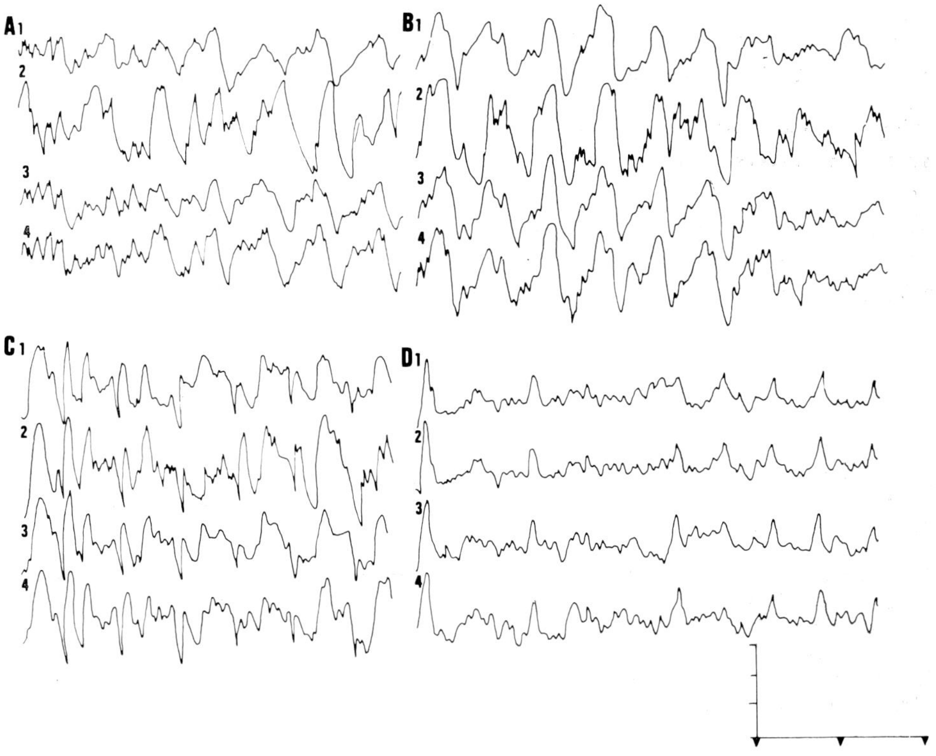

Fig. 24. Hypersynchronized cerebral EEG rhythms occurring during recovery from *hypothermia* (to 30°C). Simultaneous monopolar recordings from the right (1–2) and left (3–4) hemispheres, at medial (1, 3) and lateral (2, 4) points on the dorsal surface.
A. The onset of the synchronized slow waves.
B. The termination of the slow waves, showing the abrupt transition to an essentially normal pattern (10 sec break between A and B).
C. Return of the 'hypersynchronization', with high amplitude surface negative 'spikes' superimposed at regular intervals.
D. Small synchronized slow waves shortly before apparently full recovery of normal activity. *Calibrations*: horizontal, 1 sec per division; vertical, 50 μV per division.

which are synchronous over both hemispheres (A). After several minutes, during which the amplitude waxes and wanes at some of the leads, the EEG abruptly reverts to its usual pattern (B). When synchronous slow waves appear for a second time they are less regular and have high amplitude surface negative waves of less than 100 msec duration superimposed, at a rate of ca. two per second (C). The last sign of abnormal activity is the synchronization of slow waves over both hemispheres (D), which gives way gradually to the normal spatial pattern.

Hyperthermia of only 2–3°C quickly produces abnormalities in the electrical activity of the brain in a newly hatched chick. The effect is to reduce the number of slow waves in the cerebral hemispheres and to eliminate the high frequency waves in the optic lobes (Peters *et al.*, 1964). The remaining spontaneous cerebral slow waves become more consistent, resembling visual-evoked potentials, and are synchronous with

References p. 189–192

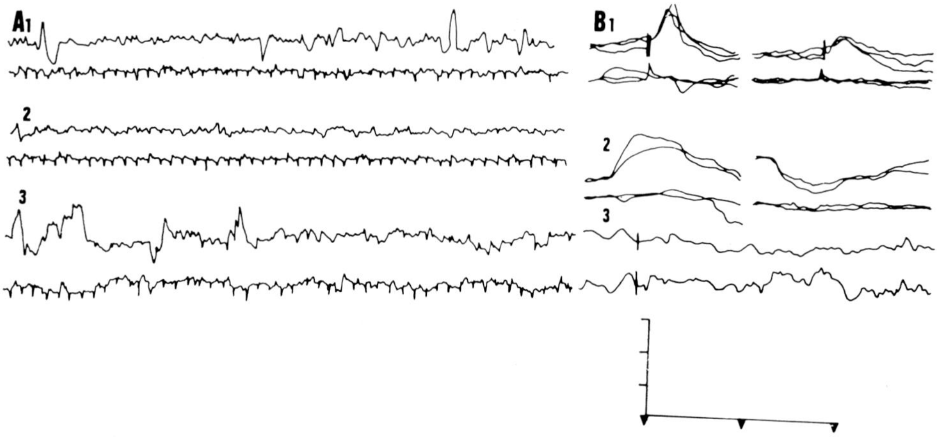

Fig. 25. Cerebral electrical activity during *hypoxia*.
A. Changes in the spontaneous EEG of a *stage-44* embryo. The large amplitude slow waves (1) which are normally present disappear (2). Shortly before electrical silence a short stretch (less than one-half minute) of augmented activity occurs (3). A simultaneous registration from the trunk is included below each cerebral record (monopolar).
B. Electrical responses to flash stimulation (1) at the *posterior* pole of the hemisphere (1 mm from the midline) during hypoxia in a *stage-45* embryo. The lower trace shows the absence of any response at a point *4 mm* from the midline and 3 mm further anterior. (There was a break of 1 min between the first set of responses and the second.) *On-* and *off-* responses are also illustrated (2). When the spontaneous EEG returns several minutes later, responses can no longer be evoked at this point (3).
Calibrations: horizontal, 2 sec per division in A, 1 sec in B; vertical, 50 μV per division in A, 100 μV in B.

smaller, more variable slow potentials in the optic lobe. Prolonged heating causes disappearance of spontaneous waves in both structures but typical evoked potentials still occur at the onset and termination of illumination. In older chicks (2–20 days old: Peters *et al.*, 1964) the only effect for a relatively long time is a reduction in slow waves, similar to that produced by normal sensory stimulation. A return to continuous slow wave activity follows, now in the optic lobe as well as in the cerebrum, together with a rapid disappearance of low amplitude fast waves. A train of fairly consistent wave complexes finally appears which resembles those evoked by visual stimulation. Although this last phase is reached much more slowly than in newly hatched and one-day old chicks, the overall EEG *survival time* is actually less than half.

Hypoxia produces certain changes in the cerebral EEG which are similar at all stages (Fig. 25A). The high amplitude surface positive waves first largely disappear, accompanied or quickly followed by an overall amplitude reduction in the remaining slow waves. A brief period of higher amplitude activity, synchronous over the entire surface, is sometimes seen just before electrical silence occurs. The faster waves usually disappear earlier than the slow ones. It has also been reported that 'spike' discharges may accompany these augmented slow waves (Garcia-Austt, 1954). Complete loss of activity may require considerable time in a deteriorating preparation but less than one minute if a large blood vessel is severed. The typical changes are also seen following local cerebral bleeding and are sometimes reversible in older embryos. In one such case a light-evoked potential was present on the posterior-medial surface of the (contralateral) hemisphere and disappeared gradually as the spontaneous electrical activity returned (Fig. 25B). Considering that pulmonary respiration begins before hatching and that an hypoxic cerebral record resembles the normal EEG of an earlier stage, it is thus possible that increasing aerobic metabolism partly determines the changing pattern of brain activity in the chick embryo.

Topical application of concentrated *potassium salts* causes, similarly to hypoxia, first a reversible reduction in amplitude and then a 'smoothing' of the cerebral slow waves (also Sedláček, 1964). It has been reported, however, that no effect can be obtained earlier than about *stage 43* and that the amplitude reduction at later stages goes only so far as a return to the *stage-43* level (Sedláček, 1966). In embryos just prior to hatching moreover, the amplitude climbs slowly back to its original level after several minutes of depression, despite continued direct application of the concentrated KCl. Drying of the brain produces irregular high voltage spikes in the cerebrum from the earliest stage at which spontaneous activity is present (Garcia-Austt, 1954). These potentials increase periodically in frequency and regularity throughout as long as 24 hours.

The *convulsant drugs* strychnine and metrazol also produce high amplitude potentials in the cerebrum of the embryo when applied topically (Garcia-Austt, 1954, 1957; Pisareva, 1965). Strychnine spikes are usually biphasic, but are reported to have in any case a surface negative phase, and are consistent in waveform in a given preparation. The duration of the negative wave is also individually consistent, averaging 250 msec in *stage-41* embryos and only ca. 100 msec thereafter. The positive wave is always longer but lasts only 150–200 msec in the late embryonic stages (Garcia-Austt, 1954) and in the adult (Bremer *et al.*, 1939). The potentials usually occur irregularly but there are periods of increased frequency similar to those seen after drying (Garcia-Austt, 1954) and after intense direct electrical stimulation (Bremer *et al.*, 1939). Young embryos are characterized by latencies up to 50 min and by low frequencies of "spike" discharge (once in *ca.* five minutes on the average) but the corresponding values at the time of hatching are five minutes latency and 20–25 wave complexes per minute. Topical metrazol application elicits similar complexes but at a rate varying between 3 and 15 per second and sometimes grouped in successive clusters (Garcia-Austt, 1957). As with strychnine, they are strongest at the point where the drug has been applied but are synchronous over much of the hemisphere and sometimes on the opposite side as well. The spontaneous activity is not clearly affected by these treatments and persists as a background for the 'spikes'. The light-evoked potential in the cerebrum is also not altered but becomes followed consistently on the treated side by a typical large amplitude negative wave (Rougeul, 1957). *Cocaine* applied topically for a few seconds completely blocks the strychnine spikes (Bremer *et al.*, 1939), an effect duplicated by *γ-aminobutyric acid (GABA)* (Pisareva, 1965), but it eliminates spontaneous and visual-evoked potentials only after a much longer treatment.

Strychnine has a similar effect upon the cerebrum of the embryo when injected as when applied topically (Katori, 1962). Waves are also elicited in the optic lobes which are not necessarily synchronous with those in the hemisphere and have a higher threshold and lower amplitude. Subconvulsive doses administered after hatching

References p. 189–192

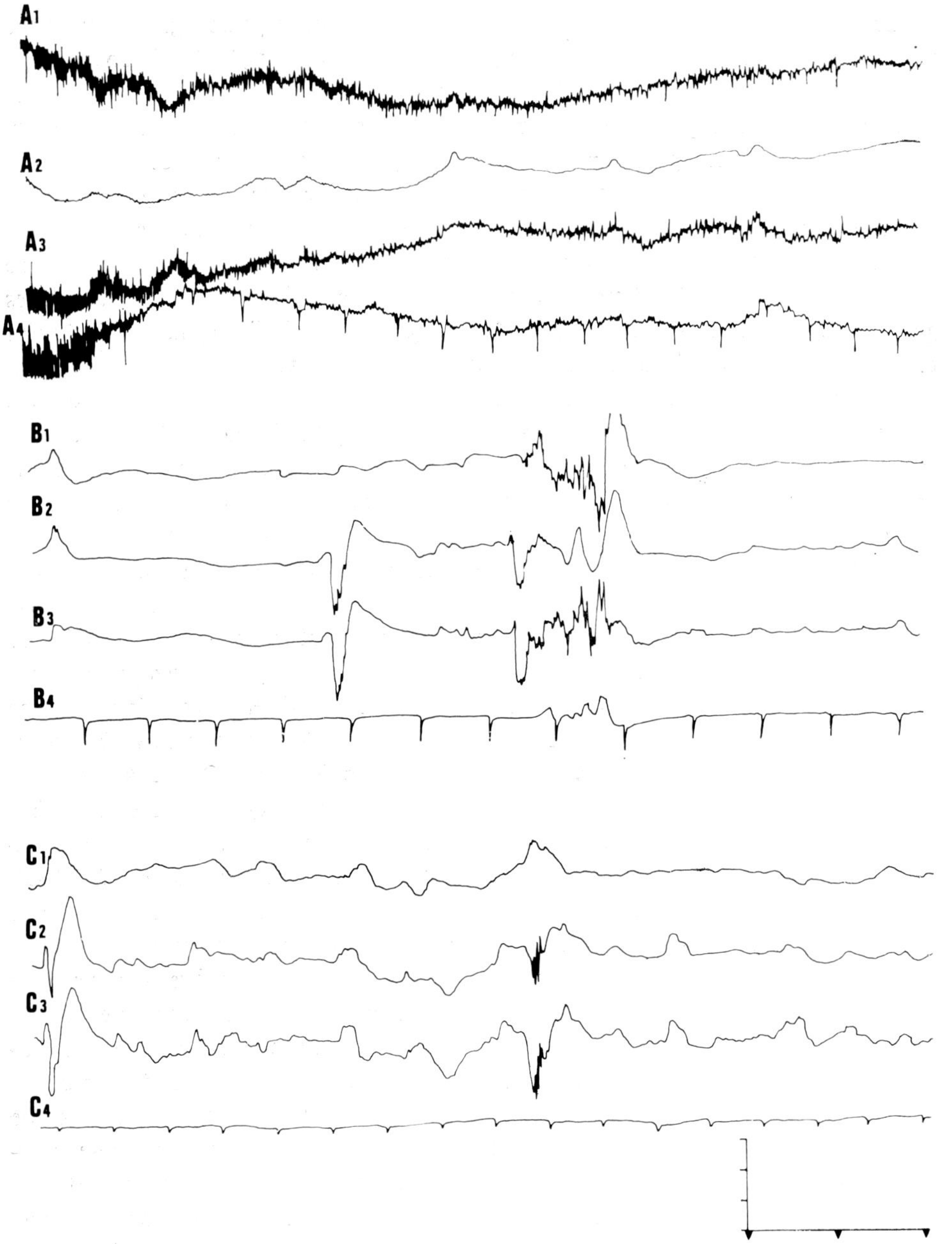

Fig. 26. Typical changes in the cerebral activity of the chick embryo following injection of *cardiazol*. Line 1 is a monopolar recording from the left side, line 2 the differential between left and right hemispheres, and line 3 monopolar from the right side; the ECG recorded simultaneously from the trunk is shown in line 4.

A. Tonic seizure, with muscle potentials and small movement artifacts appearing at each cerebral lead but not in the *differential* recording (line 2).

B. Variable unilateral wave complexes and bilateral waves accompanied by body movements in the period after disappearance of the background EEG.

C. Brief return of normal-appearing background waves with continuation of the large drug-induced potentials.

(The preparation used for illustration was at *stage 43* of development.)

Calibrations: horizontal, 1 sec per division; vertical, 50 μV per division.

cause simply a slight amplitude increase in the cerebral EEG, accompanied by decreased muscle tone (Spooner, 1964; Spooner and Winters, 1966). *Picrotoxin* too gives similar large 'spikes' after injection from the stage of earliest cerebral EEG onwards (Katori, 1962) but which are synchronous over the hemisphere and optic lobe. The amplitudes and the spike intervals are generally highly variable in an irregular sequence but high frequency bursts of regular waves occur periodically. Spikes sometime appear in the optic lobes at an even earlier stage than the appearance of the normal EEG. Injection of *GABA* in the embryo reversibly reduces the drug-elicited waves in both brain structures studied (Katori, 1962). It also eliminates flash-evoked potentials and spontaneous spikes from the optic lobe at all stages after hatching without affecting the slow waves (Scholes and Roberts, 1964). Cerebral slow waves increase in amplitude in the typical way, together with general muscular relaxation (Spooner, 1964).

Wave complexes which resemble sensory-evoked potentials are elicited in the cerebral hemispheres, in addition to the ways already mentioned, by the injection of other commonly used drugs. *Metrazol*, a convulsant, *nembutal*, a general anesthetic, and *succinyl choline*, a paralyzing agent, despite their evidently different action upon the central nervous system produce certain common effects (Figs. 26 to 28). There is a qualitatively similar picture at all embryonic stages following injection of a convulsive dose of metrazol. Little or no change occurs in the EEG until the first *tonic* muscular seizure (within a few minutes), which is accompanied by a suddenly isoelectric cerebral record save for a few small waves and continuous muscle potentials (Fig. 26A; also Peters *et al.*, 1956). Subsequent tonic phases produce this same effect but the time for recovery of the cerebral activity varies greatly. After several tonic seizures, complex potentials of large amplitude begin to accompany the *clonic* muscle contractions and the background EEG starts to decay gradually. The clonic wave complexes may be more than three times the maximal amplitude normally observed and are bilaterally synchronous, although rarely identical (Fig. 26B). Many smaller, mostly unilateral wave complexes occur throughout, with wide variation in their amplitudes, shapes and intervals. In the cases where the highest doses of the drug had been given, or following several successive injections, almost all of the large waves are surface positive. They range from 200–500 msec in duration and are often followed by a longer negative wave. Sometimes there is also a negative prepotential of less than 100 msec duration and 50 μV amplitude. Brief bursts of small high frequency oscillations appear after the above pattern has become established, usually riding upon a slow wave and conceivably representing eyeball movements (Paulson, 1964). As the cerebrum approaches an isoelectric state, these various phenomena become less and less frequent but a brief period (less than one-half minute) of return of the normal EEG often occurs (Fig. 26C). A subconvulsive dose of metrazol produces a typical electrical slow wave response in the five days old chick. Larger amounts elicit wave complexes identical to those evoked by selected thalamic stimulation (Spooner, 1964; Spooner and Winters, 1966) and resembling the large potentials just described for the embryo.

A sub-paralyzing dose of *succinyl choline* in the embryo quickly causes almost complete disappearance of the fast cerebral rhythm (Fig. 27A). The EEG may remain un-

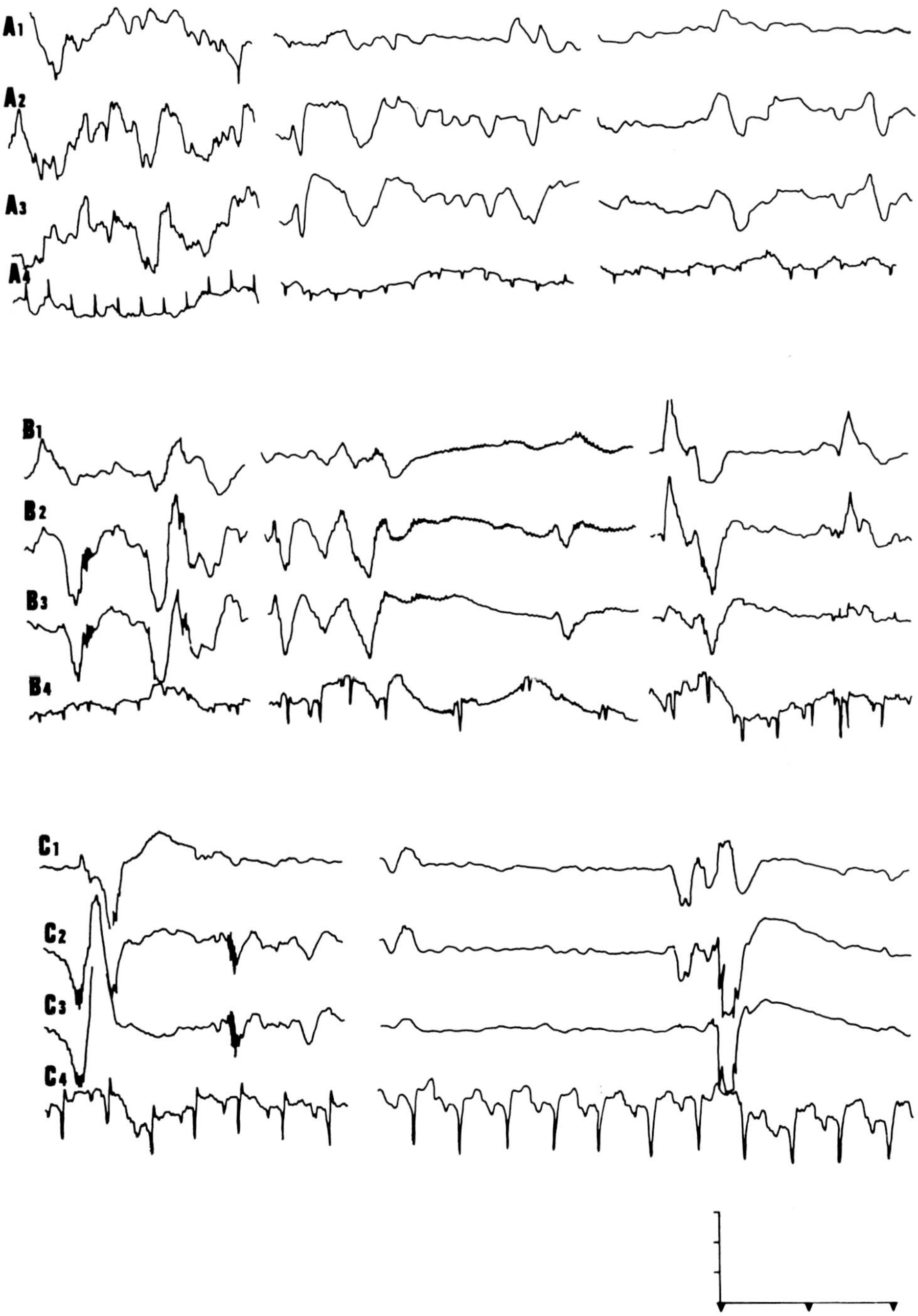
A1
A2
A3
A4
B1
B2
B3
B4
C1
C2
C3
C4

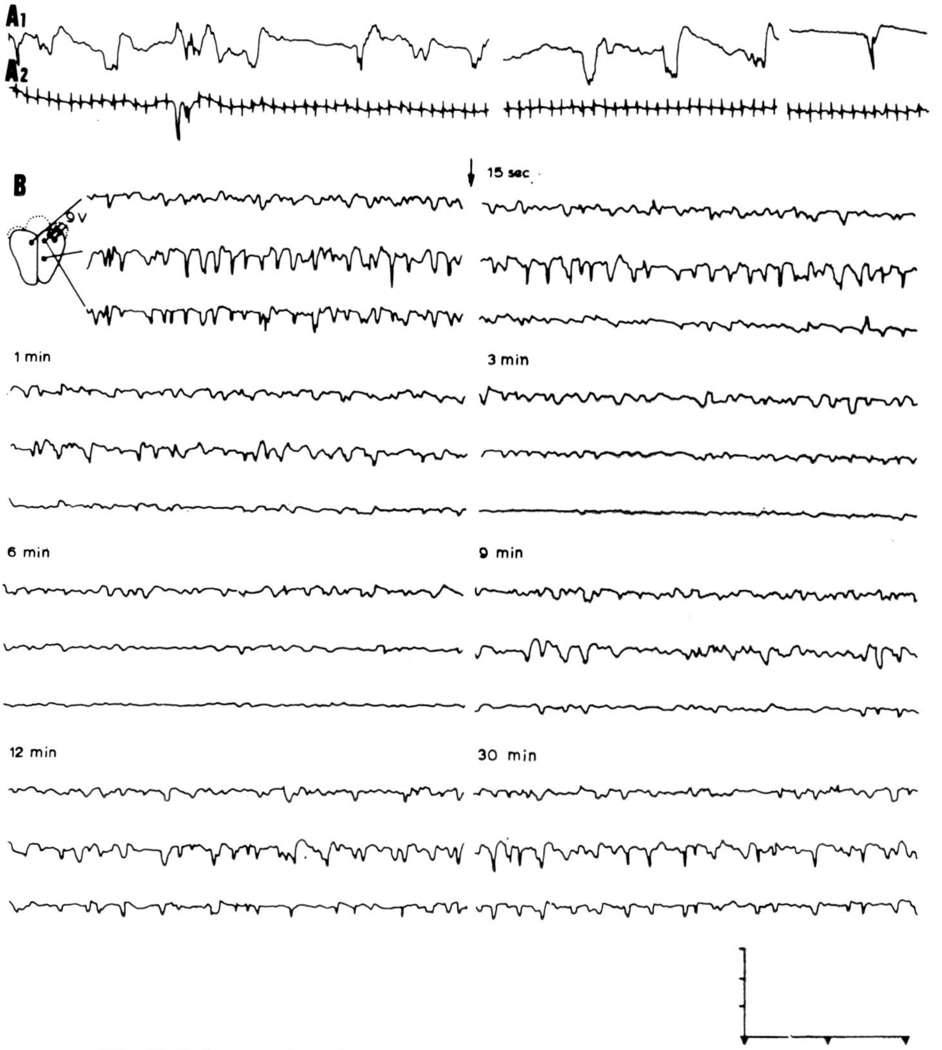

Fig. 28. Influence of *nembutal* on the cerebral electrical activity in the chick.
A. Three stretches taken respectively ½ min, 1 min, and 2 min after injection of 5 mg nembutal in a *stage44* embryo. A monopolar cerebral recording (line 1) is shown simultaneously with ECG and trunk movements (line 2).
B. Slow *spreading depression* of the 'spontaneous' electrical activity in a one week old chick under moderate anesthesia (2.5 mg). It begins several seconds after D.C. stimulation at the point indicated by the double arrow and spreads over the surface at a rate of ca. 5 mm/min. Recovery starts about 9 min after the stimulus.
Calibrations: horizontal, 2 sec per division; vertical, 100 μV per division in A and 200 μV in B.

Fig. 27. The influence of *succinyl choline* on the cerebral EEG of the chick embryo. Monopolar (lines 1 and 3) and differential recordings (line 2) from a *stage-45* preparation; the simultaneous ECG is given in line 4.
A. Three stretches showing respectively the normal pattern, the activity within one-half minute of injection (50 μV), and the activity 1 min later.
B. Three stretches showing respectively the beginning of large wave complexes against the background EEG, sudden depression later of slow electrical activity, and partial restoration 2–3 min afterwards.
C. Two stretches ca. one-half hour later, showing continuation of the large amplitude potentials with much reduced background activity.
Calibrations: horizontal, 1 sec per division; vertical, 50 μV per division.

changed for some time thereafter except for sudden periods of slow wave activity and variable bursts of irregular low amplitude oscillations. Wave complexes of high amplitude then appear, frequently bilaterally synchronous, and become more prominent as the background activity declines (Fig. 27B,C). The largest peaks are mostly surface positive and often occur in pairs, usually followed by a negative wave which is less consistent in duration. The frequency of these complexes ultimately decreases and there is a brief return of a more normal EEG shortly before the recorded electrical activity stops in the cerebrum. The records from embryos treated with *d*-tubocurarine (Katori, 1962) indicate that similar potentials may occur in both the hemisphere and the optic lobe even earlier than the onset of the normal 'spontaneous' electrical waves.

Nembutal in a minimal dose produces simply a typical large amplitude slow wave pattern in the chick after hatching (Key and Marley, 1962; Spooner, 1964; Spooner and Winters, 1966). It is also capable, however, of causing the disappearance of fast components from the cerebral EEG and silent intervals between the slow waves (Fig. 28A). Similar to the drug effects described in previous paragraphs, these intervals often become progressively longer and wave complexes of increased amplitude appear. Such potentials have a variable waveform, but are predominantly surface positive with a negative afterpotential if a large enough dose has been injected (also Ookawa and Gotoh, 1965). (Mapping of the dorsal surface of the hemisphere in the young chick (Spooner, 1964) has shown that this is actually true only up to the lamina hyperstriatum, lateral to which (neostriatum) the polarity reverses.) Spontaneous activity in the optic tectum is reduced or eliminated save for 'spikes' which are roughly synchronous with the wave complexes in the cerebrum (Ookawa and Gotoh, 1965). Visual-evoked potentials are altered so that eventually only the initial negative spike persists (Scholes and Roberts, 1964). Phenobarbital can elicite large amplitude waves in the cerebrum already at embryonic *stages 41* to *42*, and in the optic lobe slightly earlier (Katori, 1962). A striking difference from later stages of development is that the waves may build up rapidly into a high amplitude 'seizure'-like pattern before breaking up into the usual predominantly biphasic complexes. The frequency of these latter potentials undergoes periodic fluctuation at all stages, independently in the two brain structures which have been studied, but never reaches the intensity seen during the initial period of drug sensitivity. *Chlorpromazine* has an almost identical effect at these stages as phenobarbital, thus producing electrical seizures earliest in the optic lobes and slightly later in development in the cerebrum (Katori, 1962), but in older embryos it causes only a reduction of the EEG in both regions. In the five day old chick, on the contrary, typical cerebral slow waves accompanied by body relaxation result (Spooner, 1964; Spooner and Winters, 1966). A final effect of barbiturate anesthesia is to facilitate the production of *spreading depression* following electrical, chemical, or mechanical stimulation of the hemisphere surface (Fig. 28B). This phenomenon has never been observed earlier than five days after hatching and the probability of its occurrence increases with the depth of the drug effect (Ookawa and Gotoh, 1964). Its characteristics have been extensively studied in the cerebrum of adult birds (Bureš *et al.*, 1960; Shima and Fifková, 1963; Shima *et al.*, 1963).

The 'hallucinogenic' agent *d-lysergic acid diethylamide* (LSD) has also been studied

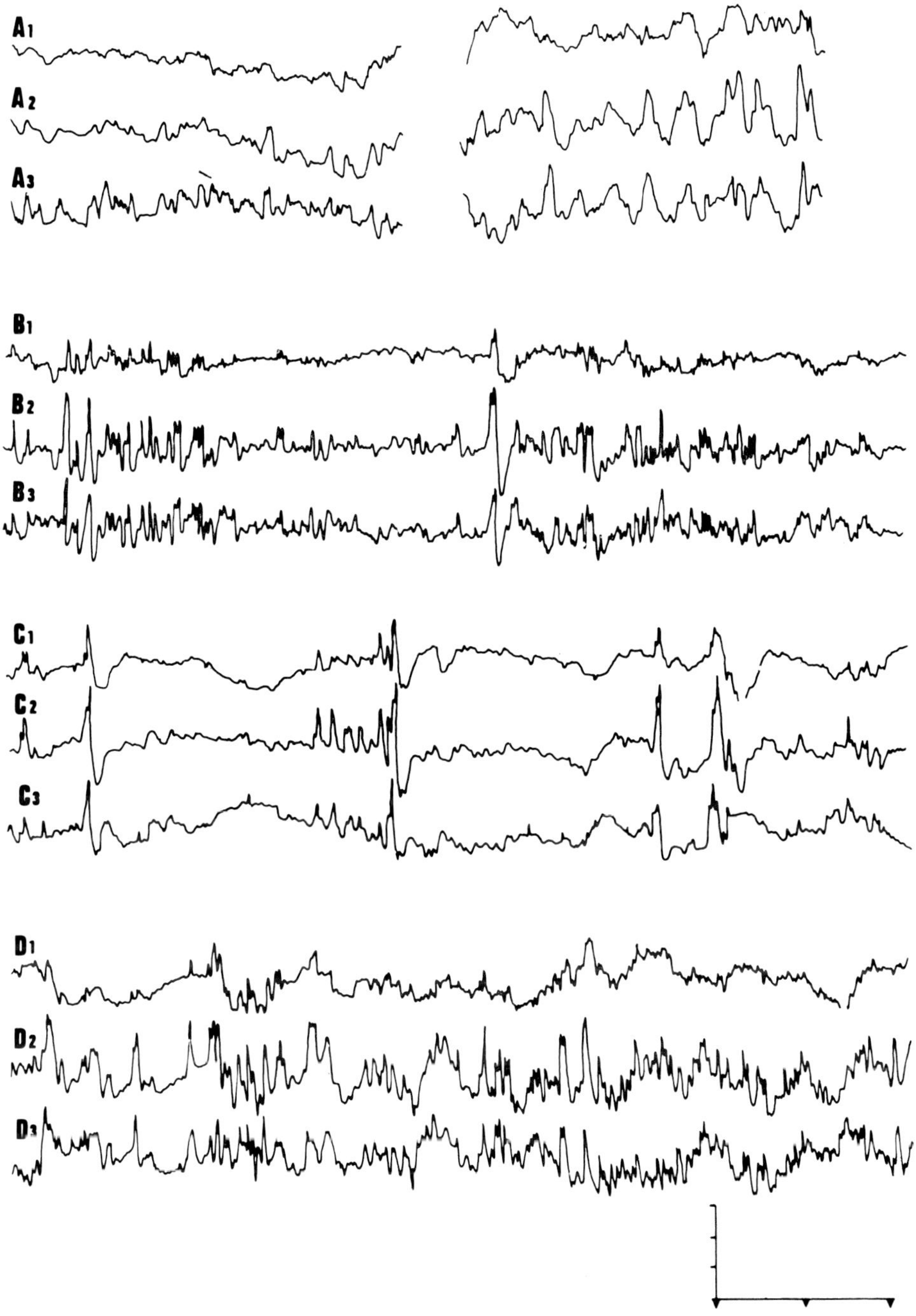

Fig. 29. Influence of *LSD* on the cerebral EEG in a *stage-45* chick embryo. Simultaneous monopolar recordings several millimeters below (line 1) and just at the dorsal surface of the hemisphere (line 3). The differential between the two points is shown in line 2.
A. Two stretches of the pre-injection activity showing respectively low and high amplitude phases.
B–D. Variable patterns of high frequency barrages and large wave complexes occurring continually after injection. (C–D is a continuous record.)
Calibrations: horizontal, 1 sec per division; vertical, 50 μV per division.

References p. 189–192

in the chick embryo (Katori, 1962). Potentials similar to those described in preceding paragraphs are elicited in the cerebrum, as a rule synchronous over a wide area, at a stage prior to the earliest EEG. At all later stages the optic lobe responds as well, in a similar way but not necessarily simultaneously with the cerebral waves. In our experience a minute amount of LSD (5 μg injected intraperitoneally) duplicated in a *stage-45* embryo the effects of a moderate dose of nembutal (Fig. 29). Changes in the cerebral EEG began about 15 min after injection and persisted for at least three hours. Stretches of low amplitude alternated with variable duration barrages of 'spike'-shaped waves and high amplitude complexes. An electrode several millimeters below the surface registered synchronous waves which were mostly smaller and often of the opposite polarity. LSD and several other hallucinogens have been found to produce in the five day old chick first a long-lasting low amplitude cerebral EEG which seems identical to that following sensory stimulation. This occurs despite a relaxed body position and often closed eyes but may be succeeded by typical large slow waves (Spooner, 1964; Spooner and Winters, 1966). In the optic lobe these drugs all eliminate the 'spontaneous' electrical waves while leaving visually evoked potentials and spike discharges unchanged (Fig. 17).

The effect upon the cerebral EEG of a large number of *catechol-*, *indole-*, and *phenylethyl*-amines has been studied in the chick at different ages after hatching. Three groups of drugs could be distinguished on the basis of the physiological effects during the first month of life, which proved to be clearly related to the chemical structure (Key and Marley, 1962; Dewhurst and Marley, 1965a, b). *Central depressant* amines produce typical slow waves together with relaxation and decreased responsiveness and activity (i.e. *sleep*). Chemicals of this class are distinguished by the presence of substituted groups (chlor-, methoxy-, or 3,4 hydroxy-) on a phenyl or indole ring with an aliphatic side chain. Adrenaline is the most potent member and nor-adrenaline and dopamine are also included. *Central excitant* amines are devoid of substituted groups on both the ring structure and the β-carbon of the side chain; they produce a typical *alert* behavior and EEG. The most potent members are tryptamine and amphetamine. Drugs of one group antagonize the effects of the other, and for both groups the most potent effect is obtained with an N-methylated two-carbon side chain. Most of the structurally-intermediate chemicals (*i.e.* with a single hydroxyl group, either on the aromatic ring or on the β-carbon) have equivocal effects or none at all, but some fall unpredictably into either the 'depressant' or the 'excitant' class. From four weeks of age the chicks enter a transitional phase lasting two to three weeks wherein previously depressant amines elicit episodes of low voltage activity alternating with the slow wave stretches. After this phase the response is identical to that of the adult, *i.e.* low amplitude cerebral activity associated as usual with alert and active behavior.

In addition to confirming the above results in the five day old chick, Spooner (1964) and Spooner and Winters (1965) have investigated the effects upon this preparation of several other neurologically important chemicals. *Acetyl choline* and other parasympathetically acting substances produce electrical slow waves and body relaxation when injected in the lowest effective doses but may have opposite effects in larger quantities or if injected intracerebrally. The indole amine *serotonin* (5-hydroxytryptamine) and *reserpine* also produce at first a typical electrical slow wave pattern. Increasing doses of serotonin, however, cause an abnormal EEG (Hehman *et al.*, 1961) which differs from that seen following any of the treatments described up till now. The rapid rhythm disappears but the slow waves, rather than breaking up into short complexes, become abnormally large and regular (reminiscent of the initial effect of hyperthermia). Irregular positive spikes appear with still larger doses, at a mean frequency of 12–16 per second and independently in each hemisphere, while the slow waves gradually disappear. The spikes are variable but do not exceed 50 msec in duration or 50 μV in amplitude.

F. Impedance changes in chick brain

In recent years a considerable number of investigations have been reported on impedance measurements in the central nervous system (van Harreveld, 1966). The electrical resistance of brain tissue is determined mainly by the interstitial or extracellular electrolytes, since most of the intracellular electrolytes enclosed by high impedance cell membranes cannot readily participate in the transport of the measuring current. The specific resistance of brain tissue is therefore a good indication of its extracellular space. Since changes and shifts of electrolytes are of primary importance for neural function a systematic study was made of the impedance changes during development of the chick brain.

High and low frequency impedance measurements (10–40 Mc/sec and 400 c/sec respectively) show characteristic changes during development of various brain areas. High frequency impedance of the cerebellum and optic lobes is relatively low between the 11th and 16th day of incubation and its values are about 1–4 kΩ (Fig. 30). The same results are found in the hemispheres. There exists a sudden change in high frequency impedance on the 17th day of incubation in all parts of the brain. This change

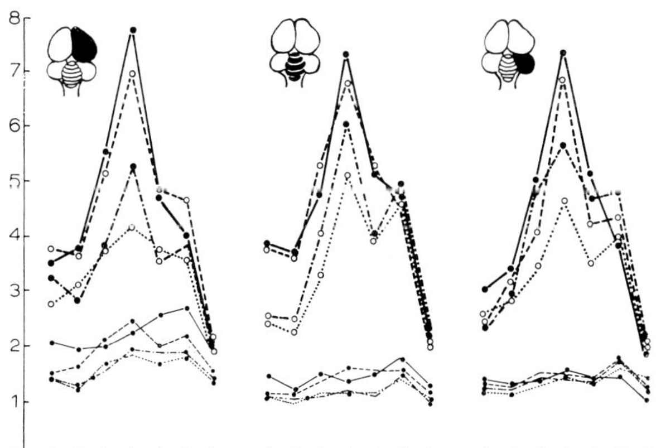

Fig. 30. Development of high frequency impedance of some brain areas in chick embryos. Abscissa: frequency in Mc/s; ordinate: impedance in kΩ. Thin lines: dotted line–13 th day of incubation, dot dash line–14th day, broken–15th day, full–16th day. Thick lines: dotted–17th day, dot and dash–18th day, broken line–20th day, full–21st day.

References p. 189–192

is very marked and amounts on the 17th day to 4–5 kΩ and on the 21st day of incubation to 7–8 kΩ. The impedance now becomes frequency dependent. Two peaks appear at 25 and at 35 Mc/sec. The second peak, however, gradually disappears as impedance values at 25 Mc/sec increase further. Maximum values of high frequency impedance thus increase between the 17th and 21st day by a factor of 4 in the hemispheres, by a factor of 5.5 in the cerebellum, and by a factor of 5 in the optic lobes.

Changes in low frequency impedance have a rather similar course. Between the 13th and 15th day of incubation the low frequency impedance is about 1.5 kΩ. A considerable increase occurs starting from the 17th day and continuing up to the 21st day of incubation.

Without going into details about the theoretical considerations concerning impedance changes in the brain, it is interesting to note that during a relatively short period of the development major changes in the impedance have been found. It seems safe to assume (van Harreveld, 1966) that the specific impedance is a measure for the extracellular space in the brain, at least as far as adult brain tissue is concerned.

Apparently the period between the 17th and 21st day of incubation is characterized by major shifts in the electrolytes between the cellular and extracellular compartments of the brain. The brain seems to reach an adult situation as far as the distribution of electrolytes is concerned. Whether these changes are due to the maturation of membrane properties or to some other factors has to be determined by potential measurements of the neuronal and glial membranes. (This research is in progress at present.)

SUMMARY

(1) A review has been made, including results obtained by the authors, of the known electrophysiological parameters which define normal brain development in the chick. Spontaneous electroencephalograms, steady potential levels, and potentials evoked in the brain by sensory or direct electrical stimulation have been described. The modifications produced by various environmental alterations and by the administration of certain chemicals have also been reviewed.

(2) Spontaneous slow waves appear in the hyperstriatum, optic tectum and cerebellum at the beginning of the third (last) week of incubation. Potentials can be elicited still earlier by a number of commonly used drugs.

(3) The early electric activity is similar in all three structures and consists of apparently randomly patterned waves. The cerebral hemispheres and optic lobes each subsequently develop a distinctive pattern of electrical activity. The cerebrum shows large amplitude, predominantly surface positive slow potentials while the tectum, beginning at a later stage, shows bursts of 'spikes'.

(4) The tectal spontaneous activity matures over the first three days after hatching to a pattern of continual but irregular spikes, with periods of superimposed slower potentials. The latter occur simultaneously with the slow waves in the cerebral hemispheres but are much smaller in amplitude.

(5) The cerebral slow waves increase rapidly during *stage 43* both in mean and peak amplitudes and in the frequency of their occurrence, and reach almost mature levels

already at two to three days before hatching. Brief flattening of the electrical record then begins to occur intermittently (*stage 44*) during periods lasting several minutes, alternating with periods of continuous slow waves whose regularity fluctuates. This is also the pattern seen after hatching during behavioral sleep but the periods of flattening are much less extensive than during late embryonic development (*stage 45*).

(6) The optic lobe is the first brain structure studied to respond to sensory stimulation (light). This occurs only in the last day or two before hatching (*stage 45*) and is followed shortly by similar responses in the cerebral hemisphere (hyperstriatum). Polyphasic potentials are evoked by light in both of these structures and by sound in a different region of the cerebrum. The latency, duration and recovery time of these responses decrease with maturation. Slow fluctuations in excitability occur, sometimes simultaneously in the two regions of the brain.

(7) Sensory stimulation in all modalities causes disappearance of the large cerebral slow waves, beginning several hours after hatching. At about the same time, the spontaneous cerebral electrical activity begins a cyclic disappearance and reappearance of these waves, correlated with behavioral *waking* and *sleeping* respectively. The percentage of time spent in the waking state increases rapidly throughout the first day. The corresponding electrical record shows a continually fluctuating level of small slow waves which then increase progressively in amplitude with the transition to the sleeping state.

(8) Electrical stimulation of the cerebral hemisphere, high temperature or treatment with strychnine, nembutal and many other drugs can elicit trains of large amplitude waves resembling sensory evoked-potentials. These waves are generally irregular in timing and variable in their consecutive amplitudes and intervals, and they undergo furthermore wide fluctuations in the *mean* values of all these variables. They are abolished by γ-aminobutyric acid.

(9) Shocks can elicit a *direct cerebral response* long before the onset of spontaneous electrical activity. This is a very brief surface negative wave until shortly after the time of the earliest EEG, whereupon a longer negative wave follows the short one. The amplitude increases progressively during *stage 43* and several additional components appear shortly before hatching. No spreading of excitation over the hemisphere surface occurs until late in embryonic development (*stage 45*).

(10) High and low frequency impedance measurements have shown characteristic shifts in the electrical properties of brain areas between the 17th and 21st day of incubation, indicating major shifts in the distribution of electrolytes.

REFERENCES

BREMER, F., DOW, R. S., AND MORUZZI, G., (1939);Physiological analysis of the general cortex in reptiles and birds. *J. Neurophysiol.*, **2**, 473–487.

BUREŠ, J., FIFKOVÁ, E., AND MARŠALA, J., (1960); Leão's spreading depression in pigeons. *J. comp. Neurol.*, **114**, 1–10.

BUSER, P., AND ROUGEUL, A., (1954); La réponse électrique du cervelet de pigeon à la stimulation de la voie optique et son analyse par microélectrodes, *J. Physiol.*, **46**, 287–291.

CASTRO, G. DE OLVEIRA, (1963); Effects of reduction of nerve centers on the development of residual ganglia and nerve patterns in the wing of the chick embryo. *J. exptl. Zool.*, **152**, 279–294.

CORNER, M. A., PETERS, J. J., AND RUTGERS VAN DER LOEFF, P., (1966); Electrical activity patterns in the cerebral hemispheres of the chick during maturation, correlated with behavior in a test situation. *Brain Res.*, **2**, 274–292.

CRAGG, B. G., EVANS, D., AND HAMLYN, L. H., (1954); The optic tectum of *Gallus domesticus*: a correlation of the electrical responses with the histological structure. *J. Anat. (London)*, **88**, 292–306.

DELONG, G. R., AND COULOMBRE, A. J., (1965); Development of the retinotectal topographic projection in the chick embryo. *exptl. Neurol.*, **13**, 351–363.

DEWHURST, W. G., AND MARLEY, E., (1965a); The effects of α-methyl derivatives of noradrenaline, phenylethylamine and tryptamine on the central nervous system of the chicken. *Brit. J. Pharm.*, **25**, 682–704.

DEWHURST, W. G., AND MARLEY, E., (1965b); Action of sympathomimetic and allied amines on the central nervous system of the chicken. *Brit. J. Pharm.*, **25**, 705–727.

ERULKAR, S. D., (1955); Tactile and auditory areas in the brain of the pigeon. *J. comp. Neurol.*, **103**, 421–440.

GARCIA-AUSTT, E., (1954); Development of electrical activity in the cerebral hemispheres of the chick embryo. *Proc. Soc. exptl. Biol. Med.*, **86**, 345–352.

GARCIA-AUSTT, E., (1957); Ontogenetic evolution of the electroencephalogram in humans and animals. In: *Proc. IV Int. Congr. Electroenceph. clin. Neurophysiol.*, pp. 173–177.

GARCIA-AUSTT, E., AND PATETTA-QUEIROLO, M. A., (1961); The electroretinogram of the chick embryo. I. Onset and development. *Acta Neurol. latinoamer.*, **7**, 179–189.

GOGAN, P., (1963); Projections sensorielles au niveau du télencéphale chez le pigeon sans anesthésie générale. *J. Physiol.*, **55**, 248–259.

HAMBDI, F. A., AND WHITTERIDGE, D., (1954); The representation of the retina on the optic tectum of the pigeon. *Quart. J. exptl. Physiol.*, **39**, 111–118.

HAMBURGER, V., (1956); Developmental correlations in neurogenesis. In D. Rudnick (Ed.), *Cellular Mechanisms in Differentiation and Growth*. Princeton Univ. Press, pp. 191–212.

HAMBURGER, V., (1958); Regression versus peripheral control of differentiation in motor hypoplasia. *Amer. J. Anat.*, **102**, 365–409.

HAMBURGER, V., (1961); Experimental analysis of the dual origin of the trigeminal ganglion in the chick embryo. *J. exptl. Zool.*, **148**, 91–124.

HAMBURGER, V., AND HAMILTON, H. L., (1951); A series of normal stages in the development of the chick embryo. *J. Morphol.*, **88**, 49–92.

HARA, K., (1961); Regional neural differentiation induced by prechordal and presumptive chordal mesoderm in the chick embryo. *Thesis Utrecht Univ.*, 44 pp.

HEHMAN, K. N., VONDERAHE, A. R., AND PETERS, J. J., (1961); Effect of serotonin on behavior, electrical activity of the brain, and seizure threshold of the newly hatched chick. *Neurology*, **11**, 1011–1016.

HUGHES, A., (1955); Ultra-violet studies on the developing chick nervous system. In H. Waelsch (Ed.), *Biochemistry of the Devléoping Nervous System*. Academic Press, New York, pp. .166–168.

JONES, A. W., AND LEVI-MONTALCINI, R., (1958); Patterns of differentiation of the nerve centers and fiber tracts of the avian cerebral hemispheres. *Arch. Ital. Biol.*, **96**, 231–284.

JOUVET, M., (1965); Paradoxical sleep — a study of its nature and mechanisms. In K. Akert, C. Bally, and J. P. Schadé (Eds.), Sleep Mechanisms. *Progr. in Brain Research, vol. 18*. Elsevier, Amsterdam, pp. 20–57.

KAMP, A., KOK, M. L., AND QUARTEL, F. W. DE (1965); A multiwire cable for recording from moving subjects. *Electroenceph. clin. Neurophysiol.*, **18**, 422–423.

KATORI, M., (1962); The development of the spontaneous electrical activity in the brain of a chick embryo and the effects of several drugs on it. *Japan. J. Pharm.*, **12**, 9–25.

KEY, B. J., AND MARLEY, E., (1962); Effects of the sympathomimetic amines on behaviour and electrocortical activity of the chicken. *Electroenceph. clin. Neurophysiol.*, **14**, 90–105.

KLEIN, M., (1963); Étude polygraphique et phylogènique des états de sommeil. *Thèse, Fac. De Médicine de Lyon*, 101 pp.

KLEIN, M., MICHEL, F., AND JOUVET, M., (1964); Étude polygraphique du sommeil chez les oiseaux. *C. R. Soc. Biol.*, **158**, 99–103.

LAVELLE, A., (1965); Critical periods of neuronal maturation. In W. A. Himwich and H. E. Himwich (Eds.), The Developing Brain. *Progr. in Brain Research, vol. 9*. Elsevier, Amsterdam, pp. 93–96.

LEVI-MONTALCINI, R., (1958); Chemical stimulation of nerve growth. In W. D. McElroy and B. Glass (Eds.), *A Symposium on the Chemical Basis of Development*. Johns Hopkins Univ. Press, Baltimore, pp. 645–664.

LEVI-MONTALCINI, R., (1964); Events in the developing nervous system. In D. P. Purpura and J. P. Schadé (Eds.), Growth and Maturation of the Brain. *Progr. in Brain Research, vol. 4.* Elsevier, Amsterdam, pp. 1–26.

MOTTET, K., AND BARRON, D., (1954); Effects of the peripheral field on the cytochemical differentiation of neurones. *Yale J. Biol. Med.*, **26**, 275–292.

O'LEARY, J. L., AND BISHOP, G. H., (1943); Analysis of potential sources in the optic lobe of duck and goose. *J. cell. comp. Physiol.*, **22**, 78–87.

OOKAWA, T., AND GOTOH, J., (1964a); Spreading EEG depression in chickens. *Poultry Sci.*, **43**, 1294–1296.

OOKAWA, T., AND GOTOH, J., (1964b); Electroencephalographic study of chickens: periodic recurrence of low voltage and fast waves during behavioral sleep. *Poultry Sci.*, **43**, 1603–1604.

OOKAWA, T., AND GOTOH, J., (1965); Electroencephalogram of the chicken recorded from the skull under various conditions. *J. comp. Neurol.*, **124**, 1–14.

PAULSON, G. W., (1964); The avian EEG: an artifact associated with ocular movements. *Electroenceph. clin. Neurophysiol.*, **16**, 611–613.

PAULSON, G. W., (1965); Maturation of the evoked responses in the duckling. *Exptl. Neurol.*, **11**, 324–333.

PETERS, J. J., CUSICK, C. J., AND VONDERAHE, A. R., (1961); Electrical studies of hypothermic effects on the eye, cerebrum, and skeletal muscles of the developing chick. *J. exptl. Zool.*, **148**, 31–40.

PETERS, J. J., CUSICK, C. J., AND VONDERAHE, A. R., (1963); Influence of photic stimulation and hypothermia on the electromyogram of the developing chick. *Amer. J. Physiol.*, **204**, 304–308.

PETERS, J. J., VONDERAHE, A. R., AND MCDONOUGH, J. J., (1964); Electrical changes in brain and eye of the developing chick during hyperthermia. *Amer. J. Physiol.*, **207**, 260–264.

PETERS, J. J., VONDERAHE, A. R., AND POWERS, T. H., (1956); The functional chronology in the developing chick nervous system. *J. exptl. Zool.*, **133**, 505–518.

PETERS, J. J., VONDERAHE, A. R., AND POWERS, T. H., (1958); Electrical studies of functional development of the eye and optic lobes in the chick embryo. *J. exptl. Zool.*, **139**, 459–468.

PETERS, J. J., VONDERAHE, A. R., AND POWERS, T. H., (1960); Chronological development of electrical activity in the optic lobes, cerebellum, and the cerebrum of the chick embryo. *Physiol. Zool.*, **33**, 225–231.

PETERS, J. J., VONDERAHE, A. R., AND SCHMID, D., (1965); Onset of cerebral electrical activity associated with behavioral sleep and attention in the developing chick. *J. exptl. Zool.*, **160**, 255–262.

PETERSON, E., AND MURRAY, M., (1955); Myelin sheath formation in chick spinal ganglion cultures. *Amer. J. Anat.*, **96**, 319–353.

PHILLIPS, R. E., (1966); Evoked potential study of connections of the avian archistriatum and caudal neostriatum, *J. comp. Neurol.*, **127**, 89–100.

PISAREVA, N. L., (1962); The influence of γ-aminobutyric acid on the electrical activity of the brain in birds in embryogenesis (in Russian, English summary). *J. higher nerv. Activ.*, **12**, 734–739.

PISAREVA, N. L., (1965); Bioelectrical responses from midbrain tectum evoked by photic stimuli in chick embryos (in Russian, English summary). *J. Evol. Biochem. Physiol.*, **1**, 175–182.

RAMON Y CAJAL, S., (1960); *Studies on Vertebrate Neurogenesis* (transl. by L. Guth). Charles Thomas, Springfield, Ill., 432 pp.

ROGERS, K. T., (1960); Studies on chick brain of biochemical differentiation related to morphological differentiation and onset of function. II. Histochemical localization of alkaline phosphatase. *J. exptl. Zool.*, **145**, 49–60.

ROUGEUL, A., (1957); Exploration oscillographique de la voie visuelle du pigeon: projections mésencéphaliques, télencéphaliques et cérébelleuses. *Thèse, Fac. de Médicine de Paris*, 114 pp.

ROUGEUL, M. B., AND BUSER, P., (1953); Données sur la topographie des projections visuelles dans l'encéphale du pigeon. *C.R. Soc. Biol.*, **147**, 1750.

SCHADÉ, J. P., (1959); Maturational aspects of EEG and of spreading depression in rabbit. *J. Neurophysiol.*, **22**, 245–257.

SCHADÉ, J. P., CORNER, M. A., AND PETERS, J. J., (1965); Some aspects of the electro-ontogenesis of sleep patterns. In K. Akert, C. Bally and J. P. Schadé (Eds.), Sleep Mechanisms. *Progr. in Brain Research, vol. 18.* Elsevier. Amsterdam, pp. 70–78.

SCHOLES, N. W., (1964); The optic system of the chick: a tool for the study of drugs acting within the central nervous system. *Proc. West. Pharm. Soc.*, **7**, 45.

SCHOLES, N. W., (1966); Pharmacological definition of neuronal components generating spontaneous and evoked potentials in the tectum of the chick: effect of γ-hydroxybutyrate (GOHBA). *J. Pharm. exptl. Therap.* (in press).

SCHOLES, N. W., AND ROBERTS, E., (1964); Pharmacological studies of the optic system of the chick: effect of γ-aminobutyric acid and pentobarbital. *Biochem. Pharm.*, **13**, 1319–1324.

SEDLÁČEK, J., (1963); The problems of the ontogenetic origin of the mechanism of temporary connection (in Russian, English summary). *Acta Univ. Carol. Med.*, **4**, 265–317.

SEDLÁČEK, J., (1964); Effect of EEG depression on the temporary connection in chick embryos. *Physiol. Bohemoslov.*, **13**, 510–514.

SEDLÁČEK, J., (1966); Development of the steady potential of the brain of chick embryos. *Physiol. Bohemoslov.*, **15**, 111–116.

SEDLÁČEK, J., AND MAČEK, O., (1966); The development of brain impedance in chick embryos. *Physiol. Bohemoslov.*, **15**, 104–110.

SHARMA, K. N., DUA, S., SINGH, B., AND ANAND, B. K., (1964); Electro-ontogenesis of cerebral and cardiac activities in the chick embryo. *Electroenceph. clin. Neurophysiol.*, **16**, 503–509.

SHEFF, A. G., AND TUREEN, L. L. (1962); EEG studies of normal and encephalomalacic chicks. *Proc. Soc. exptl. Biol. Med.*, **111**, 407–409.

SHIMA, I., AND FIFKOVÁ, E., (1963); Remote effects of striatal spreading depression in pigeon brain. *Japan. J. Physiol.*, **13**, 630–640.

SHIMA, I., FIFKOVÁ, E., AND BUREŠ, J., (1963); Limits of spreading depression in pigeon striatum. *J. comp. Neurol.*, **121**, 485–492.

SPOONER, C. E., (1954); Observations on the use of the chick in the pharmacological investigation of the central nervous system. *Ph. D. thesis, Univ. of Calif., Los Angeles, Univ. microfilms*, no. 64–6387, Ann Arbor, Mich., 222 pp.

SPOONER, C. E., (1965); Preparation and implantation of brain electrodes in the young chick. *Electroenceph. clin. neurophysiol.*, **18**, 419–421.

SPOONER, C. E., AND WINTERS, W. D., (1965); Evidence for a direct action of monoamines on the chick central nervous system. *Experientia*, **21**, 256–258.

SPOONER, C. E., AND WINTERS, W. D., (1966); Neuropharmacological profile of the young chick. *Int. J. Neuropharmacol.*, **5**, 217–236.

STEFANELLI, A., (1954); Autonomous differentiation of some chick neurons isolated in chorion-allantoic grafts. *Nature*, **174**, 974.

SZÉKELY, G., AND SZENTÁGOTHAI, J., (1962); Reflex and behavior patterns from implanted supernumerary limbs in the chick. *J. Embryol. exptl. Morphol.*, **10**, 140–151.

TUGE, H., KANAYAMA, Y., AND YUEH, C. H., (1960); Comparative studies on the development of the EEG. *Japan. J. Physiol.*, **10**, 211–220.

VAN HARREVELD, A., (1966); *Brain tissue electrolytes.* Butterworths, Washington, 171 pp.

Developmental Patterns in the Central Nervous System of Birds

II. Some Biochemical Parameters of Embryonic and Post-Embryonic Maturation

J. VOS, J. P. SCHADÉ AND H. J. VAN DER HELM

Central Institute for Brain Research, Amsterdam (The Netherlands)

INTRODUCTION

The study of the relationship between physiological events and structure has been greatly aided by results of biochemical investigations at the cellular and subcellular level. Although an overwhelming number of papers on neurochemical subjects have been published in recent years, we are still very far from drawing causal relationships between, e.g. enzymatic patterns and synaptic potentials.

A detailed and thorough investigation of the developing brain may shed some light on these problems, because structural, physiological and biochemical changes occur in a developing organ in established sequence and chronology and can be studied under normal and altered conditions.

The next decade may bring great progress in explaining the basic chemical changes accompanying the neurophysiological events observed in the growing brain. We are inclined to look at correlations at the molecular level, but before we can work at such a high magnification, we have to assemble the building stones for gross correlations.

The present report deals with changes found in nitrogen and water content as well as in protein composition and enzyme activities during the latter part of embryonic life of the chick brain. A number of post-hatched stages are also included in the analyses. The investigations reported here will provide a basis for further study of events at the microchemical level.

1. Brain weight

The results of measurements of brain weight are represented in Fig. 1. A single cerebral hemisphere increases in weight from about 30 mg at 10 days of incubation to 250 mg at 10 days post-hatching. The largest increase occurs between 12 days

---

* This research was supported in part by grants from the National Institute of Neurological Diseases and Blindness (NB 3048) and from the National Institute of Mental Health (MH 6825), Public Health Service, Bethesda, U.S.A.

References p. 210–213

(49 mg) and 20 days of incubation (250 mg). The optic lobe increases only from 30 mg at 10 days of incubation to 90 mg at 10 days post-hatching. The period of rapid increase in this case also occurs between 12 and 20 days of incubation.

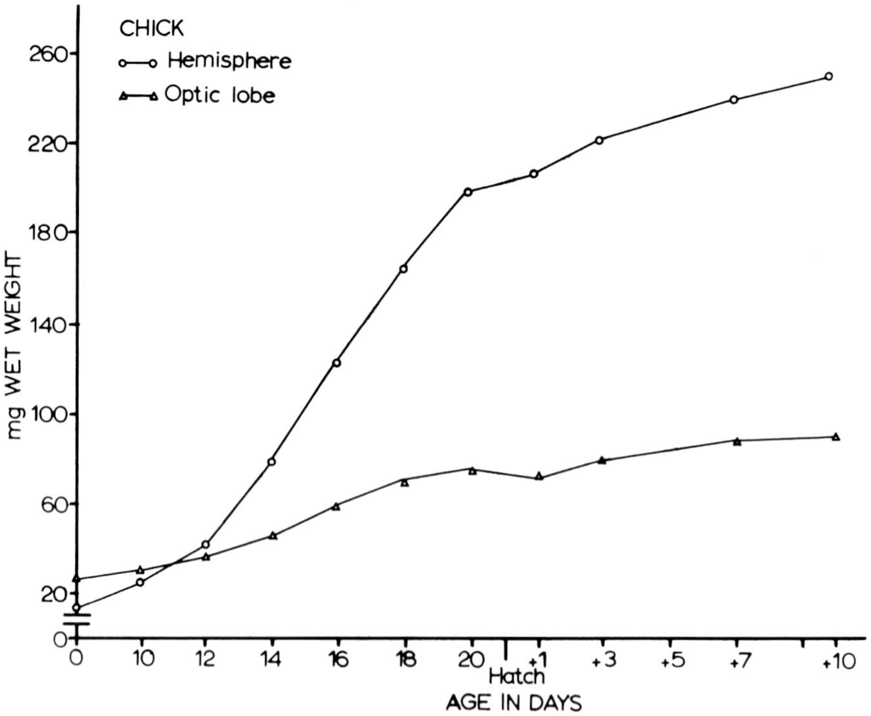

Fig. 1. Growth of chick hemisphere and optic lobe.

2. *Water content*

In 1913 Koch and Koch already showed that in the rat the water content of the brain decreased markedly from birth to maturity. This is a common finding which has been shown for a number of species, e.g. rabbit (Graves and Himwich, 1955; Davison and Wajda, 1959), mouse (Uzman and Rumley, 1958), guinea pig (Flexner and Flexner, 1950), dog (Himwich and Fazekas, 1941), cat (Yannet and Darrow, 1938) and chick (Mandel *et al.*, 1947). This change in water content poses a specific problem in expressing biochemical parameters per unit of wet weight. It is generally observed that the water concentration decreases from approximately 90% to about 80% in whole brain of different species from the onset of the rapid growth phase to the adult stage. The concentration of solids nearly doubles in a relatively short time. It has therefore been assumed that small increases in constituents or enzyme concentrations in the developing brain may represent only the decrease in water concentration (Sperry, 1962). For this reason biochemical parameters of the developing and maturing brain have often been expressed on a dry weight basis or using protein content or DNA as a reference. However, values based on a wet weight of tissue reflect the actual functional amount of constituents present in the tissue in a better way.

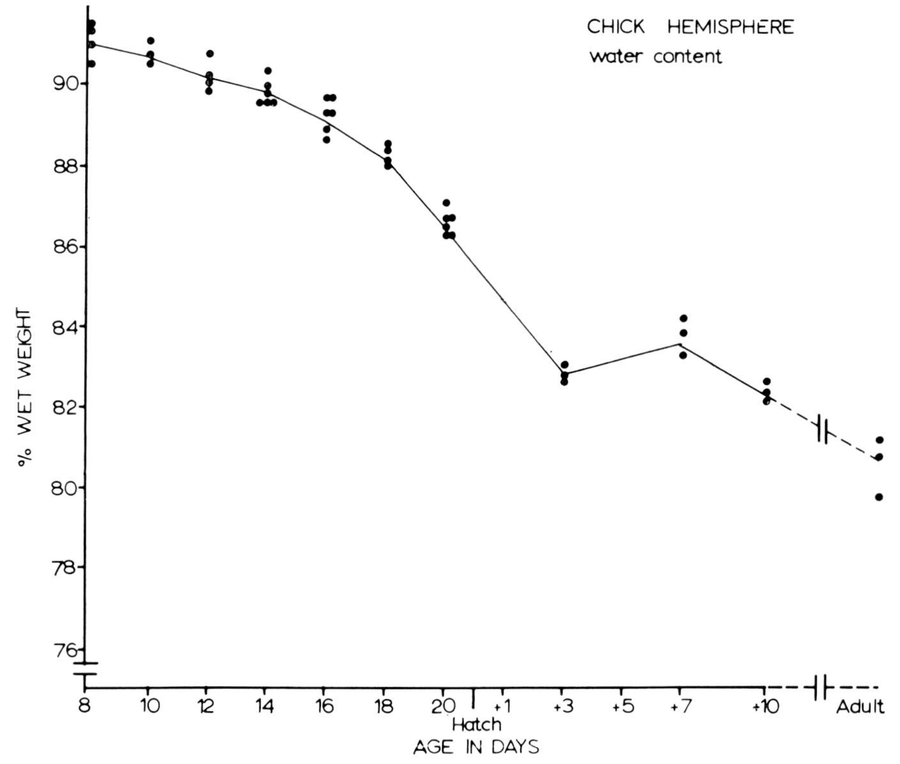

Fig. 2. Changes with age in water content of chick hemisphere.

Measurements of the water content of chick brain are shown in Figs. 2 and 3. In the hemisphere the water content decreases from 91% at 8 days of incubation to 82.4% at 10 days post-hatching. A rapid decrease occurs from 89.2% to 82.8% between 16 days of incubation and 3 days post-hatching. The hemisphere of the adult brain contains 80.5% of water. It should be noted that from 3 to 10 days post-hatching only a very slight decrease occurs.

In the optic lobe (Fig. 3) a decrease is found from 90.6% at 8 days of incubation to 81.1% at 10 days post-hatching. Here the rapid decrease occurs from 89.2% at 18 days of incubation to 82.3% at 3 days of age. This change is followed by a slight decrease to 81.1% at 10 days. A further decrease is found until the mature level of 76.0% is reached.

While in the hemisphere a slight but significant decrease is found from 8 to 16 days of incubation, the water content of the optic lobe appears to remain at an approximate constant level until 18 days of incubation.

The results obtained for chick hemisphere and optic lobe are in good agreement with those of Mandel *et al.* (1947) who studied the water content of whole brain from 10 to 19 days of incubation. Their values of the whole brain are in general 1 to 2% lower, which is probably caused by the relatively low water content of the brain stem (Graves and Himwich, 1955).

From the review by Himwich (1962) it is evident that a decrease in water concentra-

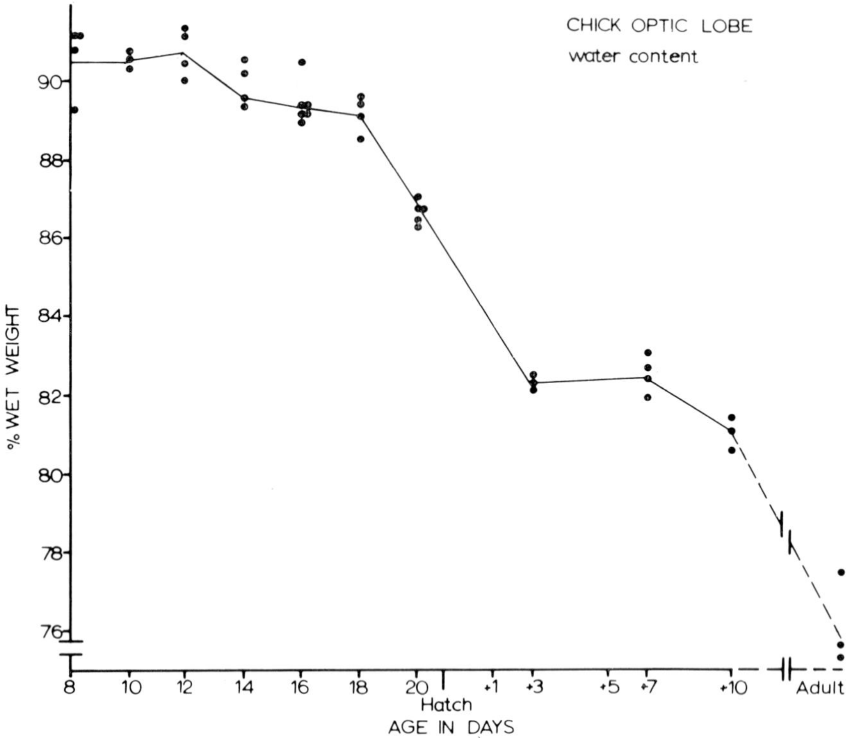

Fig. 3. Changes with age in water content of chick optic lobe.

tion occurs in the brains of all species studied, and that the pattern of decrease is usually the same as that found in rabbit pallium. A number of explanations have been offered about the drop in water concentration.

In the mouse (Uzman and Rumley, 1958) and rat (Clouet and Gaitonde, 1956; Laatsch, 1962) this decrease is preceded by a slight increase in water concentration during 3–5 days after birth.

Several authors have tried to explain this drop in water concentration. Donaldson and Haita (1931) concluded from their findings that cell bodies, dendrites and unmyelinated axons suffer only a slight loss of water between birth and maturity. According to these authors, the progressive decrease in water of the entire brain or brain parts is mainly due to the accumulation of myelin having a water content of about 50%.

Uzman and Rumley (1958), studying the mouse brain, found a decrease in DNA content per unit wet weight. They assumed that a decrease in cell population might be related to the decrease in water. There are, however, no data in the literature recording a loss of cells occurring at 14 to 16 days after birth. However, the data of these authors indicate a process which is more likely to cause a decrease in water concentration. Coinciding with a decrease in water they found an increase in total lipids before they could detect any myelin. This is in agreement with the findings of Folch-Pi (1955) who found an early rise in total lipids in the developing mouse brain. The discrepancy between the rapid increase in lipids before myelination starts needs some further comment. The failure to demonstrate myelin by histological techniques does not mean that myelination does not take place. Luse (1962) showed by electron microscopy that myelination occurs before it can be detected by ordinary histological techniques, while Waelsch *et al.* (1941) found that the synthesis of lipids is so great during early development that it is more likely to be involved in growth processes than in myelination. This means that the rapid lipid synthesis during early development is mainly involved in the formation of membranes while in later stages the increase of lipid content parallels myelination. Vernadakis and Woodbury (1962) showed in developing rat brain that the decrease in water concentration is almost inversely proportional to the increase in proteins and lipids. Comparing the results about decrease in water and increase in proteins and lipids in the literature (Graves and Himwich, 1955; Folch-Pi, 1955; Waelsch, Sperry and Stoyanoff, 1941; Davison and Wajda, 1959; Uzman and Rumley, 1958) with our data, we could also calculate that the increase in proteins and lipids parallels the decrease in water concentration.

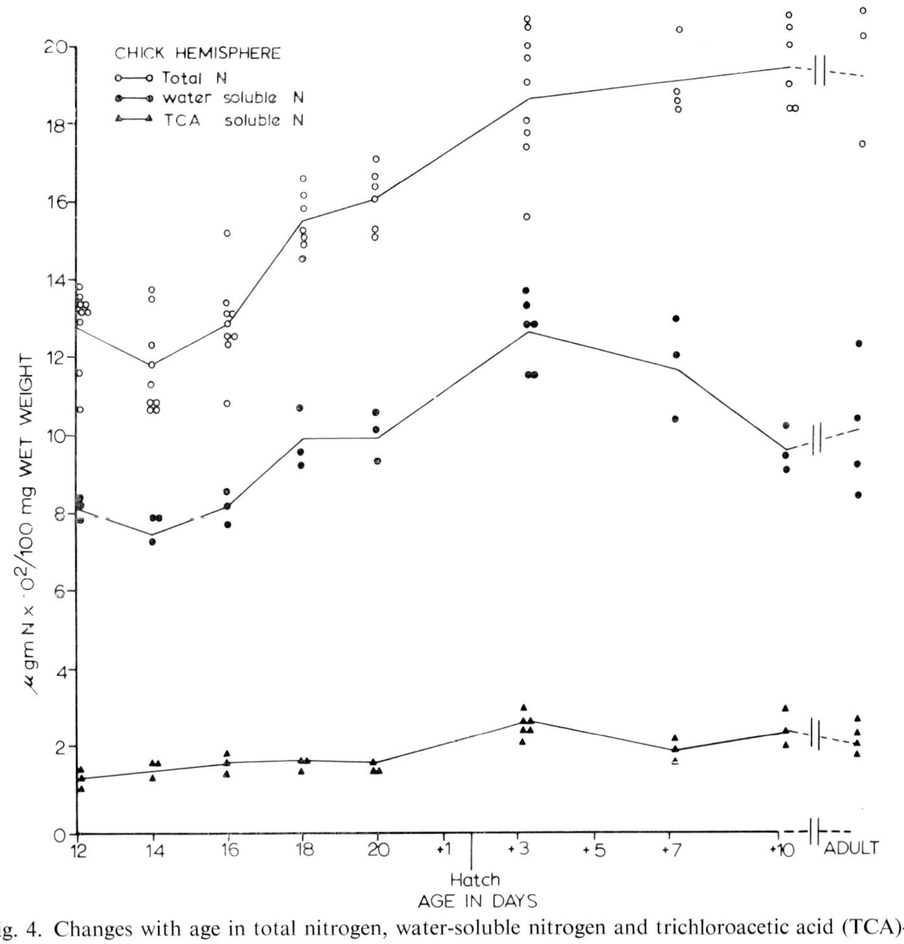

Fig. 4. Changes with age in total nitrogen, water-soluble nitrogen and trichloroacetic acid (TCA)-soluble nitrogen of chick hemisphere.

This decrease occurs at a time when myelination is only present at a submicroscopic level in phylogenetic early parts of the brain. It seems therefore, that myelination will contribute only very little to the water decrease observed in early stages, although it may be responsible for a further decrease in water content in later stages.

3. Nitrogen content

In the chick hemisphere total nitrogen increases from 1280 μg per 100 mg wet weight at 12 days of incubation to 1980 μg at 10 days post-hatching, which is about the adult level (Fig. 4). The decrease from 12 to 14 days of incubation is not significant ($p = 0.1$). It is evident that a rapid increase in total N occurs from 1180 μg at 14 days of incubation to 1880 μg at 3 days post-hatching.

In contrast to the pattern of changes in the soluble nitrogen content of, e.g. the rabbit (Vos, 1966), in the chick an increase is found from 810 μg at 12 days of incubation to a peak (1280 μg) at 3 days after hatching. This increase is followed by decrease

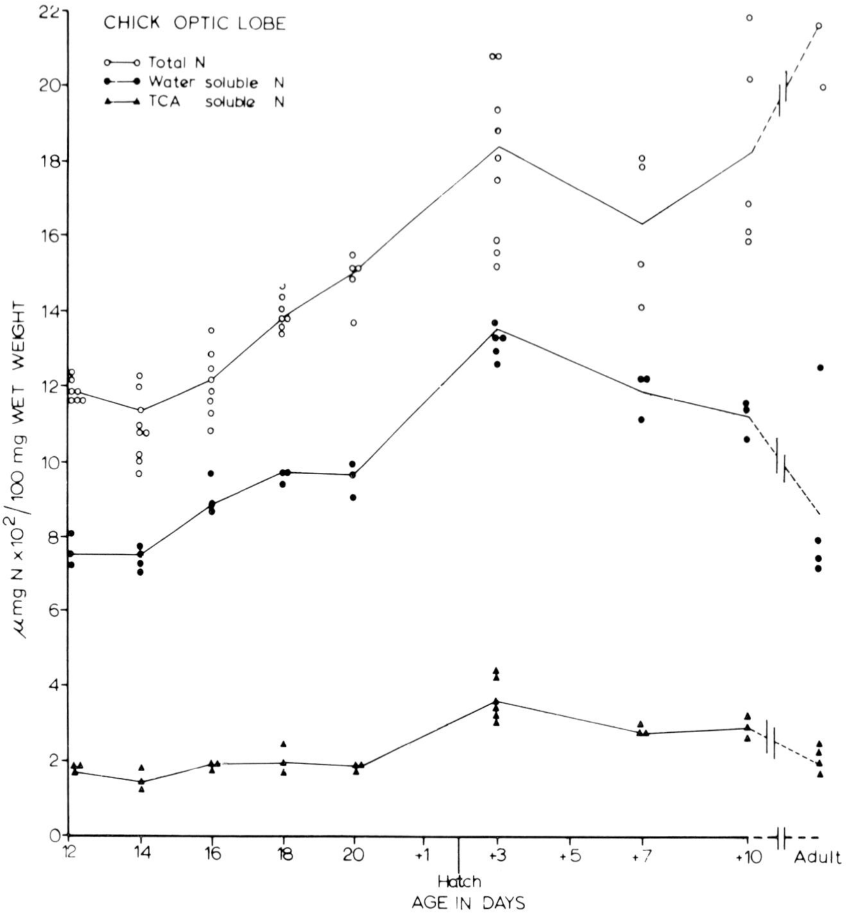

Fig. 5. Changes with age in total nitrogen, water-soluble nitrogen and trichloroacetic acid (TCA)-soluble nitrogen of chick optic lobe.

to a significantly lower level (990 μg) at 10 days post-hatching. The observed peak is partly due to a peak in TCA-soluble nitrogen present at the same age. It is remarkable that the TCA-soluble nitrogen content remains at a rather constant level until hatching (about 170 μg per 100 mg wet weight) then continuing at a much higher level after hatching and showing a slight but significant peak at 3 days post-hatching (280 μg).

Changes in nitrogen content of the optic lobe are shown in Fig. 5. Total nitrogen rises from 1180 μg per 100 mg wet weight at 12 days of incubation to 1830 μg at 10 days post-hatching. The adult level is much higher (2200 μg). The period of rapid increase occurs from 14 days of incubation to 3 days post-hatching.

The nitrogen content at 7 days post-hatching lies somewhat lower as compared to that of 3 and 10 days (significance level $p = 0.05$). Increase in soluble nitrogen from 740 μg at 12 and 14 days of incubation to a highest value (1360 μg) at 3 days post-hatching is more pronounced in the optic lobe than in the hemisphere. The high level at 3 days is followed by a decrease to 1130 μg at 10 days of age. The adult value is much lower (880 μg). This parallels the behavior of TCA-soluble nitrogen content which rises from its low level before hatching (about 180 μg) to a highest value at 3 days of age (370 μg). Thereafter, the level remains high until 10 days (300 μg) followed by a slight decline to the adult level (220 μg).

Our data on total nitrogen content agree well with those of Gayet and Bonichon (1961) who studied the developmental changes in optic lobe from 5 to 20 days of incubation.

With regard to the TCA-soluble nitrogen content there is an important difference between rabbit and chick brain (Vos, 1966). Contrary to the findings in rabbit pallium an increase is found showing a highest value at 3 days of age.

At the moment it is not quite possible to give an explanation for this increase. An increase in free aminoacids cannot be ruled out although Roberts *et al.* (1958) found no increase, except for γ-aminobutyric acid, in the amounts of other aminoacids until hatching. Another difference in comparison to the rabbit is the increase in water-soluble nitrogen which exceeds that caused by the increase in TCA-soluble nitrogen. If we assume that the difference between water-soluble and TCA-soluble nitrogen roughly represents the soluble proteins, the soluble protein nitrogen increases in the hemisphere from 670 μg at 12 days of incubation to 1000 μg at 3 days post-hatching, while, in the optic lobe, this increase is from 570 μg to 990 μg. In this respect an interesting observation is the fact that distinct changes could be demonstrated in the composition of water-soluble proteins in the chick hemisphere when studied by means of electrophoresis techniques (see below).

4. *Electrophoretic patterns of proteins*

Proteins constitute some 10–20% of the wet weight of the adult brain (LeBaron and Folch-Pi, 1959; Folch-Pi, 1955; Laatsch, 1962). They occur partly in soluble form (about 50%) while the remainder consists of proteins which are not soluble in aqueous solutions, e.g. proteolipids, neurokeratin and phosphatidopeptides (LeBaron and

References p. 210–213

Folch-Pi, 1956). The soluble proteins can be separated by several techniques in a number of fractions. Electrophoresis has been most frequently used for this purpose.

It has been shown that different turnover rates exist between young and adult animals (Lajtha, 1964), which may suggest that changes will take place in protein composition of the developing brain. Chick hemispheres of various age groups were analysed by means of polyacrylamide disc gel electrophoresis (Vos and van der Helm, 1964).

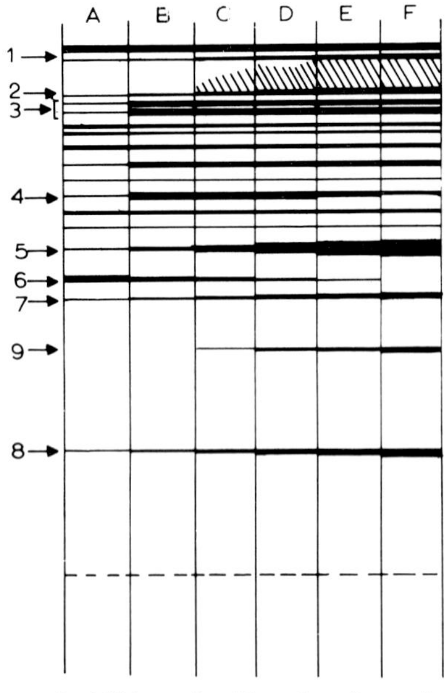

Fig. 6. Electrophoretic patterns, in 15% acrylamide gels, of proteins extracted from chick hemispheres. A, at 6 days of incubation; B, C, D, E at 12, 14, 16 and 19 days of incubation; F at 7 days after hatching.

Fig. 6 shows the electrophoretic patterns in 15% acrylamide gels. Several changes can be noticed. A gradual increase in the relative amounts of fractions 5, 7 and 8 were found. At 3, two sharp bands are found which stained very weakly at 6 days of incubation, while at 12 days these two bands were very much pronounced. After 12 days of incubation almost no change was observed in these 2 fractions. At 6 days, fraction 4 also stains very weakly and is more pronounced at 12 days. This fraction showed increased staining up till 14 days, whereafter it decreased towards 7 days after hatching. Fraction 6 is strongly stained at 6 days of incubation and gradually decreases in staining intensity until it seems to have disappeared at 7 days post-hatching. Fraction 9 appears at 14 days of incubation as a weak fraction and increases slightly to 7 days post-hatching. It must be emphasized that it is not quite certain whether fractions like 9 and 6 actually appear or disappear at a certain stage. It might be possible that their concentration is merely too low at a certain stage to become visible.

Fig. 7 shows the protein pattern in a 6% gel at 6 and 12 days of incubation only, since after 12 days of incubation only minor changes are found. The most obvious

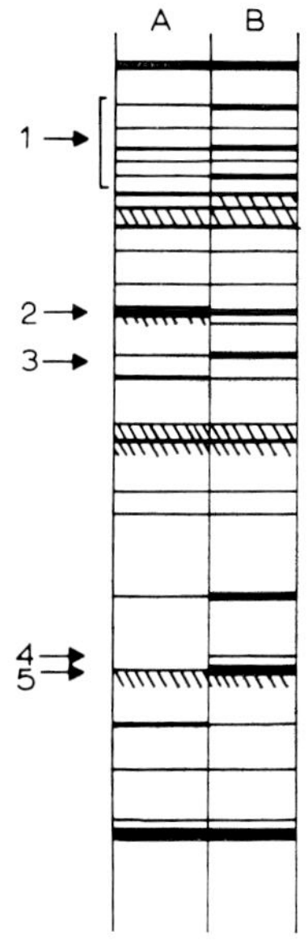

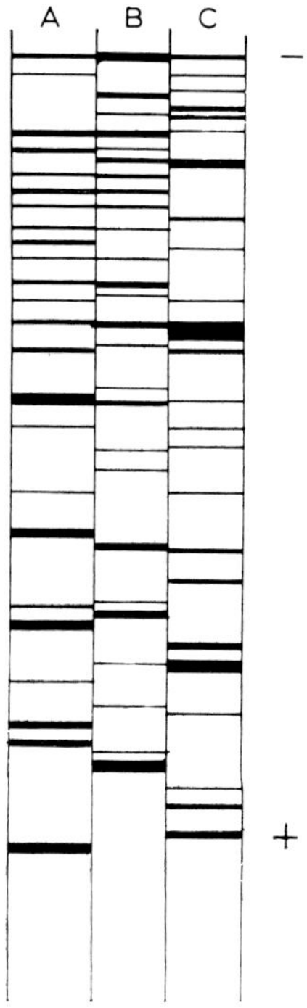

Fig. 7. Electrophoretic patterns, in 6% acrylamide gels, of proteins extracted from chick hemispheres. A, 6 days of incubation; B, 12 days of incubation.

Fig. 8. Electrophoretic patterns, in 7.5% acrylamide gels, of proteins extracted from 12 day old chick embryos. A, heart; B, hemisphere; C, skeletal muscle.

changes are a gradual increase of the color intensity of the fractions at 1, which were shown to be lipid and PAS positive, and a decrease of fraction 2, which becomes almost invisible at 19 days of incubation. Fraction 3 on the other hand becomes gradually stronger. Fraction 4 could not be seen in gels at 6 days, but was present at 12 days of incubation, whereafter it did not change any more. Also fraction 5 was more heavily stained at 12 days of incubation and subsequent stages than it was at 6 days. It seems surprising that the chick hemisphere at 6 days of incubation shows almost all the fractions present in later stages in about the same quantities. That this similarity in protein pattern does not exist among other tissues is shown in Fig. 8. There can be no doubt that the protein patterns of heart, hemisphere and skeletal muscle are completely different at 12 days of incubation, except for fraction 1 and 2, which shows the same mobility as serum albumin of the chick.

In an attempt to localize some of the fractions found in extracts, at the subcellular level, the protein patterns in the rat brain were studied (Vos, 1966). Comparing the protein patterns of homogenate, crude mitochondrial fraction, nuclear fraction and supernatant (11.500 g), we have not been able to find any differences in the relative amounts of the various fractions. Since it might be expected that these subfractions were contaminated with cytoplasmic proteins, a crude mitochondrial fraction was separated in 30 fractions by centrifugation into a continuous sucrose gradient

(0.8–1.7 *M* sucrose). The results have indicated that the protein patterns in the different fractions are very similar up to 1.6 *M* sucrose to the pattern of the crude mitochondrial fraction. However, fraction 1 increased in intensity up to 1.3 *M* sucrose and decreased again and disappeared above 1.6 *M* sucrose.

Since the present techniques do not enable us to analyse the composition of each of the protein fractions, a detailed discussion of the results is still premature.

The results are in agreement with the data of Schalenkamp (1963) who studied brain proteins by means of agar gel- and immunoelectrophoresis in chick embryos. He also found a similarity between embryonic and post-hatched chicks with regard to their protein patterns. Considering the fact that the number of fractions do not show major changes during the development of the chick brain, one must assume that during the characteristic morphological changes the composition of the soluble proteins remains almost unaltered. This probably means that the soluble protein composition forms a basic characteristic of the brain of a certain species. Unfortunately our knowledge of the non-soluble proteins during development is very scanty. The results obtained on subcellular fractions, prepared from a crude mitochondrial preparation by sucrose density centrifugation, also indicate that a rather constant pattern of soluble proteins is present. The similarity of the protein patterns in 0.8 to 1.6 *M* sucrose poses a special problem. It has been shown for instance by Gray and Whittaker (1962) and Johnson and Whittaker (1963) that in the sucrose gradient several particles can be separated, e.g. membrane fragments, mitochondria and pinched-off nerve endings. As judged from the electrophoretic experiments, it is suggestive to assume that the different particles have a similar soluble protein composition. This means as far as these protein bands become visible after staining, because it may be assumed that these particles differ in their enzyme composition. It remains not clear what the origin of the different protein bands may be, whether they are structural proteins, built into membranes and other cytoplasmic organelles, or are composed of different enzymes migrating in the gel as one fraction. It remains to be investigated whether the apparent similarity of the protein patterns in the developing brain as well as in its subcellular fractions indicates a basic characteristic of nervous tissue, which is already present at early stages of development and changes only little with age. In that case the rapid growth of the brain and its cellular constituents will not be accompanied by the formation of completely new proteins, but by the synthesis of already existing proteins at a higher speed.

5. *Levels of glutamate decarboxylase (GAD) and γ-aminobutyric transaminase (GABAT)*

The activities of a great many enzymes increase during the rapid growth period. Very few studies deal with the behavior of closely related enzymes in this period of brain development. In view of the current opinion on the important function of γ-aminobutyric acid (GABA) in nervous activity, an investigation was made on the levels of GAD and GABAT during the development of chick and a comparison was made with rats.

TABLE I

ACTIVITY OF GAD AND GABAT AND THE GABAT/GAD RATIO IN DEVELOPING CHICK BRAIN

Age (days)	*GAD*	*GABAT*	*GABAT/GAD ratio*
12	3.4	13	3.4
14	5.4	18	3.3
16	8.4	27	3.0
18	15.3	34	2.2
20	25.5	52	2.0

Homogenates of chick brain in 0.32 *M* sucrose were prepared, and Triton X-100 (final concentration 0.5%) added before enzyme determination. Activities in μmoles/g wet wt./h. Age in days after incubation. (Mean values of four experiments.)

The levels of GAD, GABAT and the GABAT/GAD ratio in all experiments are presented in Table I. There is a sharp increase of both enzyme activities in the chick after the 14th day following incubation and in the rat after the 5th day.

The GABAT/GAD ratio is fairly constant during the whole period studied in the rat brain. This was also found to be true when the activities of both enzymes were determined in water homogenates (van den Berg and van Kempen, 1964). A later study revealed, however, that the activities of both enzymes could be raised by adding Triton X-100 (van Kempen *et al.*), the effect of this detergent being fairly constant during the development. The measurements are more reliable when Triton X-100 is used. The GABAT/GAD ratio falls in the chick brain (Table I).

Intracellular localization. It was found earlier that the activities of GAD and GABAT were lower in sucrose homogenates from immature and mature rat brain than in water homogenates, the enzymes appearing to be particle bound (van Kempen *et al.*, 1965; van den Berg *et al.*, 1965). There is only one important difference: namely that GAD from the immature brain sediments more slowly. This result was also established for rat brain (van den Berg *et al.*, 1965). It is possible that GAD-containing particles from immature brains are damaged during the separation, resulting in a different sedimentation behavior. The changes in some properties of the GAD-containing particle may suggest a change in GABA metabolism during development The increases of the glutamate and GABA levels during the development in rat (Vernadakis and Woodbury, 1962), rabbit (Schadé and Baxter, 1960) and cat brain (Berl, 1963) are different. Information on the possible developmental changes in glutamate and GABA turnover is needed for an interpretation of the changes in the GAD-containing particle.

6. *Developmental changes in lactate dehydrogenase (LDH) activity*

A major increase of LDH in the developing chick hemisphere is preceded by a decrease from 8 to 14 days following incubation. This decrease from 74 to 48 units is most rapid from 8 to 10 days followed by a less rapid phase from 10 to 14 days, reaching a level of 43 units (Fig. 9). From 14 to 20 days following incubation a fast increase occurs from 43 to 86 units, which is followed by a less rapid increase to 10 days post-hatching (108 units). The overall increase between 14 days of incubation and 10 days post-hatching is about 2.5-fold.

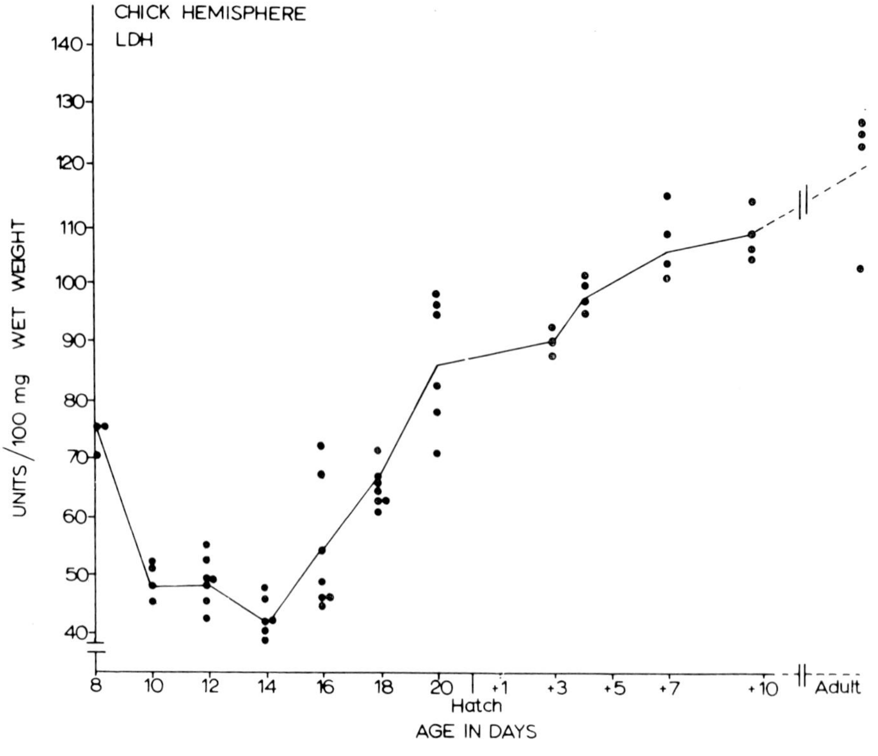

Fig. 9. Lactate dehydrogenase activity in the chick hemisphere as a function of age.

In the optic lobe (Fig. 10) no significant change is found between 8 days (51 units) and 14 days (58 units) of incubation. From 14 to 20 days of incubation a rapid increase is, however, found from 58 to 114 units. This is followed by a small but significant increase to 10 days post-hatching (143 units). The overall increase between 14 days of incubation and 10 days post-hatching is also about 2.5-fold. It should be noted that the LDH concentration tends to be higher in the optic lobe. The period of rapid increase in both brain parts lies between 14 and 20 days of incubation and is of the same order of magnitude. The increases from 20 days of incubation to 10 days post-hatching in both brain parts run parallel to each other.

The results obtained in investigating the LDH isozyme pattern of the developing chick brain were disappointing because only one single fraction was found after agar gel electrophoresis (Fig. 11), while the other fractions could not or in some cases only very vaguely be visualized. This indicates that the changes in LDH isozyme pattern of chick brain predominantly involves one fraction only.

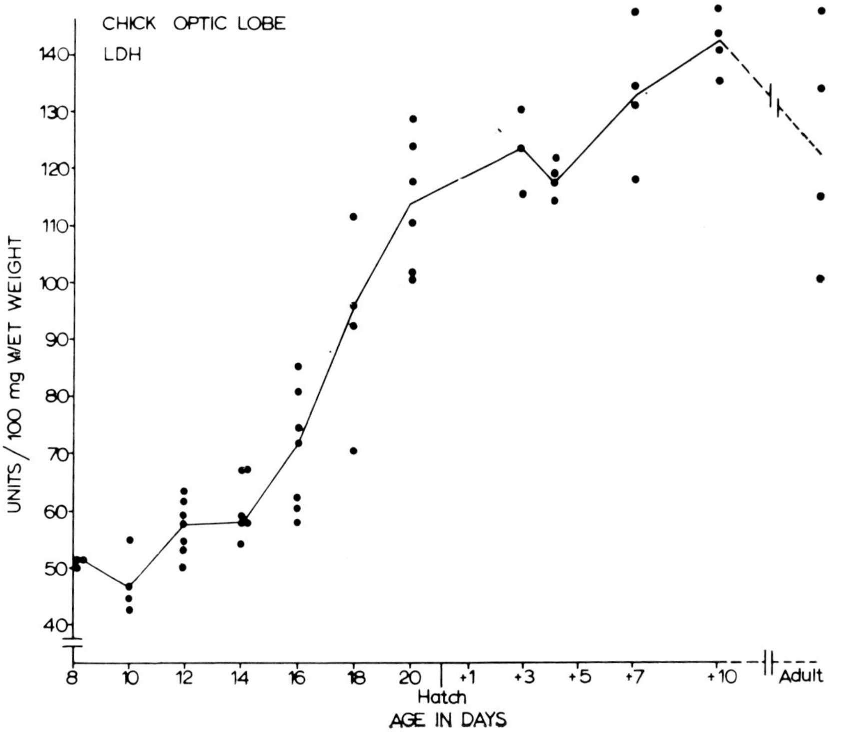

Fig. 10. Lactate dehydrogenase activity in the chick optic lobe as a function of age.

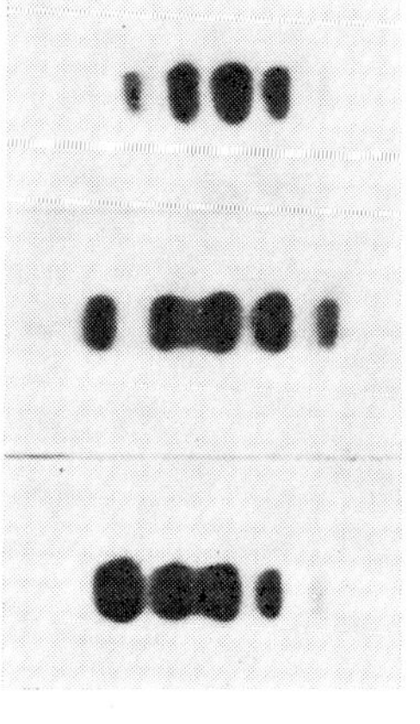

Fig. 11. Lactate dehydrogenase isozyme pattern of the chick hemisphere after 12 days of incubation.

References p. 210–213

LDH plays a major role in pyruvate metabolism. In brain tissue it is normally present in considerable concentration reaching values many times those of the enzymes involved in the initial stages of glycolysis (McIlwain, 1959; Lowry and Passaonneau, 1964). It is capable of transforming pyruvate into lactate at a very high speed. Even during convulsive activity a slight increase in pyruvate is found as compared to an enormous increase in lactate.

LDH has been studied in the brain of developing animals of a number of species. Kuhlman and Lowry (1956) found a two-fold increase in whole rat brain from birth to maturity. Similar results were obtained from mouse and guinea pig (Flexner *et al.*, 1960). In our results the high level of LDH activity in the hemisphere of the chick at 8 days following incubation is remarkable. This may be corelated with the large amount of cell division found at this stage of development (O'Connor, 1950).

LDH isozymes. As is now well known LDH occurs in different molecular forms. These molecular entities being constituted of different proteins showing common catalytic properties have been called isozymes (Markert and Møller, 1959). In vertebrate tissues LDH exists mostly as 5 isozymes. It was shown by Markert and Møller (1959) that the relative concentrations of the isozymes may change during development. This phenomenon has been studied more extensively in different organs of developing animals (Bonavita, 1964; Lindsay, 1963; Markert and Ursprung, 1962). From these studies it can be concluded that various organs have a different isozyme pattern, that is, the chemical properties of the isozymes differ from organ to organ, while during development, moreover, definite changes occur in the relative proportions of the isozymes. No data are available on isozyme patterns in developing brain of chick.

Bonavita (1964), studying the isozyme patterns of LDH in various parts of the developing rat brain, observed a rather specific pattern of development. The main characteristic is an increase in concentration of the two slow moving isozymes I and II (agar gel electrophoresis). In the brain of the chick no definite pattern could be found by means of agar gel electrophoresis since only one fraction could be made clearly visible (Fig. 11). By means of starch gel electrophoresis it was shown that in the chick organs one fraction primarily predominates and also that the mobility of the different isozymes differs largely from those of other animals (Vessell and Bearn, 1962; Lindsay, 1963). The LDH isozymes of the chick brain parts either were probably not sufficiently separated in our experiments on agar gels, or the one fraction predominates in the brain to such an extent that the remaining isozymes cannot be made visible.

7. *Glutamate-oxaloacetate transaminase (GOT) levels*

In the hemisphere of the chick similar changes, as previously observed in the rabbit, were found. From 14 days following incubation to 4 days following hatching a steady increase from 810 to 3640 units was determined. Between 4 and 10 days post-hatching the concentration remained the same (significance level $p = 0.1$). The GOT concentration is significantly higher as compared to the value found in 10 day old animals (Fig. 12). The overall increase between 14 days following incubation and 10 days

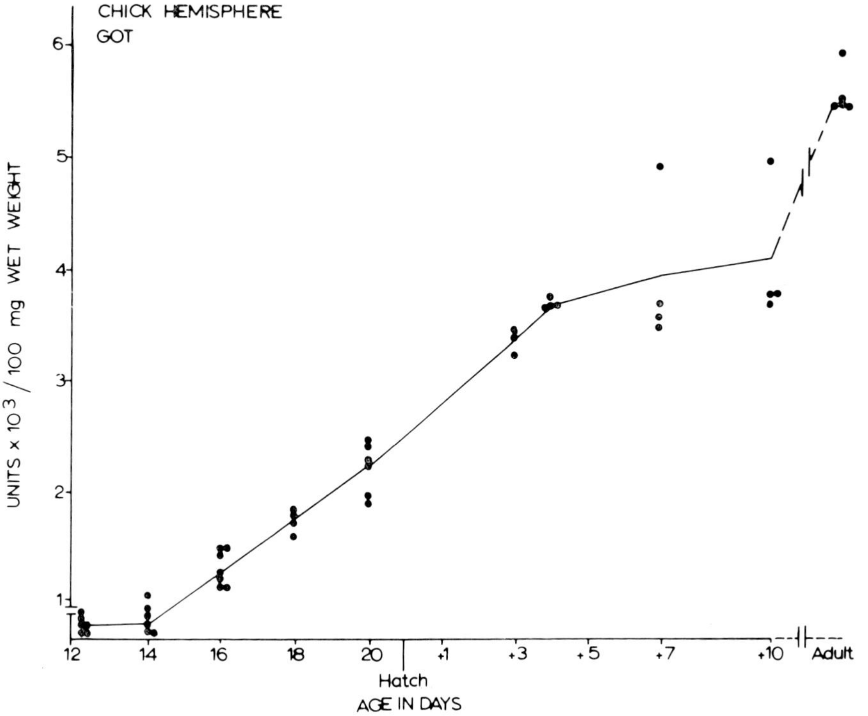

Fig. 12. Aspartate transaminase activity in the hemisphere of the chick as a function of age.

following hatching is about 5-fold. In contrast to the observations in the chick hemisphere, an increase in GOT concentration in the optic lobe could be demonstrated from 12 to 14 days following incubation. This increase shows an almost linear course up to 4 days following hatching. Between 4 and 10 days post-hatching only a slight increase was observed (from 4500 to 5290 units). Similar to the results obtained in the LDH determinations, a higher activity was found in the optic lobe during the period of rapid morphological differentiation. The GOT activity, however, increases about 5-fold, which is 2 times the value found for the increase in LDH activity during the same developmental period. It also appears that the period of rapid increase lasts shorter for LDH.

In this respect it is interesting to note that enzymes involved in glutamine metabolism and in the formation or breakdown of GABA show a very steep rise during development. This increase, being among the highest observed in the developing brain, is in the order of 5–10 times per unit wet weight, in contrast to the enzymes involved in oxidative metabolism and glycolysis, which increase about 2–3 times generally (Sisken *et al.*, 1960, 1961; Rudnick *et al.*, 1954; Baxter *et al.*, 1960; van den Berg and van Kempen, 1964; Rudnick and Waelsch, 1955; McMurray and Bayer, 1965; Berl, 1965; Pitts, 1965). In our laboratory observations were made in the rabbit brain; between 5 and 30 days of age a 5-fold increase was found in rabbit pallium. It should be noted that, so far, no relationship has been found between an increase in enzyme activity and substrate level. This was clearly shown in the case of glutamo-

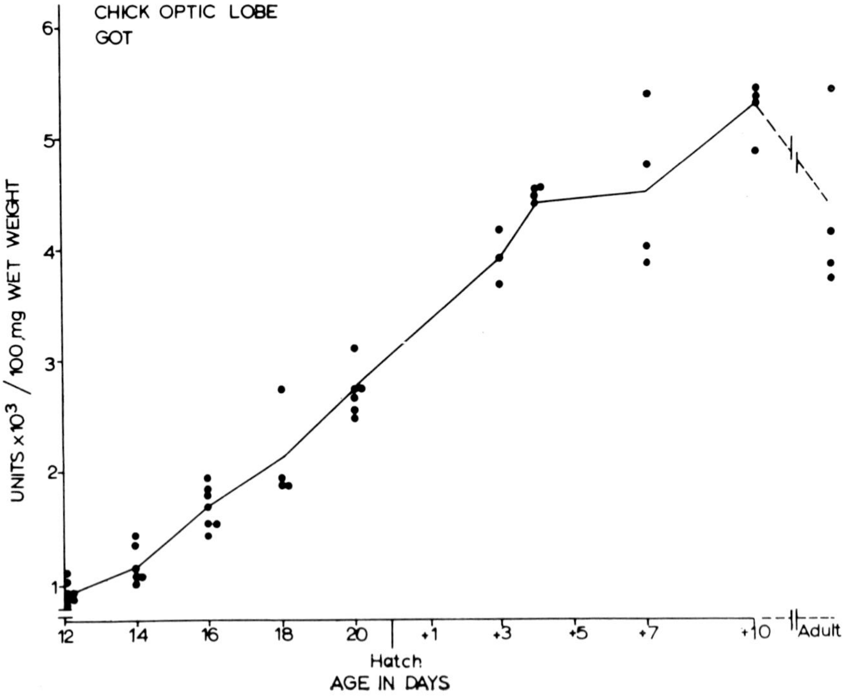

Fig. 13. Aspartate transaminase activity in the optic lobe of the chick as a function of age.

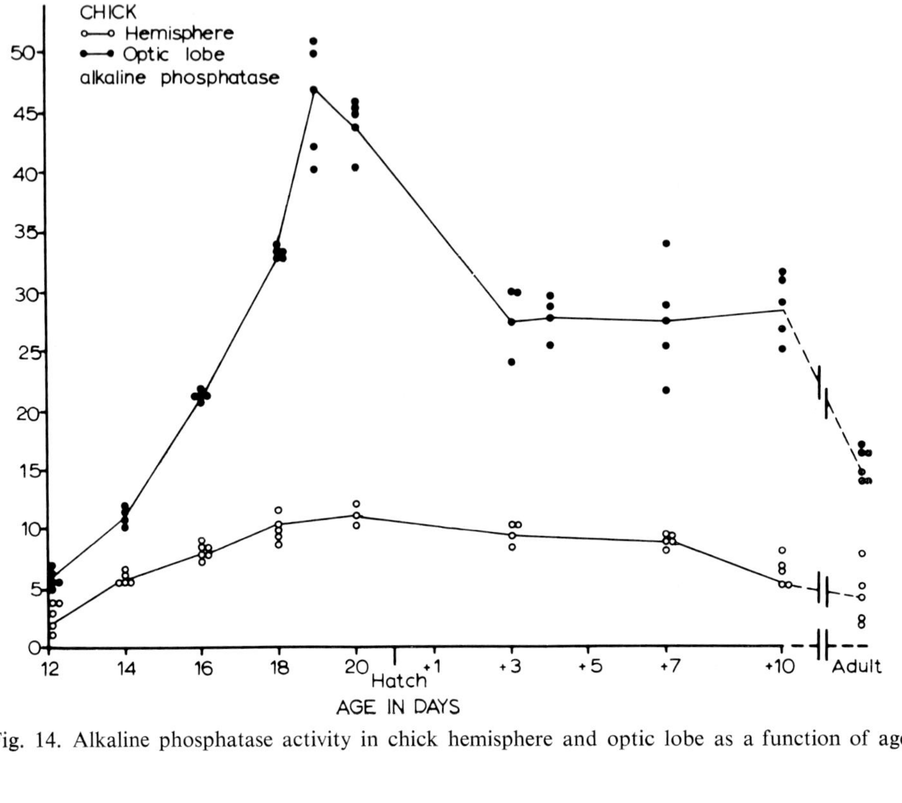

Fig. 14. Alkaline phosphatase activity in chick hemisphere and optic lobe as a function of age.

transferase, which rose 5- to 6-fold in parallel with a decrease in glutamine concentration. Glutamate dehydrogenase and GOT increased 6- to 8-fold while glutamate content remained fairly constant (McMurray and Bayer, 1965).

DISCUSSION

As to the general pattern of increase of enzymatic activities it should be pointed out that enzymes like acetylcholinesterase (Gayet and Bonichon, 1961) and enzymes involved in glutamine and GABA metabolism show their most rapid increase during the period of characteristic morphological differentiation. This increase is some 5- to 10-fold in comparison to the starting levels and shows a sigmoidal curve. On the other hand, enzymes involved in energy metabolism show a smaller increase, between 2 and 5 times the initial level. The rather uniform way, in which a large number of enzymes change the concentration levels during development and maturation, has led several authors to speculate on their role in neuronal activity. For instance, great emphasis has been laid on the coincidence between increase of enzymatic activity and the development of sustained electrical activity (see for review Himwich, 1962). But the energy involved in the ionic shifts responsible for EEG activity are rather small compared to the energy necessary for maintenance of a steady membrane potential of about 60–80 mV. It is, therefore, necessary to consider a few points related to enzyme activities measured during development. Firstly, it is well known that there exists an enormous excess in enzyme concentration. *In vitro* measurements of enzymes involved in cerebral glucose metabolism indeed showed that these concentrations are greatly in excess in relation to the activities needed for glucose metabolism *in vivo* (McIlwain, 1959; Lowry, 1955; Lowry and Passaonneau, 1964). Furthermore it might be expected that the development of the blood-brain barrier will play an essential role, especially with regard to substrate induction of enzyme synthesis. Compartmentation of the metabolism of some compounds may also be of importance in the developing brain as shown by Berl (1965). It is, therefore, important to consider that measured activities *in vitro* may be deceptive in regard to the needs *in vivo*. One should also be aware of the fact that the tissue investigated is extremely heterogeneous. Neurons, glial cells and mesodermal cells such as e.g. endothelial cells are ground in homogenates. The glia/neuron index is about 3.5 in the adult rat and changes with age (Brizzee *et al.*, 1964). Therefore, in studying the pattern of enzymatic activities during development, the interpretation of the results is complicated by several parameters changing with age.

Nevertheless, the general pattern of increase in concentrations of enzymes is more or less the same in different regions of the brain and also in different animals. This brings us to the question whether some fundamental general principle is involved. On the surface of the neuronal membrane several thousands of excitatory and inhibitory synapses end, influencing the membrane potential. The changes in membrane potential which are caused by them are small, however, compared to the membrane potential itself. This potential, which is about 60–80 mV, is maintained by the active transport of Na^+ and K^+ ions through the cell membrane, a process which requires

References p. 210–213

energy supplied by energy-rich phosphates. Keesey and Wallgren (1965) calculated that about one quarter of the energy available from respiration is required for sodium and potassium transport. If we now consider a full-grown neuron with its large dendritic area, it is quite obvious that over a large surface an ionic gradient must be maintained. This surface area is much smaller at the beginning of the rapid developmental period (Schadé *et al.*, 1964). It is, therefore, likely that enzymes involved in energy metabolism will increase per unit area of cell surface to keep pace with the increased need for energy-rich phosphates to maintain the membrane potential over a larger surface area, and also to deliver energy for the increased synthetic activities.

In this respect an important observation has been made by Samson *et al.* (1964, 1965), who studied the Mg^{++} dependent, Na^{+} and K^{+} stimulated ATPase of brain during development. The concentration of this enzyme, which is most probably localized in or near the cell membrane, was found to increase during development according to a sigmoidal curve, while its increase was some 8- to 10-fold. This large increase resembles that of acetylcholinesterase concentration during development, an enzyme which is certainly related to surface phenomena of the nerve cell. In this respect, it is remarkable that the same increase occurs in the concentration of enzymes related to the metabolism of GABA, a substance which is generally believed to play a role in modulatory mechanisms. Unfortunately, only few data are available on the surface area of dendrites in the developing brain per wet weight unit also taking into account the decrease in cell density. Schadé and Baxter (1960) and Schadé (1965), who studied the surface area of dendrites during development, found a 2- to 3-fold increase in surface area of the apical dendrites and a 6- to 7-fold increase in surface area of the basal dendrites in the rabbit pallium. As was mentioned before, the enzyme concentrations found are no absolute measure for their activity *in vivo*, and several changing parameters also interfere in the activities measured during development of the brain. Still, it remains very attractive to relate the increase in enzyme activities measured during development to the increase in surface of the neuron. We may not expect to find a 1 to 1 relationship between enzyme activity and cell surface, but the expression of enzymatic activity in surface area may give us a better understanding of the phenomena related to development and maturation of the brain. The surface area of the mature neuron probably does not exhibit any important differences in chemical composition as compared to immature neuron.

The present investigations have permitted an initial inventory-taking of the distribution and concentration of a small number of enzymes. The electron microscope has shown us a glimpse of the enormous complexity of the intraneuronal space: the neuron is filled with membranes. The beginning of an understanding has been made, but only the close cooperation of many disciplines will bridge the gap between enzymology and morphology.

REFERENCES

Baxter, C. F., Schadé, J. P., and Roberts, E., (1960); *Maturational changes in cerebral cortex.* II. Levels of glutamic acid decarboxylase, γ-aminobutyric acid and some related amino acids.

Inhibition in the Nervous System and γ-aminobutyric acid. E. Roberts, Editor. New York-London, Pergamon Press (p. 214–218).

BERL, S., (1965); The determination and distribution of glutamine synthetase in developing cat brain. *Internat. Neurochem. Confer., Oxford*, 25–30 July.

BERL, S., (1965); Compartmentation of glutamic acid metabolism in developing cerebral cortex. *J. biol. Chem.*, **240**, 2047–2054.

BONAVITA, V., (1964); Molecular evolution of lactate dehydrogenase in developing nervous tissue. Growth and Maturation of the Brain. *Progress in Brain Research*, *Vol.* 4. D. P. Purpura and J. P. Schadé, Editors. Amsterdam-New York, Elsevier (p. 254–272).

BRIZZEE, K. R., VOGT, J., AND KHARETCHKO, X., (1964); Postnatal changes in glia/neuron index with a comparison of methods of cell enumeration in the white rat. Growth and Maturation of the Brain. *Progress in Brain Research, Vol. 4.* D. P. Purpura and J. P. Schadé, Editors. Amsterdam-New York, Elsevier (p. 136–149).

CLOUET, D. H., AND GAITONDE, M. K., (1956); The changes with age in the protein composition of the rat brain. *J. Neurochem.*, **1**, 126–133.

DAVISON, A. N., AND WAJDA, M., (1959); Metabolism of myelin lipids: Estimation and separation of brain lipids in the developing rabbit. *J. Neurochem.*, **4**, 353–359.

DONALDSON, H. H., AND HAITA, S., (1931); On the weight of the parts of the brain and on the percentage of water in them according to brain weight and age in albino and in wild Norway rats. *J. comp. Neurol.*, **53**, 263–308.

FLEXNER, J. B., AND FLEXNER, L. B., (1950); Biochemical and physiological differentiation during morphogenesis. XI. The effect of growth on the amount and distribution of water, protein and fat in the liver and cerebral cortex of the fetal guinea pig. *Anat. Rec.*, **106**, 413–427.

FLEXNER, L. B., FLEXNER, J. B., ROBERTS, R. B., AND DE LA HABA, G., (1960); Lactic dehydrogenase of the developing cerebral cortex and liver of the mouse and guinea pig. *Developmental Biol.*, **2**, 313–328.

FOLCH-PI, J., (1955); *Composition of the brain in relation to maturation.* Biochemistry of the developing nervous system. H. Waelsch, Editor. New York. Academic Press Inc. (p. 121–136).

GAYET, J., AND BONICHON, A., (1961); *Morphological differentiation and metabolism in the optic lobes of the chick embryo.* Regional Neurochemistry. S. S. Kety and J. Elkes, Editors. London, Pergamon Press (p. 135–150).

GRAVES, J., AND HIMWICH, H. E., (1955); Age and water content of rabbit brain parts. *Am. J. Physiol.*, **180**, 205–208.

GRAY, E. G., AND WHITTAKER, V. P., (1962); The isolation of nerve endings from brain: An electron-microscopic study of cell fragments derived by homogenization and centrifugation. *J. Anat. Lond.*, **96**, 79–88.

HIMWICH, W. A., (1962); *Biochemical and neurophysiological development of the brain in the neonatal period.* Intern. Rev. Neurobiology. Vol. 4. C. C. Pfeiffer and J. R. Smythies, Editors. New York-London, Academic Press (p. 117–158).

HIMWICH, H. E., AND FAZEKAS, J. F., (1941); Comparative studies of the metabolism of the brain of infant and adult dogs. *Am. J. Physiol.*, **132**, 454–459.

HIMWICH, W. A., AND HIMWICH, H. E., (1965); The developing brain. Editors. *Progress in Brain Research. Vol.* 9. New York-Amsterdam. Elsevier

JOHNSON, M. K., AND WHITTAKER, V. P., (1963); Lactate dehydrogenase as a cytoplasmic marker in brain. *Biochem. J.*, **88**, 404–409.

KEESEY, J. C., AND WALLGREN, H., (1965); Movements of radioactive sodium in cerebral cortex slices in response to electrical stimulation. *Biochem. J.*, **95**, 301–310.

KOCH, W., AND KOCH, M. L., (1913); Contributions to the chemical differentiation of the central nervous system. III. The chemical differentiation of the brain of the albino rat during growth. *J. biol. Chem.*, **15**, 423–448.

KUHLMAN, E., AND LOWRY, O. H., (1956); Quantitative histochemical changes during the development of the rat cerebral cortex. *J. Neurochem.*, **1**, 173.

LAATSCH, R. H., (1962); Glycerol phosphate dehydrogenase activity of developing rat central nervous system. *J. Neurochem.*, **9**, 487–492.

LAJTHA, A., (1964); *Alteration and pathology of cerebral protein metabolism.* Intern. Rev. Neurobiology. Vol. 7. C. C. Pfeiffer and J. R. Smythies, Editors. New York, Academic Press (p. 1–40).

LEBARON, F. N., AND FOLCH-PI, J., (1956); The isolation from brain tissue of a trypsin-resistant protein fraction containing combined inositol and its relation to neurokeratin. *J. Neurochem.*, **1**, 101–108.

LEBARON, F. N., AND FOLCH-PI, J., (1959); The effect of pH and salt concentration on aqueous extraction of brain proteins and lipoproteins. *J. Neurochem.*, **4**, 1–18.

LINDSAY, D. T., (1963); Isozymic patterns and properties of lactate dehydrogenase from developing tissue of the chicken. *J. exp. Zool.*, **152**, 75–89.

LOWRY, O. H., (1955); *A study of the nervous system with quantitative histochemical methods*. Biochemistry of the developing Nervous System. H. Waelsch, Editor. New York, Academic Press (p. 350–357).

LOWRY, O. H., AND PASSAONNEAU, J. V., (1964); The relationships between substrates and enzymes of glycolysis in brain. *J. biol. Chem.*, **239**, 31–42.

LUSE, S. A., (1962); *Membrane and myelin*. D. B. Tower and H. Grundfest, Editors. Properties of Membranes. p. 55–66.

MANDEL, P., STOLL, R. AND BIETH, R., (1947); Sur le développement biochimique du cerveau de l'embryon de poulet durant la seconde partie de l'incubation. *C.R. Soc. Biol.*, **141**, 416.

MARKERT, C. L., AND MØLLER, R., (1959); Multiple forms of enzymes: tissue ontogenetic and species specific patterns. *Proc. nat. Acad. Sci., (Wash.)*, **45**, 753–763.

MARKERT, C. L., AND URSPRUNG, H., (1962); The ontogeny of isozyme patterns of LDH in the mouse. *Developmental Biol.*, **5**, 363.

MCILWAIN, H., (1959); *Biochemistry and the central nervous system*. London, J. and A. Churchill (p. 80).

MCMURRAY, W. C., AND BAYER, S. M., (1965); Amino acid metabolism in developing rat brain. *Internat. Neuroch. Conf., Oxford*, 25th–30th July.

O'CONNOR, R. J., (1950); The metabolism of cell division. *Brit. J. exp. Path.*, **31**, 390–396.

PITTS, F. N., (1965); Succinic semialdehyde dehydrogenase of brain. *Internat. Neuroch. Conf., Oxford*, 25th–30th July.

PURPURA, D. P., AND SCHADÉ, J. P., (1964); Growth and maturation of the brain. Editors. *Progress in Brain Research. Vol. 9*. New York-Amsterdam, Elsevier.

ROBERTS, E., LOWE, I. P., GUTH, L., AND JELINCK, B., (1958); Distribution of γ-aminobutyric acid and other amino acids in nervous tissue of various species. *J. exp. Zool.*, **138**, 313–328.

RUDNICK, D., MELA, P., AND WAELSCH, H., (1954); Enzymes of glutamine metabolism in the developing chick embryo: A study of glutamotransferase and glutamine synthetase. *J. exp. Zool.*, **126**, 297–321.

RUDNICK, D., AND WAELSCH, H., (1955); *Development of glutamotransferase in the nervous system of the chick*. Biochemistry of the Developing Nervous System. H. Waelsch, Editor. New York, Academic Press (p. 335–338).

SAMSON, F. E., DICK, H. C., AND BALFOUR, W. M., (1964); Na^+–K^+ stimulated ATP-ase in brain during neonatal maturation. *Life Sciences*, **3**, 511–515.

SAMSON, F. E., QUINN, D., AND DAHL, D., (1965); Maturation of the rat brain and Na^+–K^+ ATP-ase. *Internat. Neuroch. Conf., Oxford*, 25th–30th July.

SCHADÉ, J. P., (1965); Correlative morphology, physiology and biochemistry of the developing nervous system. *Internat. Neuroch. Conf., Oxford*, 25th–30th July.

SCHADÉ, J. P., AND BAXTER, C. F., (1960a); *Maturational changes in cerebral cortex*. I. Volume and surface determinations of nerve cell components. Inhibition in the nervous system and GABA. E. Roberts, Editor. New York-London, Pergamon Press (p. 207–213).

SCHADÉ, J. P., AND BAXTER, C. F., (1960b); Changes during growth in the volume and surface area of cortical neurons in the rabbit. *Exp. Neurol.*, **2**, 158–178.

SCHADÉ, J. P., AND PASCOE, E. G., (1965); Maturational changes in cerebral cortex. III. Effects of methionine sulfoximine on some electrical parameters and dendritic organization of cortical neurons. *Progress in Brain Research, Vol. 9*. New York-Amsterdam, Elsevier (p. 132–154).

SCHADÉ, J. P., VAN BACKER, H., AND COLON, E., (1964); Quantitative analysis of neuronal parameters in the maturing cerebral cortex. Growth and Maturation of the Brain. *Progress in Brain Research, Vol. 4*. D. P. Purpura and J. P. Schadé, Editors. Amsterdam-New York, Elsevier (p. 150–175).

SCHALEKAMP, M. A. D. H., (1963); *Immunologische aspecten van de orgaanontwikkeling*. Thesis, Utrecht.

SISKEN, B., ROBERTS, E., AND BAXTER, C. F., (1960); *Gamma aminobutyric acid and glutamic decarboxylase activity in the brain of the chick*. Inhibition on the Nervous System and γ-aminobutyric acid. E. Roberts, Editor. New York-London, Pergamon Press (p. 219–225).

SISKEN, B., SANO, K., AND ROBERTS, E., (1961); γ-Aminobutyric acid content and glutamic decarboxylase and γ-aminobutyrate transaminase activities in the optic lobe of the developing chick. *J. biol. Chem.*, **236**, 503–507.

SPERRY, W. M., (1962); *The biochemistry of the brain during early development. Neurochemistry.* K. A. C. Elliott, I. H. Page and J. H. Quastel, Editors. Springfield, Illinois, C. C. Thomas (p. 55–84).

UZMAN, L. L., AND RUMLEY, M. K., (1958); Changes in the composition of the developing mouse brain during early myelination. *J. Neurochem.*, **3**, 170–184.

VAN DEN BERG, C. J., (1964); *Glutamaat decarboxylase: Isolering en niveau in hersenweefsel tijdens de ontwikkeling.* Thesis, Leyden.

VAN DEN BERG, C. J., AND VAN KEMPEN, G. M. J., (1964); Glutamate decarboxylase and γ-aminobutyrate transaminase in developing rat brain. *Experientia*, **20**, 375–377.

VAN DEN BERG, C. J., VAN KEMPEN, G. M. J., SCHADÉ, J. P., AND VELDSTRA, H., (1965); Levels and intracellular localization of glutamate decarboxylase and γ-aminobutyrate transaminase and other enzymes during the development of the brain. *J. Neurochem.*, **12**, 863–869.

VAN KEMPEN, G. M. J., (1964); *γ-Aminobutyraat transaminase: Een onderzoek over eigenschappen en localisatie in hersenweefsel.* Thesis, Leyden.

VAN KEMPEN, G. M. J., VAN DEN BERG, C. J., VAN DER HELM, H. J., AND VELDSTRA, H., (1965); Intracellular localization of glutamate decarboxylase, γ-aminobutyrate transaminase and some other enzymes in brain tissue. *J. Neurochem.*, **12**, 581–588.

VERNADAKIS, A., AND WOODBURY, D. M., (1962); Electrolyte and amino acid changes in rat brain during maturation. *Am. J. Physiol.*, **203**, 748–752.

VESSELL, E. S., AND BEARN, A. G., (1962); Variations in the lactic dehydrogenase of vertebrate erythrocytes. *J. gen. Physiol.*, **45**, 553–565.

VOS, J., (1966); Some biochemical aspects of the developing rabbit and chick brain. Thesis, Amsterdam.

VOS, J., AND VAN DER HELM, H. J., (1964); Electrophoresis of brain proteins in polyacrylamide gel. *J. Neurochem.*, **11**, 209–210.

WAELSCH, H., (1951); Glutamic acid and cerebral function. *Adv. Protein Chem.*, **6**, 299–341.

WAELSCH, H., SPERRY, W. M., AND STOYANOFF, V. A., (1941); The influence of growth and myelination on the deposition and metabolism of lipids in the brain. *J. biol. Chem.*, **140**, 885–897.

YANNET, H., AND DARROW, D. C., (1938); The effect of growth on the distribution of water and electrolytes in brain, liver and muscle. *J. biol. Chem.*, **123**, 295–305.

Developmental Patterns in the Central Nervous System of Birds

III. Somatic Motility during the Embryonic Period and its Relation to Behavior after Hatching*

M. A. CORNER AND A. P. C. BOT

Central Institute for Brain Research, Amsterdam (The Netherlands)

INTRODUCTION

The development of somatic motility ('behavior') in bird embryos has been studied extensively in certain respects (for a general review of the earlier literature, see Carmichael, 1954). The *chronology of functional innervation* of the muscles has been worked out for the chick (Orr and Windle, 1934; Kuo, 1932a, 1938), for the pigeon (Tuge, 1937) and for the duck (Gottlieb and Kuo, 1965). Much information is thus available about the muscle groups at successive stages of development which can first be observed to contract 'spontaneously' or be made to do so by sensory stimulation ('reflex'). The close correspondence which has been reported between the times of appearance of the first spontaneous movements and the earliest histologically demonstrated neuro-muscular connections (Windle and Orr, 1934; Visintini and Levi-Montalcini, 1939) suggests that close approximations to the true innervation times have been obtained. No information is available, however, from the ideal method of direct stimulation of motor nerves and electrical recording from the muscles. There is in any case little likelihood that the skeletal muscles begin to contract *prior* to innervation in birds ('myogenic'), since all spontaneous motility can be eliminated by the neuromuscular blocking agent *curare*, leaving the muscles still excitable by direct electrical stimulation (Kuo, 1939a, c; Visintini and Levi-Montalcini, 1939; Hamburger, 1963). Furthermore, a shock produces only a single twitch of the surrounding muscle fibers, in contrast to the prolonged generalized twitching usually occurring spontaneously (Visintini and Levi-Montalcini, 1939; also Szepsenwol, 1946).

The general chronology which has emerged is the same in all four studies cited above. The muscles for elevation of the head are the first to show contractions, from the fourth day of incubation. Roughly in succession thereafter, through the remainder of

* This research was supported in part by grants from the National Institute of Neurological Diseases and Blindness (NB 3048) and from the National Institute of Mental Health (MH 6825), Public Health Service, Bethesda, U.S.A.

the first week, the following muscular actions appear: ventral head flexion, sidewards head turning, ventral flexion of the anterior trunk region, *idem* for posterior trunk, sidewards trunk flexion, tail flexion (both lateral and up-and-down), forelimb and hindlimb movements at the base. Both limbs then show through the first half of the second week a progressive extension of activity to more distal joints, including the digits. Eyelid and eyeball movements first appear early in the second week of incubation and are quickly followed by the first opening and closing of the beak and by swallowing. There thus appears to be a general cephalo-caudal sequence of motor

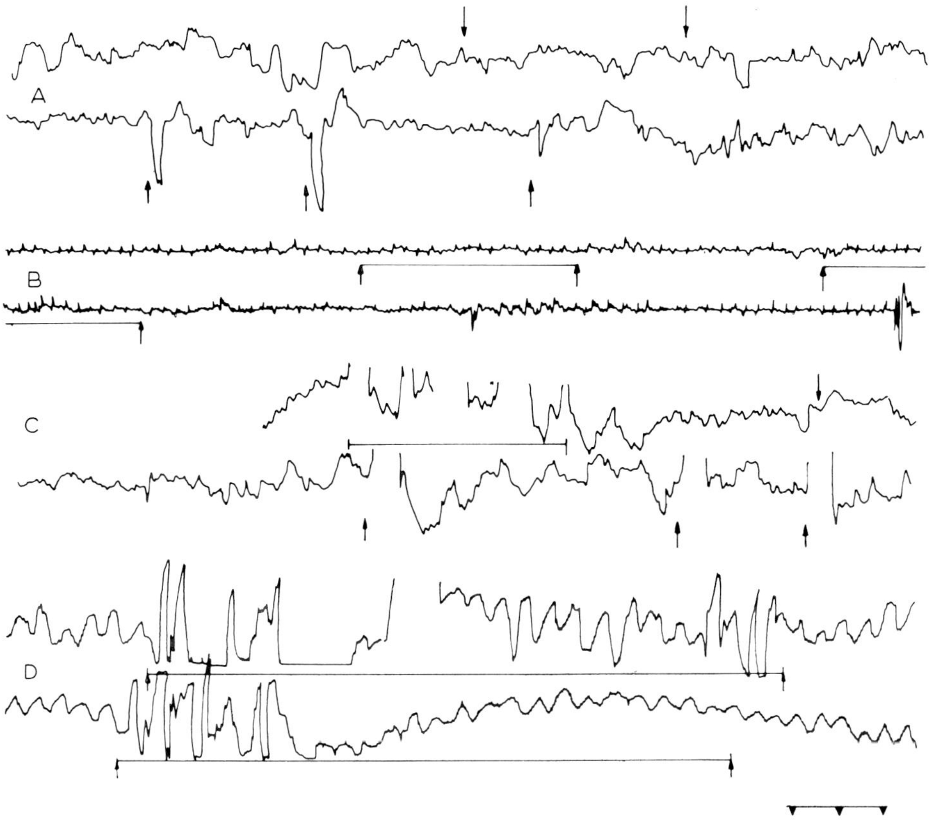

Fig. 1. The appearance of acoustic-evoked body movements in the chick.
A. A stage *43* embryo showing the absence of response to loud claps (arrows, top line) despite tactile-evoked reflex motility (arrows, bottom line).
B. An early stage *44* embryo, with frequent spontaneous movements of varying strength and duration but no somatic response to trains of loud claps (lines between the arrows; continual record).
C. Movement artifacts consistently following a loud clap (arrows, bottom line; continual record) in a stage *44* embryo. A weaker clap evoked no noticeable reaction (arrow, upper line) several seconds after a burst of spontaneous movements (line).
D. Consistent motor response to acoustic stimulation in a stage *45* embryo. Trains of handclaps (lines between arrows) evoke large body movements.
In *A* and *C* a brain lead (EEG background) is used to register the movements, whereas in *B* and *D* an upper trunk placement is used (background ECG or respiratory rhythm). Calibration, 1 sec per division.

References p. 235–236

nerve outgrowth from the spinal cord, followed by the development of the cranial motor nerves. Individual differences in chronology are evident, thus for example forelimb movements appearing prior to those of the hindlimb in some embryos, the opposite in others, and about at the same time in the rest (Kuo, 1932a).

The *chronology of sensory innervation* of the body surface has similarly been studied by attempting to elicit an observable motor response, either by tactile or by electrical stimulation of the skin. The special sensory innervation (optic, auditory, vestibular) has been followed by means of electrical recording from the sense organs as well as by observation of motor responses to stimulation. In no case has an ideal method been applied, e.g. recording the electrical activity evoked in the sensory nerves and central nervous system. Functional skin innervation begins in the pigeon (Tuge, 1937) and in the chick (Orr and Windle, 1934; Hamburger and Balaban, 1963; also Volokhov, 1961) at the end of the first week of incubation, possibly earliest in the mouth and upper neck regions (Tuge, 1937), and covers the entire body surface within 1–2 days. It is correlated not with the appearance of nerve fibers in the skin, which occurs several days earlier, but with the growth of collaterals from the dorsal column into the spinal gray matter (Windle and Orr, 1934; Visintini and Levi-Montalcini, 1939). *Proprioceptive* reflexes are reported to appear slightly later, simultaneous with the earliest monosynaptic reflex pathways (Visintini and Levi-Montalcini, 1939; also see Hamburger, 1964). Somatic motor responses to *acoustic* stimulation first appear in the chick embryo during *stage 44* (Fig. 1), i.e. from 17–18 days of incubation in most cases (Kuo, 1932a; Sedláček, 1962; also Gottlieb, 1965). This is also the time that the cochlear microphonic response attains its full ability to reproduce sounds, although an electrical response has been present from the 13th day (Vanzulli and Garcia-Austt, 1963). It is not clear therefore whether it is the limitations of the receptor organ or incompleteness of central neural connections which prevent earlier appearance of the auditory reflex. Body movements evoked by *rotation* appear at about the same stage as does the auditory reflex and *visual*-evoked movements appear slightly later, but the relative timing of these three events is individually variable (Kuo, 1932a). Vestibular stimulation (slow turning) is reported able to elicit nystagmus movements of the head already at 8 days of incubation, at which time vestibular nerve fibers first appear both in the auditory organ and in the hindbrain (Visintini and Levi-Montalcini, 1939). The optic reflex circuit might be completed by maturation of the retina rather than of the central connections, since the electroretinogram itself does not appear until early in *stage 45* (Peters *et al.*, 1958; Garcia-Austt and Patetta-Queirolo, 1963).

Patterns of sensory-evoked somatic movements

From the time of earliest sensibility, the entire functioning musculature can be activated by a single touch or scratch of adequate intensity at any sensitive spot on the body surface (Kuo, 1932a, 1938, 1939c; Orr and Windle, 1934; Tuge, 1937; Hamburger and Balaban, 1963). These evoked movements have a similar character in all cases, consisting of alternating lateral flexions of the head and trunk accompanied by movements of the limbs, digits and tail. Throughout incubation the pattern of motor

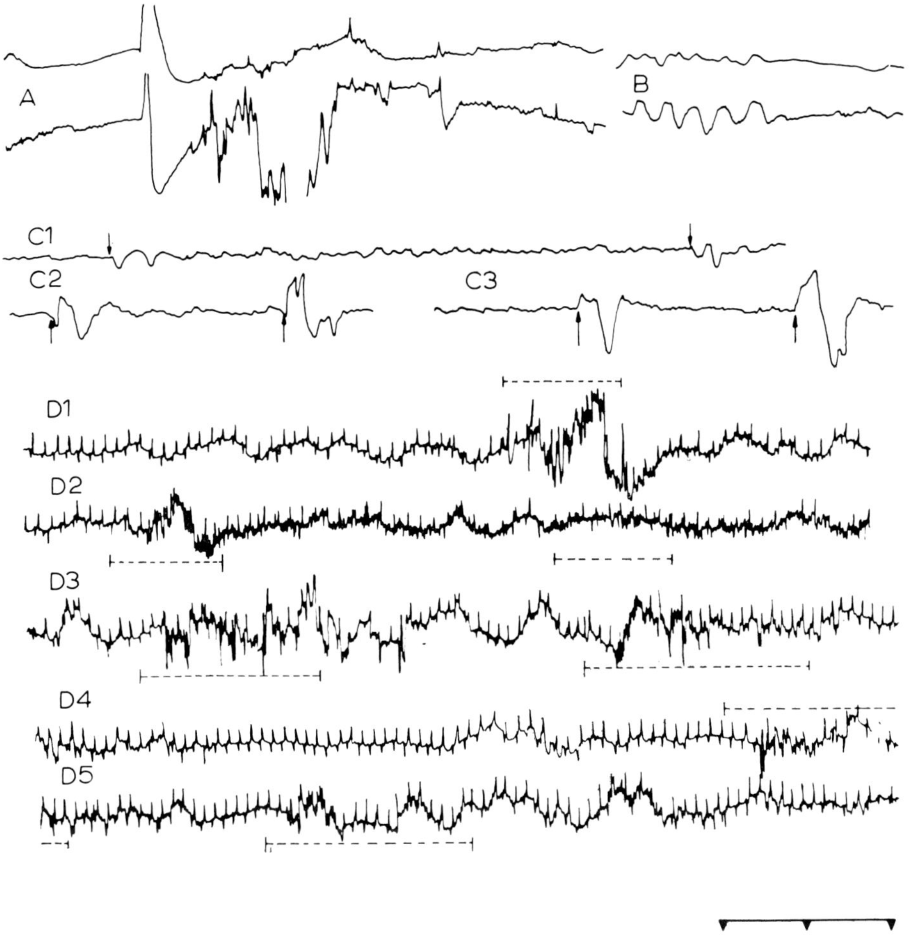

Fig. 2. Characteristics of sensory-evoked body movements in the chick embryo.
A. Burst of vigorous motility evoked by a brief tactile stimulus in a stage *39* embryo. The differential cerebral record (upper trace) shows no activity at this stage except for some simultaneous movement artifacts.
B. A still typical response to touch in a stage *45* embryo after disappearance of the cerebral EEG due to hypoxia (upper trace).
C. Increasingly vigorous responses evoked by single taps on the nostril (arrows) of progressively greater intensity (1–3). Head movement artifacts are superimposed on a monopolar cerebral record.
D. Effects of repetitive stimulation (dashed lines) in a late stage *45* embryo. In *D*1–2 (continuous record) handclaps were used, and in *D*3 and *D*4–5 (continuous record) 20 per sec stroboscope flashes. An electrode in the breast recorded ECG, EMG and movement artifacts. The onset and termination of each stimulus train were determined by means of a simultaneously-running stopwatch.
Calibration: 1 sec per division in *A* and *B*, 2 sec per division in *C* and *D*.

response appears to remain unrelated to the site of origin of sensory impulses if the stimulus intensity is high enough. When the special senses begin to function moreover, a seemingly identical type of 'total-body' response can be elicited by optic, acoustic or vestibular stimulation as by tactile (own observations). An important point to emphasize is the *triggered* nature of these reflexes, with movements lasting up to ca.

5 seconds resulting from very brief stimuli (Fig. 2A, B; also Hamburger, 1963). Repetitive stimulation can prolong the response somewhat (Fig. 1D); the excitability of a given sensory area is greatly depressed following such a response or after several normal responses in quick succession (also Visintini and Levi-Montalcini, 1939). The apparent lack of effect of sensory stimulation upon the electrical activity of higher brain centers, on the other hand, is described in the first article of this series (Corner *et al.*, this volume).

The form of the *total-motor response* to sensory stimulation changes in a characteristic way during embryonic development. Certain basic features can be easily distinguished, although objective recordings and quantitative data will be needed for further progress in this area. Lateral flexion of the head and trunk becomes progressively less evident and appears to disappear by the 10th or 11th day *in ovo*, with leg movements predominating from the 8th day (Kuo, 1932a, 1938). The co-ordinated character of the motility is lost during the second week due to the appearance of irregular twitches of the limbs and other body parts, unpredictable in sequence and not co-ordinated with each other (also see Hamburger, 1963). Moreover, in addition to waves following the usual cephalo-caudal sequence, movements now originate in the trunk region and progress anteriorly or in both directions at once (Orr and Windle, 1934; Hamburger and Balaban, 1963). Our own observations have confirmed these last points, with the additional notation that the initial movement continues to be a strong synchronous twitch, usually of the head, trunk and other muscles together. Variation exists in the exact sites of initial activity, however, regardless of the point of stimulation. Strong twitches of an entire limb, of the neck or of several parts simultaneously then occur during the motility burst, superimposed upon the irregular local twitching. A similar widespread contraction can also be elicited by an electric shock in the basal midbrain or hindbrain region, or further anterior at higher threshold (own observations). The excitability evidently fluctuates, since not every shock of equal intensity evokes a response, and irregular localized twitching sometimes follows the strong contraction. Stronger shocks increase the probability of occurrence of both the initial and the subsequent twitches, and also increase the average strength of the first movement and the duration of the after-discharge (to a maximum of about 5 seconds). Headward conduction of contractions originating in the trunk has also been observed following a single shock in any of several brain regions (Visintini and Levi-Montalcini, 1939).

During the third week of incubation there is an increasing tendency for twitches to follow each other rapidly in the same muscle, visibly resulting in briefly sustained tension (own observations). By stage *44* the movements no longer give a jerky impression but appear to flow smoothly into one another and to result in sustained flexions and twisting of the body. The sequence of contractions is still inconsistent, however, and seemingly unco-ordinated. Rhythmic respiratory and mouthing movements begin about this time to consistently accompany the general motility. When the respiratory movements become continuous shortly afterwards (also see Kuo, 1932b; Kuo and Shen, 1937; Windle and Barcroft, 1938; Windle and Nelson, 1938) there is a brief rate increase during each burst of body movements, and rhythmic vocalization is added to the pattern. (In our experience the latter can be elicited by direct stimulation of the *brain stem* earlier than is possible by even prolonged intense tactile stimulation.) By stage *45* (19–21 days) the motility pattern has become integrated into regular, alternating kicking accompanied by co-ordinated bilateral wing flapping or sustained elevation, side-to-side head and trunk movements, and usually vocalization and swallowing — often together with rhythmic opening and closing of the beak. The bursts are now more consistent in duration as well as in movement sequence, lasting about 2 seconds on the average. With *hypoxia*, they continue unchanged after the disappearance of cerebral electrical activity (Fig. 2B) but then become shorter and weaker as the threshold rises.

In addition to the 'total-motor' response, *partial activation of the musculature* is possible from the beginning of tactile sensitivity (Kuo, 1939a, b, c; Orr and Windle, 1934; Tuge, 1937; Hamburger and Balaban, 1963). According to Kuo (*op. cit.*) localized reflexes, consisting of one or more twitches, can be elicited in each muscle group of the body of the chick embryo (beak, eye and eyelid, tail, trunk and individual segments of the limbs) as soon as the corresponding skin area becomes sensitive to stimulation. These findings are supported in the case of the wing, the leg and the tail by the results of the other workers cited above, but Tuge (1937) places later the earliest local reflexes of the beak, the eyeball and the toes in the pigeon embryo—successively between 9 and 11 days of incubation. The discrepancy may lie not in a species difference but in the relative difficulty of eliciting local reflexes at early stages, especially from the more sensitive regions such as the beak (see the papers cited above). Using electric shocks to the skin of the limbs, Kuo (1939b, c) reports that in the earliest functional stages only 10% of the responses evoked at threshold intensity are localized movements. The proportion increases subsequently, following an S-shaped curve, to ca. 50% by the end of incubation. The probability of a local reflex is higher at all stages under hypoxic or hypothermic conditions, and also if the embryo is curarized (also see Kuo, 1939a) or if the amniotic movements are reduced. In addition to highly specific local reflexes, occasional anomalous responses have been reported—thus movement of one of the limbs following stimulation of the beak (Orr and Windle, 1934).

The existence of a *fluctuation of reflex excitability* is further indicated in the reports of Kuo (*op. cit.*) by the failure of some stimuli, even when carefully controlled, to evoke any visible reaction. This occurs with a higher frequency under the same conditions which favor localization of motor responses, and also if the embryo becomes dehydrated (Visintini and Levi-Montalcini, 1939). Increasing the stimulus intensity, on the other hand, *decreases* the probabilities both for obtaining only a local movement and for no-response at all. The time required for full recovery of excitability appears to be about 20 seconds, since intervals longer than this between successive stimuli do not change the results whereas progressively shorter intervals cause a linear increase in the percentage of local reflexes (Kuo, 1939b). A significantly higher proportion of the evoked movements remain localized also if each stimulus closely follows a burst of spontaneous motility. It bears mentioning at this point that, according to Kuo (1939c), many seemingly localized contractions can be found upon closer examination to be accompanied by very weak twitching in neighboring muscles. Local reflex movements occur with varying intensity moreover, the average strength being proportional to the stimulus intensity (e.g. Fig. 2C).

Other partial patterns of sensory-evoked motility are of *intermediate degrees* between the most localized and the most general types of response (Kuo, 1932a, 1939b, c; Orr and Windle, 1934; Tuge, 1937; Hamburger, 1963; and own observations). For the most part these can be classified into: (1) visible contractions which are restricted to a relatively wide area around the point of stimulation, (2) generalized muscular activity but relatively weak or infrequent in regions more distant from the stimulus (or occasionally rapid but weak twitching over the entire body), and (3) a typical generalized ('total-body') response following initial local contractions. More extensive muscular participation tends to be associated with longer response duration, ranging thus from the short-lived local reflexes to the total movement bursts lasting up to 5 seconds. The stronger the initial contraction, in turn, the less likely it is to remain localized. When respiration, beak-clapping and swallowing, and vocalization appear late in the embryonic period they constitute additional 'partial patterns', but ones which have no obvious stimulus specificity. Despite a clear fluctuation in the response threshold (Sedláček, 1962), rhythmic mouthing movements and/or vocalization can always be evoked easily by any stimulus to which the embryo is sensitive and they accompany most other reflex movements (own observations). Both the swallowing response and more generalized motor reflexes can come to be elicited by an otherwise ineffective (sub-liminal) stimulus from about the 17th day of incubation, by pairing it in the appropriate way with any of several effective 'unconditioned' stimuli (Hunt, 1949; Sedláček, 1962, 1964a, 1966). During the period up to hatching, at least *quantitative* changes occur in the ability to elaborate such a 'temporary connection'. This capacity decreases if the cerebral electrical activity is depressed by topical KCl application to one or both hemispheres during the last day of incubation, but not at earlier stages (Sedláček, 1964b, 1966).

Spontaneous motility patterns

Already several days prior to the onset of sensory-evoked movements in bird embryos, visible contractions appear in the body musculature (Kuo, 1932a, c, 1938, 1939b, c; Orr and Windle, 1934; Tuge, 1937; Visintini and Levi-Montalcini, 1939; Rhines, 1943; Volokhov, 1961; Hamburger and Balaban, 1963; Gottlieb and Kuo, 1965). This apparently *endogenous* activity—in the sense of not arising from known stimulation of sensory receptors—persists throughout incubation (also Sedláček and Votava, 1964; and own observations). It has also been reported that electrical stimulation of the brain by a single shock in the earliest stages of motility evokes patterns of movement identical to those which occur spontaneously (Visintini and Levi-Montalcini, 1939). There is agreement in the papers cited above about the main characteristics of these early behavior patterns. Head and trunk movements dominate, first consisting mostly of single or repeated lateral flexion and later of also alternating ('S') waves which originate in the neck and progress caudalwards. Head-lifting and ventral flexion of both head and trunk have been emphasized in the reports of Kuo (*op. cit.*), declining in frequency during the last part of the first week of incubation. Parallel to this development, the S-waves tend increasingly to follow each other in quick succession and to be variable in their extent. Contractions begin also to originate at more posterior levels, remaining localized or being propagated in either direction or in both simultaneously (Hamburger and Balaban, 1963). A proportion of tail and of posterior trunk movements occur from the start independently of movements in other parts of the body (Kuo, 1938; Rhines, 1943).

The *first limb movements* appear during the above-described period of increasing inconsistency of the head/trunk pattern. All authors agree that they mostly occur together with trunk movements, although by no means with all of these. There is some question about whether independent movements of the leg and wing first occur only some hours later (Orr and Windle, 1934; Tuge, 1937; Kuo, 1938) or whether a small proportion of limb movements are localized from the start (Kuo, 1939b, c; Hamburger and Balaban, 1963). The latter studies are better designed to detect small infrequent events, and it is pointed out in the most recent of them that the few independent movements all occur during the 'activity phase' of a motility cycle—which occupies less than half of the total time. Limb and tail movements increase thereafter in strength and in the frequency of independent activity, and in addition become unco-ordinated with the trunk movements and with each other during periods of generalized motility (Orr and Windle, 1934; Kuo, 1938; Hamburger, 1963). As eyelid, eyeball, beak and tongue movements are added, they complicate still further the picture of generalized, unco-ordinated and unpredictable activity of the somatic musculature. The percentage of 'independent' movements of muscle groups increases under the same conditions which favor localized responses to sensory stimulation: hypoxia, hypothermia, curarization and reduction of amniotic movements (Kuo, 1939b). The overall motility is simultaneously reduced by these treatments, to which dehydration should also be added (Visintini and Levi-Montalcini, 1939).

Spontaneous motility occurs in a clearly *periodic manner*, aspects of which have recently been studied (Hamburger and Balaban, 1963; Hamburger, 1963, 1964; Hamburger *et al.*, 1965—also Visintini and Levi-Montalcini, 1939; Rhines, 1943). There is little alteration of the periodicity during those stages just described in which the *character* of the movements are changing rapidly. Most muscular activity takes place in phases consisting of single twitches and variable bursts separated by intervals shorter than 10 seconds. The stronger a given movement the more likely it is to be followed by a burst of additional twitches, the frequencies ranging from ca. 90% for the strongest observed movements to 60% for the weakest (Kuo, 1939b). The 'activity phases' last mostly 5–15 seconds, with occasional longer values up to 30 seconds, and alternate with 'inactive phases' in which at most a few single twitches occur. The mean duration of inactivity is about 40 seconds, with values ranging from only slightly more than 10 seconds to between one and two minutes. Successive values vary irregularly for both active and inactive phases and appear to be independent of one another. The variable temporal pattern just described applies to *individual* behavior as well as to *group mean* values, but wide quantitative differences may be expected among embryos at these and later stages (Terzin *et al.*, 1963; Hamburger,

References p. 235–236

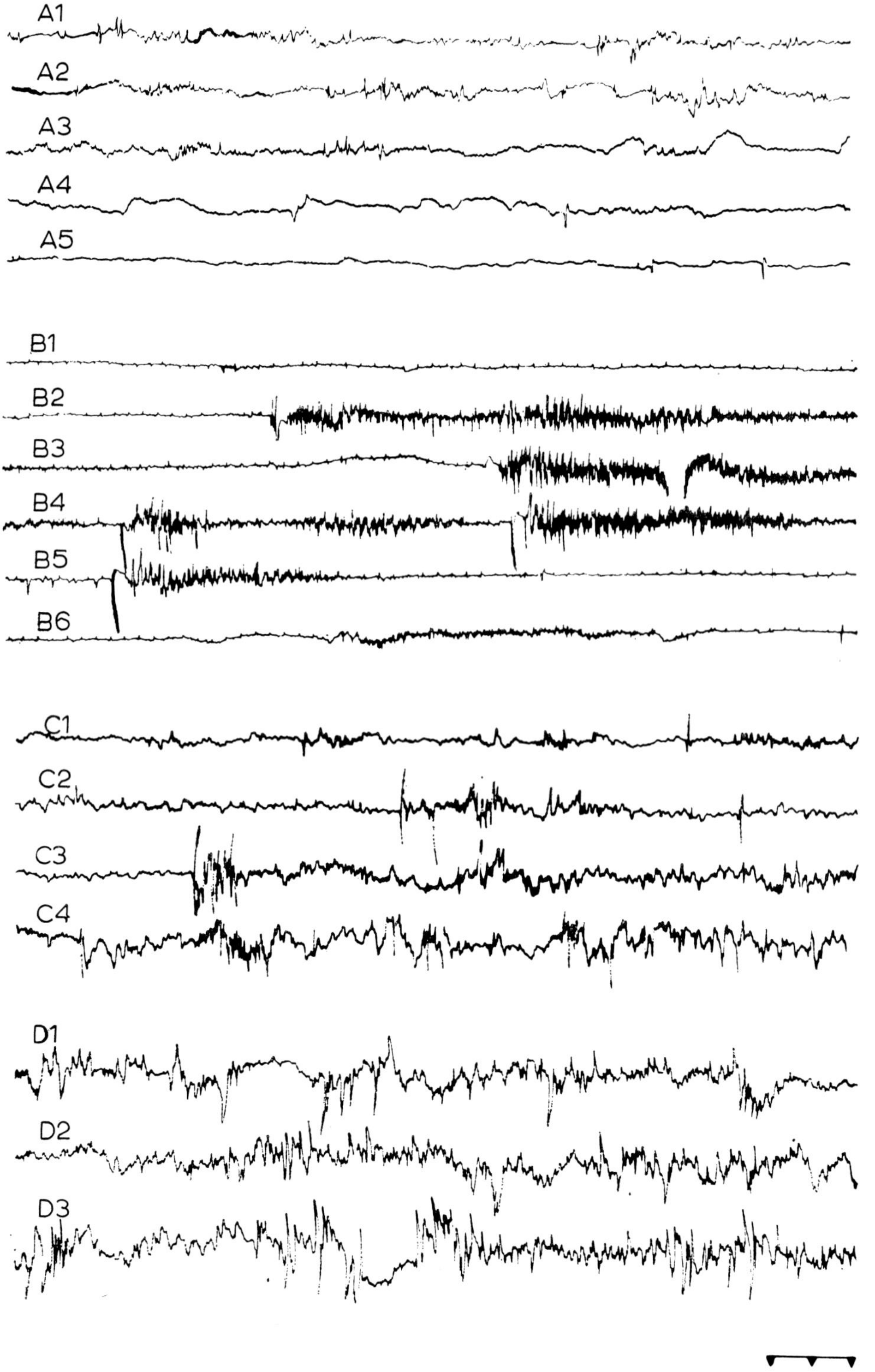
A1
A2
A3
A4
A5
B1
B2
B3
B4
B5
B6
C1
C2
C3
C4
D1
D2
D3

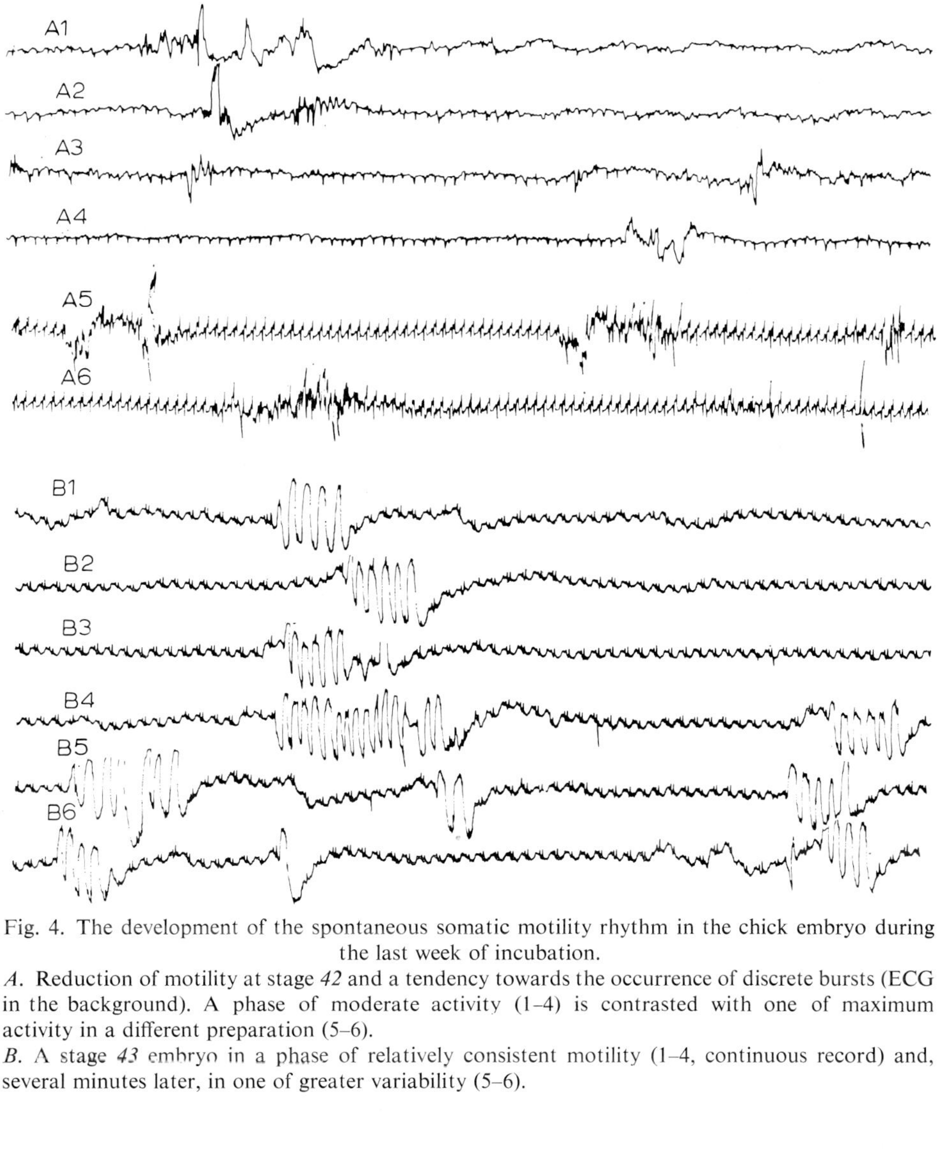

Fig. 4. The development of the spontaneous somatic motility rhythm in the chick embryo during the last week of incubation.

A. Reduction of motility at stage *42* and a tendency towards the occurrence of discrete bursts (ECG in the background). A phase of moderate activity (1–4) is contrasted with one of maximum activity in a different preparation (5–6).

B. A stage *43* embryo in a phase of relatively consistent motility (1–4, continuous record) and, several minutes later, in one of greater variability (5–6).

Fig. 3. The development of the spontaneous somatic motility rhythm in the chick embryo during the second week of incubation.

A. An *activity* phase and transition to a phase of *inactivity* in a stage *38* embryo (continuous record, 1–5).

B. Periodic fluctuations in the level of motor activity in a late stage *39* embryo, with ECG in the background (continuous record, 1–6).

C. Almost continuous activity at stage *40* but with a cyclic quantitative fluctuation in frequency and amplitude of movements (continuous record, 1–4).

D. A stage *41* embryo which shows a high level of motility without any periodic variation (continuous record, 1–4). Calibration, 1 sec per division.

References p. 235–236

1963; and own observations). Long-term fluctuations in the amount of motility have not been ruled out as contributing to the observed individual differences.

The somatic motility pattern throughout the rest of the second week of incubation retains the unco-ordinated character described earlier (own observations; also see Hamburger, 1963). Duck embryos show from about 11 days a progressively higher proportion of headturns away from the yolk (Gottlieb and Kuo, 1965) but this behavioral asymmetry reportedly exists already at 5–6 days in the chick embryo (Kuo, 1938). The periodicity of the spontaneous movements, on the contrary, changes considerably in this space of time (Hamburger and co-workers, *op. cit.*). 'Activity phases' preserve their irregular and variable pattern of bursts and twitches but, beginning at *stage 33* (about 8 days), increase steadily in their mean duration. To a lesser extent the 'inactive phases' become shorter, by *stage 39* (13 days) being few and brief and with periodicity no longer evident (also Windle and Barcroft, 1938). Electromyographic records (EMG) confirm this developmental trend (Fig. 3) and reveal in addition the presence of almost continuous weak muscular activity. This is present also during phases of relative inactivity but stops then more often and for longer periods. In our recordings, despite using the same breed of chick as Hamburger and his co-workers (White Leghorn), periodic inactivity is still present in all stage *39* embryos (6 cases) (Fig. 3B) and disappears only in the following stage (4 out of 6 cases). Even then, a cyclic fluctuation is evident in the quantitative level of the EMG and in its degree of continuity (Fig. 3C). At *stage 41* no periodicity was evident during up to 15 minutes of recording in 3 out of 6 cases (Fig. 3D). One stage *41* embryo showed the quantitative cycle characteristic of *stage 40*, while another showed periodic phases of inactivity such as are always found at stage *39* and earlier. In a third case there was an irregular slow fluctuation which contains longer stretches of inactivity than have hitherto been encountered.

An increasing level of somatic motility thus occurs during and beyond the time when amniotic movements decrease and disappear (Kuo, 1932a; Windle and Barcroft, 1938; Gottlieb and Kuo, 1965). Even at stages when these are present they are not followed consistently by body movements, while the latter frequently originate independently of amnion contractions (Rhines, 1943; Hamburger, 1963; and own observations) and continue normally in their absence (Oppenheim, 1966). There is a similar lack of a consistent or necessary relationship between motility and self-stimulation by a part of the embryo's own body (Hamburger, 1963; Gottlieb and

---

Fig. 5. Somatic motor activity of the chick embryo under hypoxic conditions (produced by bleeding).
A. Onset of augmented 'background' level of muscular contractions at stage *39* following the disappearance of visible endogenous and reflex movements (continuous record, 1–2).
B. Vigorous movements in a stage *39* embryo after a prolonged period of inactivity and shortly before complete unresponsiveness to stimulation. Gradual decline over several minutes (lines 2–4), compared with the normal motility pattern in the same preparation (line 1).
C. Increased muscular background activity in a stage *45* embryo after prolonged inactivity, leading to brief bursts of violent movements followed by a rapid decline. The largest spikes are ca. 50 μV peak-to-peak (continuous record, 1–3, with a 1 min break between lines 3 and 4). Calibration, 1 sec per division.

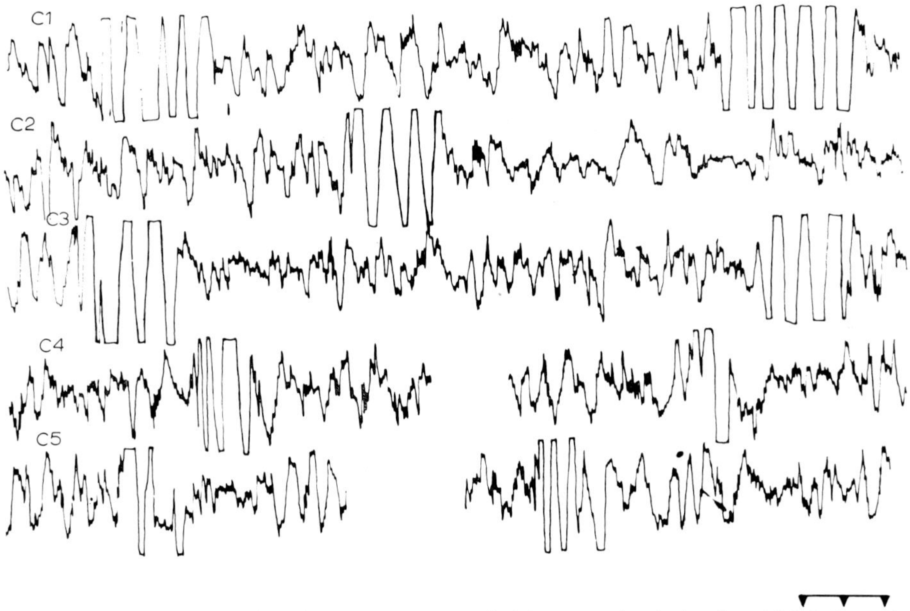

Fig. 4 *C*. Periodic bursts of body movement recorded in a restrained, sleeping chick 5 days after hatching (cerebral EEG in the background). Phases with consistently long bursts (1–3, continuous record) alternate with phases of shorter burst duration (4–5), separated by 10–15 minutes of greatly reduced activity. Calibration, 1 sec per division.

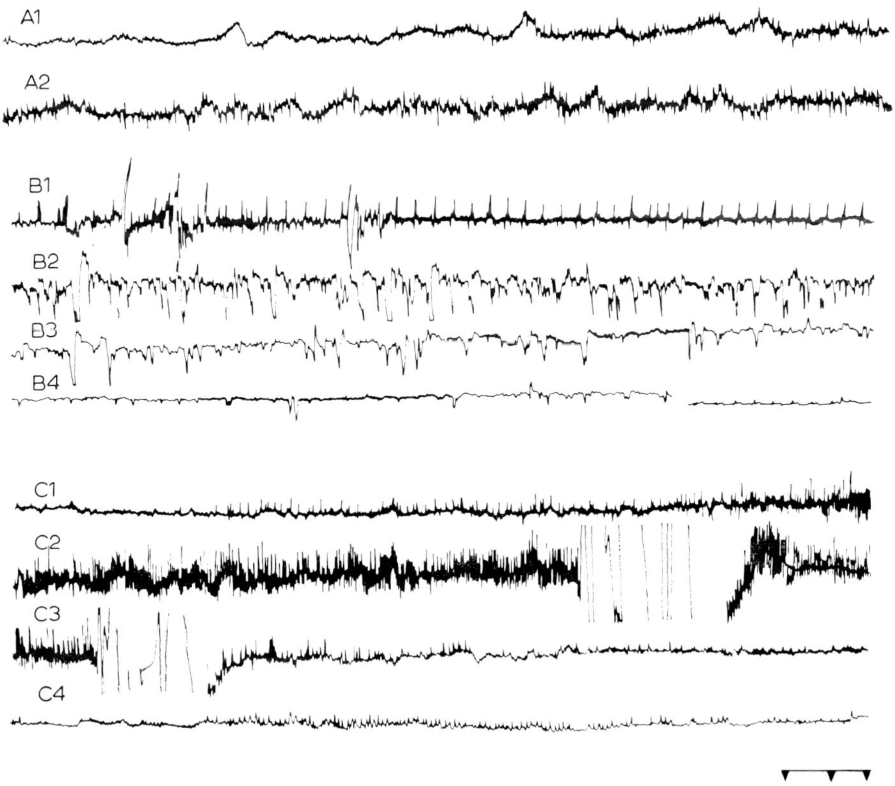

References p. 235–236

Kuo, 1965), although the latter authors have called attention to the possibility that some of the embryonic movements are evoked in this way (also Kuo, 1932c). Motility cycles are neither initiated nor reset, moreover, by tactile stimulation during inactive phases nor are they prolonged by stimulation during activity phases (Hamburger, 1963). They can be modified chemically however, the motor activity being enhanced by oxygen and depressed by carbon dioxide (Hamburger, 1963, 1964). Spontaneous motility declines and usually stops before tactile reflexes are abolished under conditions which produce hypoxia, except for continuous weak 'background' muscle activity which becomes augmented for several minutes before gradually disappearing (Fig. 5A). The reflex threshold, however, begins to rise soon after the large spontaneous movements cease and the evoked bursts become much shorter (own observations). A burst of vigorous movements lasting several seconds or a discontinuous train lasting up to ca. 3 minutes then sometimes occurs before the embryo becomes completely motionless, or recovers (Fig. 5B). The phases of increased tonus and of strong contractions followed by depression of muscular activity have been previously reported, and can moreover be duplicated by sufficiently reducing the oxygen or increasing the carbon dioxide in the atmosphere surrounding the egg (Windle and Barcroft, 1938). No initial reduction in body movements was mentioned in this study however; rhythmic respiratory movements could be provoked as early as 14 days *in ovo* by the same means.

During the third week of incubation the *character of the spontaneous movements* changes progressively, parallel with the development described earlier for sensory-evoked motility. The total-body movement pattern is *stage specific* and appears identical in a given embryo whether it occurs endogenously or following an exteroceptive stimulus (own observations). By stage *45* it therefore consists of well-co-ordinated 'struggling' which closely resembles behavior evoked under appropriate conditions after hatching (also Corner *et al.*, 1966). Series of beak movements and, a little later in development, rhythmic vocalization consistently accompany generalized motor activity—and also occur independently or simultaneously—from the time of their first appearance in stage *44* (also Kuo, 1932d; Gottlieb, 1965; Gottlieb and Kuo, 1965; Vince, 1966). The *rhythm* of the body movements also changes greatly during these stages of embryonic development (Fig. 4). At stage *42* (6 cases, ca. 16 days *in ovo*), except for the weak background twitching, much less time is spent in endogenous motor activity than at the preceding stage (also Windle and Barcroft, 1938). Large fluctuations take place in the level of activity but without any obvious indication of periodicity: sometimes short bursts of contractions occur about once per minute, sometimes the intervals are much shorter for a variable time, and sometimes stretches occur with only small movements and single twitches for more than three minutes (also Sedláček and Votava, 1964). In addition, there is clearly a reduction in the proportion of single twitches and very short bursts (Fig. 4A). Great variability still exists in the duration of the bursts, in the intervals between them and in their amplitudes in different muscle groups, but a transient period of increased consistency has been seen in one embryo.

Stage *43* embryos (3 cases) show on the whole a still greater tendency towards consistent duration of motor activity bursts and reduction in the frequency of isolated

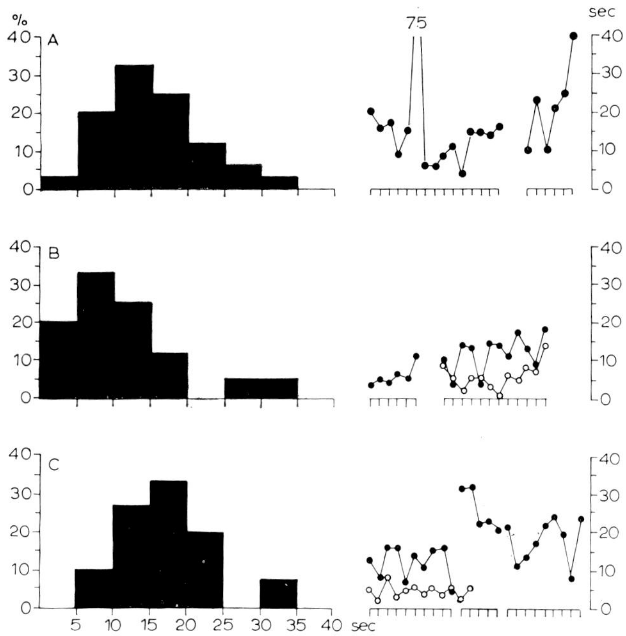

Fig. 6. The late embryonic rhythm of somatic motility in the chick.
A. *Left*, the distribution of short intervals at stage *43* (33 values from 3 normal preparations). *Right*, consecutive intervals in one embryo over a 4 min and a 2 min period, separated by a break of several minutes in the record.
B. *Left*, the distribution of short intervals at stages *44-45* (68 values from 11 normal preparations). *Right*, consecutive intervals in one normal embryo (●), with a 1 min break in the record, and in one hypoxic embryo (○) after disappearance of the cerebral EEG and until the onset of permanently reduced motility.
C. *Left*, the distribution of short intervals in a 5 day old immobilized chick (30 values). *Right*, consecutive intervals in the same bird (●) during three different periods, separated by long stretches with bursts only at intervals longer than 1 min. A stretch is also included from the movement record of an unrestrained chick just after hatching (○), showing values similar to those found in late embryos.
All intervals were measured to the nearest second from ink-writer records of electronically amplified muscle signals. The histograms are plotted as the percentage of occurrences per 5 sec period, from the left-hand value on the abscissa up to but not including the right-hand value.

movements, the extent of which is individually and/or cyclically variable (Fig. 4B). The intervals between total-body movements are distributed in a skewed manner with a peak between 10 and 15 seconds (Fig. 6A); many longer intervals also occur intermittently, as in the previous stage. Here again our material has behaved differently from that of Hamburger's group (*op. cit.*), who report only a slight reduction of overall motility from stage *39* through stage *43* (ca. 17 days *in ovo*). Both studies are at variance with the behavioral stages defined by Kuo (1938), who found a reduction of spontaneous motility to a low level, together with a steadily increasing proportion of local twitches (Kuo, 1939b), from 9 days of incubation until immediately prior to hatching. This would be accounted for by the finding that the observation technique used by Kuo (liquid vaseline applied to the shell membrane) can reduce the oxygen consumption of the egg by up to 40% (J. Sedláček, Dissert. Charles Univ. Prague, 1960—

personally communicated; also Becker, 1940). From stage *44* to hatching, the burst duration was consistently close to 2 seconds throughout up to 15 minutes of recording in most of the normal embryos studied here (4 out of 7 at stage *44*, 8 out of 11 at stage *45*). Almost all values were within one-half second from the mean value, which differed visibly from one individual record to the next. In one embryo at stage *44* and one at stage *45* most of the bursts lasted only about 1 second, while the other two stage 45 preparations showed longer and more variable bursts of movement. (One of the remaining two preparations examined gave at intervals a large total-body contraction followed by weak twitching lasting up to 2 seconds; in the second case unusually variable bursts lasting up to 2 seconds often followed each other in rapid succession.) The intervals between motility bursts tend to be shorter from stage *44* (ca. 18 days *in ovo*) through hatching (also see Vince, 1966) than at stage *43* but have a similar skewed distribution (Fig. 6B). Longer periods of inactivity are, as at stages *42* and *43*, highly variable and often last for several minutes. Single twitches of variable strength and location still occur intermittently and an almost continuous weak background activity is present which does not visibly differ from that in earlier stages.

Hypoxia produced in the last stages before hatching appears to have the same effect upon somatic motor activity as at earlier stages (Fig. 5C). Ther hythms governing spontaneous motility (durations of bursts and intervals between them) and the integrated character of the movements remain unaltered, however, for some time after the disappearance of the cerebral EEG (see Figs. 2B and 6B). Periods of maximum or of minimum motor activity each occur moreover in any phase of the slow cycle of cerebral electrical changes (see Corner *et al.*, this volume). This cerebral cycle could still conceivably have some correspondence with slow fluctuations in the *mean* duration either of motility bursts or of the intervals between them, possibilities which have not been explored here. Electrical rhythms in the optic tectum also show no obvious changes associated with total-motor activity or large single twitches, but irregular weaker movements consistently accompany endogenous or evoked bursts of large potentials (Fig. 7).

Post-hatching behavior. Periodic bursts of total-body motility continue, against a background of continuous weak twitching and occasional larger single movements, for some time after the chick has freed itself from its shell (own observations). The *distribution of intervals* between these bursts is in the same range as during the last days of incubation (see Fig. 6C—*N.B.* slightly longer intervals have been seen in other individuals and variable, long periods without bursts occur in all cases). *Durations* of successive bursts were consistent within a range of about one-half second in three chicks, with individually differing *mean* values from one to two seconds. In a fourth bird, a phase lasting at least three minutes where bursts were consistently $1\frac{1}{2}$–2 seconds in duration was succeeded some minutes later by a phase where all durations were only $\frac{1}{2}$–1 second. The *character* of these movements is similar to embryonic behavior during the last stage before hatching but now has the effect, since the chick is resting upright on its feet, of briefly elevating the body and sometimes making small steps. With the development of adequate muscle tonus to maintain an erect posture, and with the appearance of the orienting reflex and flattening of the

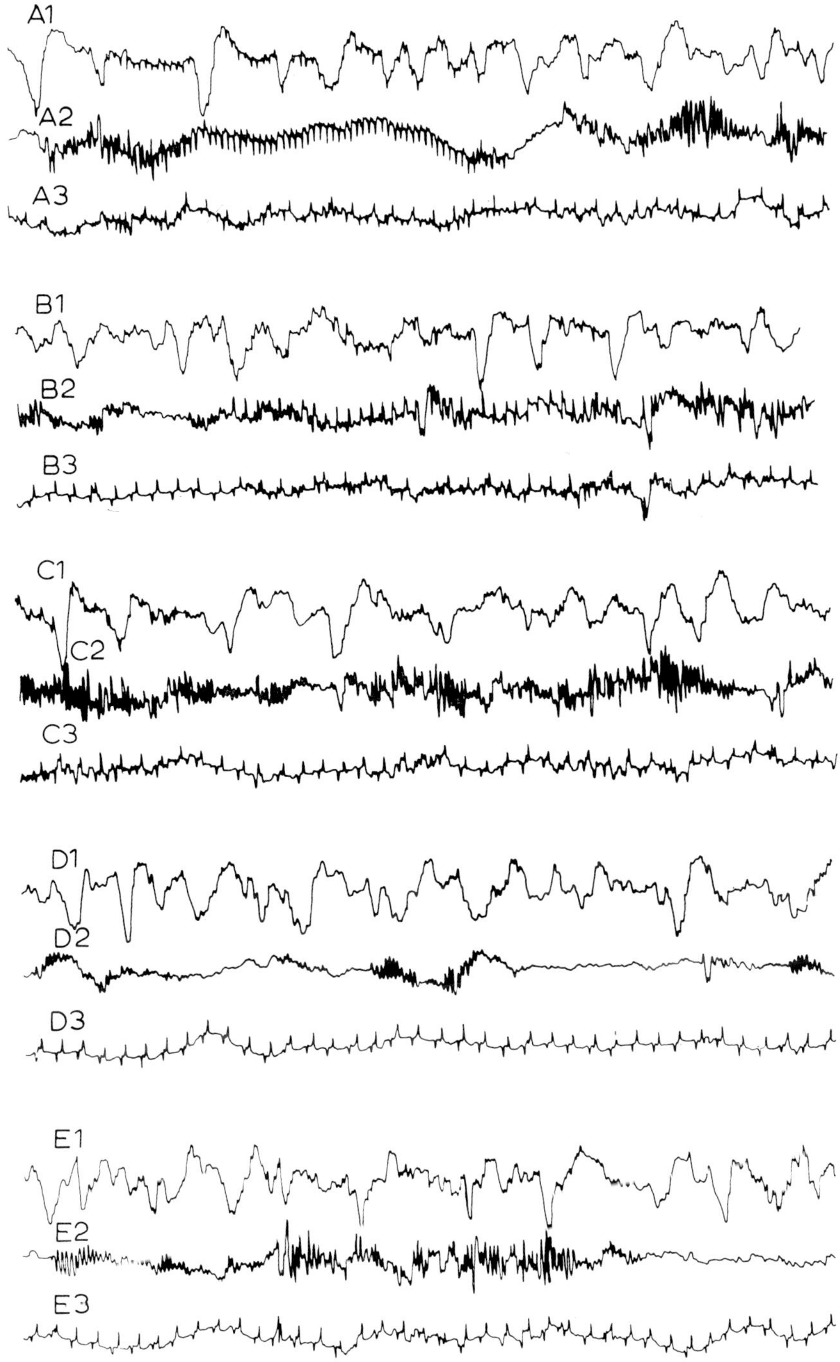

Fig. 7. Weak muscular activity (line 3: movement artifacts superimposed upon the ECG) associated with *flash-evoked* (*A* and *B*) and with *spontaneously*-occurring (*C*, *D* and *E*) large potentials in the optic lobe (line 2), compared with the absence of visible changes in the cerebral electrical rhythms (line 1). Calibration, 1 sec per division.

References p. 235–236

cerebral EEG in response to sensory stimuli (see Corner *et al.*, this volume), this periodic stereotyped struggling behavior disappears. It can re-emerge up to at least two weeks after hatching during a state of deep sleep induced by prolonged immobilization (Corner *et al.*, 1966). The intervals which have been observed are not as short overall as those during the embryonic period and their mean duration fluctuates over successive phases (Fig. 6C), which are separated by periods with much fewer bursts of struggling. The mean length of the bursts themselves also varies from one phase to the next although there is usually strong consistency within each phase (Fig. 4C—also see Corner *et al.*, 1966). A variable number of loud rhythmic cries accompanies each burst with rare exception (less than 5% of the observed occurrences) and also occurs independently with a lower frequency.

The rhythm of stereotyped motor activity does not coincide with the intermittent desynchronization of cerebral electrical activity during sleep (Fig. 4C—also see Corner *et al.*, this volume). Periods with many bursts of *struggling movements* can occur moreover during the phases of infrequent as well as of frequent electrical desynchronization. These variations in the cerebral electrical pattern are equally unrelated to the presence or absence of rhythmic *eyeball movements* (also see Paulson, 1964), which first appear along with behavioral and cerebral 'awakening' some hours after hatching (own observations). We have never seen them in records taken during the periods of highest attentiveness or behavioral activity but they may otherwise be present at all levels of alertness from waking (Fig. 8A) to deepest sleep. There also occur long stretches at all levels where these rapid eye movements fail to appear. If present, the overall frequency does not differ greatly from one situation to another but can be much increased for some time by brief electrical stimulation of the brain stem (Fig. 8B).

During the waking state, the late embryonic 'total-motor' pattern can still be

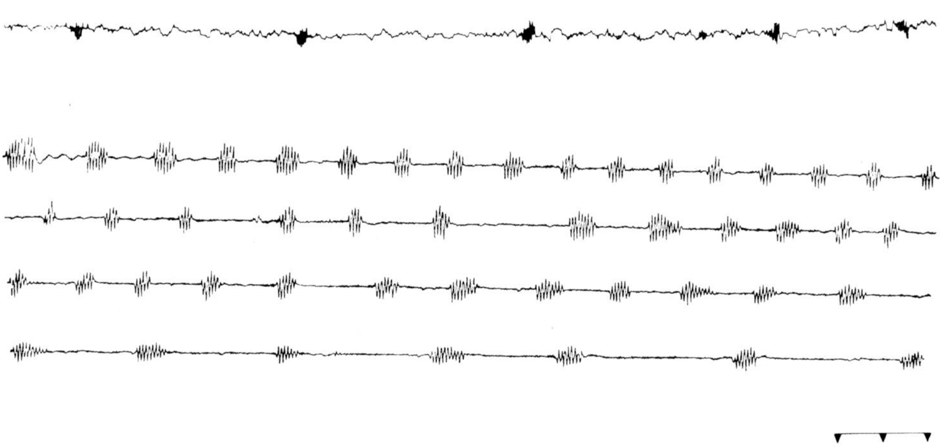

Fig. 8. Rhythmic rapid eye movements in the chick after hatching.
A. Representative normal sequence, against a background of the waking cerebral EEG.
B. Sequence in another preparation immediately following electrical stimulation of the hindbrain (continuous record, 1–4). Calibration, 1 sec per division.

clearly recognized in certain *evoked behavioral responses* (own observations). The vestibular righting *reflex*, for example, involves alternating kicking accompanied by trunk and head movements, all of comparable strength and frequency to those occurring during hatching and which can be similarly accompanied by loud rhythmic cries. The same is true of *escape* struggling behavior elicited by holding a chick fast by its leg or other part of the body. Both responses furthermore occur under maintained stimulation as a burst, not exceeding 5 seconds in duration and which is repeated at intervals. In contradistinction however to the embryonic motility bursts, which can be triggered by a brief stimulus, struggling movements evoked after hatching require continued sensory input and stop as soon as the stimulus is removed. Repetitive stimulation of adequate intensity (auditory or visual as well as tactile and vestibular) evokes long-lasting behavior of a similar character—thus *struggling* if the bird is restrained and *panic escape* if it is free-moving. This too usually stops quickly, even after more than a minute of continuous activity, as soon as the stimulation is over.

Waking behavior (own observations) consists largely of periods with continual slow and irregular stepping movements, orientation of eyes, head or body, and weak vocal pulses—apparently a *fluctuating partial activation* of the chief motor systems involved in embryonic motility. Much of this 'background' exploratory activity is clearly directed by specific sources of sensory stimulation, affecting both the direction (*approach* versus *avoidance*) and the rate of motion, and often leads to well-directed pecking reflexes. If the stimuli are appropriate, the pattern will then be interrupted by repeated *feeding* or *drinking* action sequences. Still other motor patterns which are not present prior to hatching intrude briefly upon the background activity, independently at intervals and without any evident external releasing stimuli: *defecation*, *preening* of the feathers, *stretching* of wing and leg, *scratching* at the ground, and *rubbing* the beak against the ground. The cerebral electrical pattern associated with this complex overall behavior consists of a continuous, weak high-frequency signal riding upon a fluctuating level of low amplitude slower waves (cf. Corner *et al.*, 1966; also see Corner *et al.*, this volume). Ongoing motor activities are often interrupted briefly by *attentive posture* together with a reduction in the amplitude of the cerebral slow waves, which occurs both in response to various environmental events and intermittently without any obvious stimulus. Approach or avoidance behavior of variable intensity may then follow, depending upon the stimulus characteristics, or the background pattern of activities may be resumed.

A brief and soft high-frequency *vocal pattern* ('twitter') consistently follows any stimulus which evokes attention, while intense stimuli usually evoke a sound burst of higher pitch and intensity ('shriek') (Andrew, 1964). Under certain circumstances loud, highly regular 'distress calls' are emitted while the chick is standing attentively and may continue as it begins again to walk about (own observations). Each chick differs quantitatively in this respect and furthermore has its own characteristic frequency for *steady calling*, independent of the conditions which provoke it (cold, isolation, vibration, capture, etc.). The frequency can be modified however by an imposed acoustic rhythm, individual chicks thus tending to synchronize with each other when calling in unison (unpublished results, with A.A. Verveen). The regularity

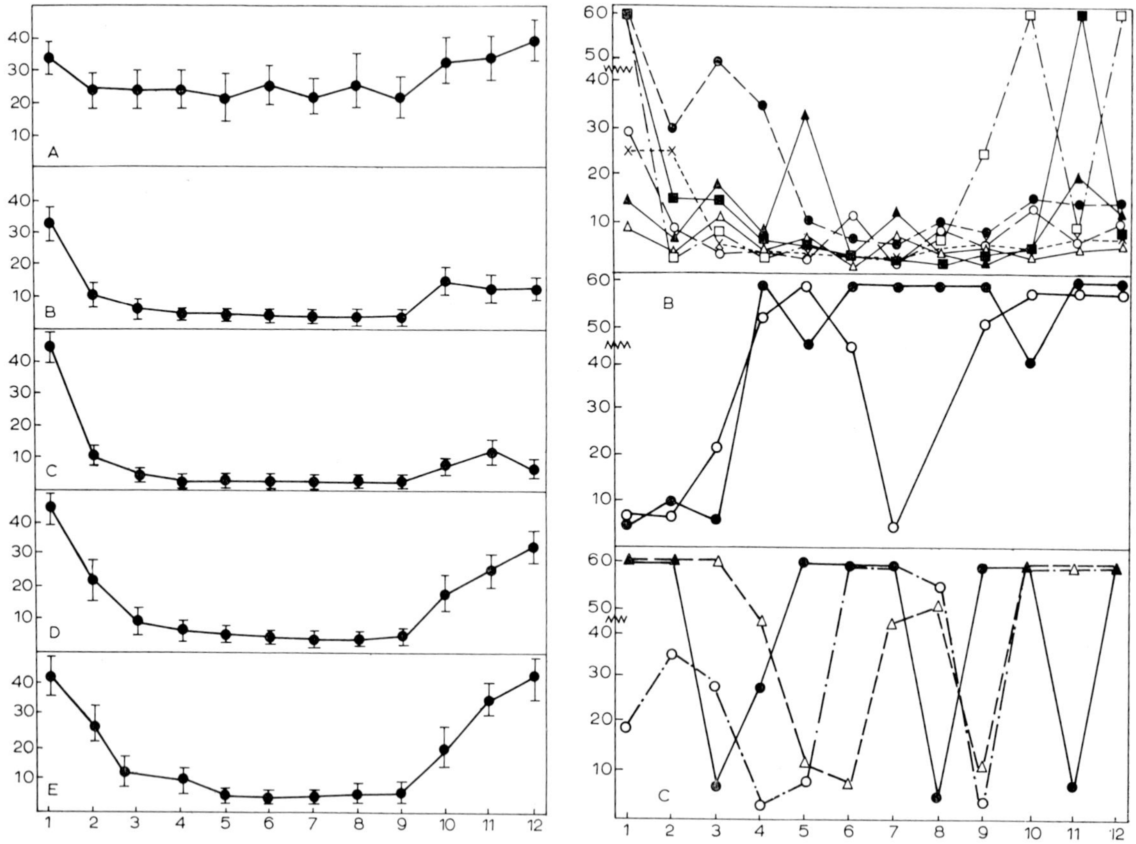

Fig. 9. Learned facilitation of approach behavior in the maturing chick. *Left*, the mean time on successive trials for jumping from a platform in order to return to a 'home' area (the height of the platform was increased after the 9th trial). *A* = 1 day; *B* = 4 days; *C* = 7 days; *D* = 10 days; and *E* = 13 days after hatching. The spread at each point gives the standard error. *Right*, the 1 day old group broken down into individual performance curves. *A* shows those chicks which behaved like the older age groups; *B* shows two individuals which responded in the opposite way; and *C* shows the birds which showed no modification with experience. '60' on the ordinate indicates *no* jump within 1 min.

and the pitch of the calls of the chick are roughly proportional to their intensity and are variable between the irregular, soft normal background vocalization and the rhythmical loud distress cries (also Andrew, 1964).

Some ways in which certain aspects of the behavioral repertoire described in the preceding two paragraphs can be controlled by *environmental situations* or *experiences* have been tested experimentally. This topic will be dealt with here only cursorily and insofar as the results reveal developmental changes. Approach responses exist already on the first day of hatching and are quickly facilitated by repeated experience (cf. Peters and Isaacson, 1963). This is achieved essentially through habituation of exploratory and attentive behavior in the situation into which the subjects are placed, but can also be contributed to by shortened hesitation if the chick must first jump from a raised platform (Corner *et al.*, 1966). In this last study it was furthermore found that the behavior in a small percentage of 1 day old chicks shows no evidence of modification by prior experience in the test environment (Fig. 9), possibly meaning that the mechanism for acquiring a 'familiarization' with a given situation appears during the first day after hatching. The *mean* rate of familiarization is fast from the start and is essentially constant throughout the first week, but shows thereafter a progressive slowing (Fig. 9). This is accounted for by the fact that about half of the birds, despite maintained alertness, begin (even on the first trial) to wait much longer before jumping or fail to do so (Corner *et al.*, 1966). In addition, going to sleep in a dark test environment—which in younger birds never occurs during the first experience and occurs within the first few seconds only by the third or fourth trial—begins, between 7 and 10 days after hatching in all cases, to appear within a few seconds even if the situation is totally unfamiliar. Approach behavior can be inhibited already in 1 day old chicks by sufficiently raising the platform after a consistent quick jumping-time has been achieved (Corner *et al.*, 1966). The effect is individually variable and can be produced as well by the *experience* of jumping from the greater height as by immediate *perception* of the change (Fig. 9). Inhibition can also be produced by means of punishing-shocks but the effect is relatively weak until 3–5 days after hatching (Peters and Isaacson, 1963). Thereafter, the identical schedule and intensity of shocks produces progressively greater inhibition (prolongation of the approach-time) through at least the middle of the second week. On the other hand, complete inhibition of the pecking reflex to a given visual stimulus can be produced already at 1 day after hatching by means of a single association with certain tastes (H. Arora, E. Lee-Teng: Progress Reports, Calif. Inst. Technol., 1965; also Lee-Teng and Sherman, 1966).

The ability to learn to make a *detour* in order to complete an approach response in a certain type of situation appears suddenly, between 5 and 9 days after hatching in different individuals of the Rhode Island Red breed, ca. 90% of them at 6–7 days (Scholes, 1965). All chicks perform perfectly or nearly so from the first successful run onwards, the day of whose occurrence cannot be altered by additional training on any number of previous days. The association persists thereafter with little loss of efficacy even in the absence of further experience. By two weeks after hatching however, only about one-third of the birds make the connection as readily as do younger ones, while the remainder fail completely to make it even after three successive days of training. In another breed (New Hampshire) it occurs in some cases even at 1 day post-hatch age and previous experience seems to have an effect, but the *optimum* learning period is still 5–9 days (Scholes and Wheaton, 1966). A 'critical period' for the formation of a highly specific association appears to exist in birds also shortly after hatching, involving persistent approach to a particular stimulus source so as to maintain close sensory contact with it ('imprinting': cf. Hess, 1964). This period shows up most clearly when the exact developmental age is used rather than the post-hatching age; it appears to last about 24 hours in ducklings and to vary slightly from bird to bird (see Gottlieb, 1961). Despite considerable plasticity in the formation of this connection, there exists a strong statistical preference for the maternal call of the same species—especially if emitted by a moving source—or, in its absence, for the species call of the siblings (Gottlieb, 1966). Both the ease of becoming imprinted and

References p. 235–236

the preference for the maternal over the sibling vocal pattern are strengthened, in the absence of any experience with the maternal call, by exposure just after hatching to additional *sibling calls* beyond those provided by the duckling itself and its natural sibs. A much more restricted period appears to exist for imprinting (6–8 hours after hatching) if the criterion is the ability of ducklings to associate pecking on a key with a brief presentation of the imprinted stimulus (Hoffman *et al.*, 1966). If such an association becomes established, the responses come in well-defined but irregular bursts with few or no distress calls in between, until the 'reward' for pecking is no longer presented ('extinction'). The response rate thereupon rises initially and then becomes replaced progressively by distress-calling.

SUMMARY

(1) The behavioral development of the chick embryo has been studied by recording spontaneous and sensory-evoked movements and muscle potentials, and by comparing detailed notes taken during the observations of selected preparations with descriptions found in the literature on this subject.

(2) There exists throughout incubation, from the time of the first somatic movements, a *motor action pattern* which involves seemingly all of the somatic musculature capable of neural activation. It can be released for several seconds by any brief sensory stimulus of adequate intensity, by direct stimulation of the brain stem, and by unknown endogenous triggers.

(3) The form which this motility takes is *stage specific*. Initially reminiscent of swimming movements in fish and amphibian embryos, it soon breaks up into a complicated but seemingly unco-ordinated and unpredictable sequence of contractions varying in extensiveness and amplitude. During the last week of incubation the separate movements become more sustained due to high-frequency repetitive twitches, finally becoming integrated into consistent bursts of stereotyped behavior which resembles post-hatching struggling movements.

(4) *Partial activation* of the body musculature occurs spontaneously throughout incubation from the earliest stages of behavioral development. With the appearance of tactile reflexes, localized movements can be evoked which are usually specific for the site of stimulation. Increasing the stimulus intensity increases the probability of eliciting a more generalized response, which can be of varying degree up to the total-pattern. There is a clear fluctuation of excitability but localized movements are favored by weak or repeated stimuli and by hypoxia, dessication, cooling or curarization.

(5) Spontaneous movements have a *rhythmic character*, with periods of frequent total-body activity alternating with periods of little or no activity. The initially relatively short periods of motility become almost continuous by two weeks of incubation. Thereafter, the spontaneous activity phase is much reduced through hatching but is not obviously periodic as in earlier stages. Motility becomes increasingly organized during the last week into consistent short bursts which, during phases of frequent activity, tend to occur at regular intervals. The quantitative values of the parameters which define this late rhythm themselves appear to fluctuate slowly.

(6) After hatching there is a cyclic return to the sleeping state the period of which is a function of environmental parameters and of age. If deep enough, the late embryonic movement pattern and rhythm re-emerge, with the latter fluctuating in a complex way until the bird reawakens. The duration and character of the motility bursts closely resemble the response evoked during the waking state by maintained strong vestibular or tactile stimulation. Repetitive stimulation (also acoustic or optic) can greatly prolong this vigorous *escape behavior* (i.e. struggling or running).

(7) The *adaptive behavior patterns* seen during waking are correlated with a desynchronized cerebral electrical rhythm (flat EEG), the quantitative variations of which reflect the level of muscle *tonus* and *attentiveness* to external stimuli. Neither the presence nor the rhythm of rapid eye movements is visibly dependent upon the cerebral activity pattern. *Stereotyped* total-body motility bursts appear only when large amplitude cerebral slow waves are present (deep sleep) but are not determined by the presence or absence of episodes of *desynchronized* sleep.

REFERENCES

ANDREW, R. J., (1964); Vocalization in chicks and the concept of 'stimulus contrast', *Anim. Behav.*, **12**, 64–76.

BECKER, R. F., (1940); Experimental analysis of the Kuo vaseline technique for studying behavior development in the chick, *Proc. Soc. Exptl. Biol. Med.*, **45**, 689–691.

CARMICHAEL, L., (1954); The onset and early development of behavior, In L. Carmichael (Ed.), *Manual of Child Psychology, 2nd ed.*, Wiley and Sons (New York), pp. 60–185.

CORNER, M. A., PETERS, J. J., AND RUTGERS VAN DER LOEFF, P., (1966); Electrical activity patterns in the cerebral hemisphere of the chick during maturation, correlated with behavior in a test situation, *Brain Res.*, **2**, 274–292.

GARCIA-AUSTT, E., AND PATETTA-QUEIROLO, M. A., (1961); The electroretinogram of the chick embryo, I. Onset and development, II. Influence of adaptation, flicker frequency and wavelength, *Acta Neurol. latinoamer.*, **7**, 179–189 and 269–288.

GOTTLIEB, G., (1961); Developmental age as a base for determination of the critical period in imprinting, *J. Comp. Physiol. Psychol.*, **54**, 422–427.

GOTTLIEB, G., (1965); Prenatal auditory sensitivity in chickens and ducks, *Science*, **147**, 1596–1598.

GOTTLIEB, G., (1966); Species identification by avian neonates: contributory effect of perinatal auditory stimulation, *Anim. Behav.*, **14**, 282–290.

GOTTLIEB, G., AND KUO, Z. Y., (1965); Development of behavior in the duck embryo, *J. Comp. Physiol. Psychol.*, **59**, 183–188.

HAMBURGER, V., (1963); Some aspects of the embryology of behavior, *Quart. Rev. Biol.*, **38**, 342–365.

HAMBURGER, V., (1964); Ontogeny of behavior and its structural basis. In D. Richter (Ed.), *Comparative Neurochemistry, Proc. 5th Internatl. Neurochem. Symp.*, Pergamon Press (London), pp. 21–34.

HAMBURGER, V., AND BALABAN, M., (1963); Observations and experiments on spontaneous rhythmical behavior in the chick embryo, *Devel. Biol.*, **7**, 342–365.

HAMBURGER, V., BALABAN, M., OPPENHEIM, R., AND WENGER, E., (1965); Periodic motility of normal and spinal chick embryos between 8 and 17 days of incubation, *J. Exptl. Zool.*, **159**, 1–14.

HESS, E. H., (1964); Imprinting in birds, *Science*, **146**, 1128–1139.

HOFFMAN, H. S., SEARLE, J., TOFFEY, S., AND KOZMA, F., (1966); Behavioral control by an imprinted stimulus, *J. Exptl. Anal. Behav.*, **9**, 177–189.

HUNT, E. L., (1949); Establishment of conditioned responses in chick embryos, *J. Comp. Physiol. Psychol.*, **42**, 107–110.

KUO, Z. Y., (1932a); Ontogeny of embryonic behavior in aves, I. The chronology and general nature of the behavior of the chick embryo, *J. Exptl. Zool.*, **61**, 395–429.

KUO, Z. Y., (1932b);Ontogeny of embryonic behavior in aves, II. The mechanical factors in the various stages leading to hatching, *J. Exptl. Zool.*, **62**, 543–487.

KUO, Z. Y., (1932c); Ontogeny of embryonic behavior in aves, III. The structural and environmental factors in embryonic behavior, *J. Comp. Psychol.*, **13**, 245–272.

KUO, Z. Y., (1932d); Ontogeny of embryonic behavior in aves, IV. The influence of embryonic movements upon the behavior after hatching, *J. Comp. Psychol.*, **14**, 109–121.

KUO, Z. Y., (1938); Ontogeny of embryonic behavior in aves, XII. Stages in the development of physiological activities in the chick embryo, *Amer. J. Psychol.*, **51**, 361–378.

KUO, Z. Y., (1939a); Studies in the physiology of the embryonic nervous system, I. Effect of curare on motor activity of the chick embryo, *J. Exptl. Zool.*, 371–396.

KUO, Z. Y., (1939b); Studies in the physiology of the embryonic nervous system, II. Experimental evidence on the controversy over the reflex theory in development, *J. Comp. Neurol.*, **70**, 437–459.

KUO, Z. Y., (1939c); Total pattern or local reflexes?, *Psychol. Rev.*, **46**, 93–122.

KUO, Z. Y., AND SHEN, T. C., (1937); Ontogeny of embryonic behavior in aves, XI. Respiration in the chick embryo, *J. Comp. Psychol.*, **24**, 49–58.

LEE-TENG, E., AND SHERMAN, M., (1966); Memory consolidation of one-trial learning in chicks, *Proc. Natl. Acad. Sci.*, **56**, 926–931.

OPPENHEIM, R., (1966); Amniotic contraction and embryonic motility in the chick embryo, *Science*, **152**, 528–529.

ORR, D. W., AND WINDLE, W. F., (1934); The development of behavior in chick embryos: the appearance of somatic movements, *J. Comp. Neurol.*, **60**, 271–286.

PAULSON, G. W., (1964); The avian EEG: an artifact associated with ocular movements, *Electroenceph. clin. Neurophysiol.*, **16**, 611–613.

PETERS, J. J., AND ISAACSON, R. L., (1963); Acquisition of active and passive responses in two breeds of chickens, *J. Comp. Phsyiol. Psychol.*, **56**, 793–796.

RHINES, R., (1943); An experimental study of the development of the medial longitudinal fasciculus in the chick, *J. Comp. Neurol.*, **79**, 107–127.

SCHOLES, N. W., (1965); Detour learning and development in the domestic chick, *J. Comp. Physiol. Psychol.*, **60**, 114–116.

SCHOLES, N., AND WHEATON, (1966); Critical period for detour learning in developing chicks, *Life Sci.*, **5**, 1859–1865.

SEDLÁČEK, J., (1962); Temporary connections in chick embryos, *Physiol. Bohemoslov.*, **11**, 300–306.

SEDLÁČEK, J., (1964a); Further findings on the conditions of formation of the temporary connection in chick embryos, *Physiol. Bohemoslov.*, **13**, 411–420.

SEDLÁČEK, J., (1964b); Effect of EEG depression on the temporary connection in chick embryos, *Physiol. Bohemoslov.*, **13**, 510–514.

SEDLÁČEK, J., (1966); Some problems of elaboration of a temporary connection in the prenatal period. *Progress in Brain Research*, Vol 22. *Brain Reflexes*. C. A. Asratyan, Editor. Amsterdam, Elsevier (in press).

SEDLÁČEK, J., AND VOTAVA, J., (1964); Significance of motor activity for development of the chick embryo, *Physiol. Bohemoslov.*, **13**, 274–280.

SZEPSENWOL, J., (1946); A comparison of growth, differentiation, activity, and action currents of heart and skeletal muscle in tissue culture, *Anat. Rec.*, **95**, 125–146.

TERZIN, A. L., ZEC, N. R., AND BOKONJIĆ, N. J., (1963); Recording of bioelectrical activities of intact chick embryos in ovo, *Brit. J. Exptl. Pathol.*, **44**, 88–100.

TUGE, H., (1937); The development of behavior in avian embryos, *J. Comp. Neurol.*, **66**, 157–175.

VANZULLI, A. AND GARCIA-AUSTT, E., (1963); Development of cochlear microphonic potentials in the chick embryo, *Acta Neurol. latinoamer.*, **9**, 19–23.

VINCE, M. A., (1966); Potential stimulation produced by avian embryos, *Anim. Behav.*, **14**, 34–40.

VISINTINI, F., AND LEVI-MONTALCINI, R., (1939); Relazione tra differenziazione strutturale e funzionale die centri e delle vie nervose nell'embrione di pollo, *Arch. Suisses Neurol. Psychiat.*, **43**, 1–45.

VOLOKHOV, A. A., (1961); On the significance of various levels of the central nervous system in the formation and development of motor reactions in embryogenesis, *Plžen. lék. Sbor.*, Suppl. 3, 141–145.

WINDLE, W. F., AND BARCROFT, J., (1938); Some factors governing the initiation of respiration in the chick, *Amer. J. Physiol.*, **121**, 684–691.

WINDLE, W. F., AND NELSON, D., (1938); Development of respiration in the duck, *Amer. J. Physiol.*, **121**, 700–707.

WINDLE, W. F., AND ORR, D. W., (1934); The development of behavior in chick embryos: spinal cord structure correlated with early somatic motility, *J. Comp. Neurol.*, **60**, 287–304.

Developmental Patterns in the Central Nervous System of Birds

IV. Cellular and Molecular Bases of Functional Activity*

M. A. CORNER AND J. P. SCHADÉ

Central Institute for Brain Research, Amsterdam (The Netherlands)

A. CELLULAR ACTIVITY PATTERNS

No direct information is presently available about synaptic activities or nerve impulse discharges in the central nervous system of bird embryos. 'Spontaneous' and evoked electrical potentials are known to reflect in many instances the summated synaptic potentials in complex networks (Anderson, 1966; Eccles, 1964; Purpura *et al.*, 1966). Endogenous membrane fluctuations in both neuronal and glial elements can conceivably also contribute to the observed potential changes. The steady potential level of brain tissue probably reflects, on the other hand, the mean level of membrane polarization in the cells of the region around the recording electrode (Bureš *et al.*, 1959; O'Leary and Goldring, 1964). With these assumptions, a begin can be made at interpreting the electrical parameters described in the first article of this series (this volume).

The potential which is evoked directly at the surface of the cerebral hemisphere by a brief shock is first seen in the chick embryo several days before any spontaneous electrical potentials can be recorded. Until about the 17th day of incubation it consists simply of a short duration, surface negative wave, which is moreover clearly discernible in all later stages. Its short duration and its stability during repetitive stimulation indicate that some type of unitary potential is responsible. The failure to record it at any distance from the stimulus site until several days later implies that new nerve fibers are being formed throughout the last week *in ovo*. The spontaneous electrical activity up to the 17th day (stage *43*) consists first solely of irregular, low amplitude slow waves and later also of a faster component. These two frequency ranges are found also in the earliest encephalograms of mammalian embryos and have been called PNII and PNI respectively for the sheep cerebral cortex, where the former is unusually prominent (Bernhard *et al.*, 1959; and this volume).

The steady potential level in all brain structures studied is low and little sensitive to inhibitors of active membrane transport up to the 17th day of incubation. One

* This research was supported in part by grants B-3048 and MH 6825 from the National Institutes of Health, Bethesda, Md. (U.S.A.)

References p. 248–250

possibility is that the number of nerve cells which are sufficiently mature to be functionally active (their activity presumably accounting for the spontaneous waves) is too small to contribute significantly to the steady polarization level. Another possible explanation is that the mean membrane potential of all excitable elements is still very low. Recordings on the single cell level would be desirable to determine the distribution of active neurons and their patterns of activity. Spontaneous firing has been encountered in cells scattered throughout the cerebral cortex of the rabbit during the earliest stages of the electrocorticogram (Schadé, 1960; Huttenlocher, 1966), similarly occurring discontinuously and simultaneously over a wide area. This is likely to be at least partly endogenous activity since bursts of spikes and slow waves occur also in isolated embryonic cerebral tissue, both of mammals and of birds (Crain, 1964, 1966; Cunningham, 1962). Later, changes in the firing rate of many cells are synchronous with spontaneous slow waves (Garma and Verley, 1965), whose duration range corresponds closely to that of cortical synaptic potentials in the kitten (Purpura *et al.*, 1965).

The 17th day *in ovo* appears to be a critical stage in the functional development of the chick brain. The polarization level and the susceptibility to certain treatments (KCl, ouabain, etc.) increase simultaneously in all of the structures studied. Interference with circulation or oxygen supply then results in the return of all known electrical parameters to the condition existing prior to the 17th day. This development implies that a general metabolic change, such as the improvements in extra-embryonic blood circulation which are taking place at this time, makes it possible for already present neurons to become functionally active. If the foregoing supposition is correct, one would expect that the functional changes at this stage are not necessarily correlated with morphological changes but with changes in the metabolic activity of the neuronal elements. This point is also suggested by the essentially mature histological organization achieved long before electrical activity has been able to be recorded from the brain (Jones and Levi-Montalcini, 1958), and is presently being studied further using Golgi-stained sections. The direct-evoked surface potentials and the spontaneous electrical pattern in the cerebral hemisphere both show a significant development in stage *43* (*i.e. ca.* 17th day). The former rapidly develops a relatively long duration, surface negative wave which immediately follows the initial deflection and which is relatively sensitive to anoxia or repetitive stimulation. The latter shows a progressive increase in large amplitude slow potentials, which become almost continuous by the end of this stage. Neither the spontaneous nor the direct-evoked negative waves then change visibly in subsequent embryonic or in post-hatching development.

The often widespread synchronization of electrical activity in one or both hemispheres, taken together with the failure of evoked foci of activity to propagate over large surface areas or to the opposite side, indicates the participation of intricate circuits between cortical and sub-cortical regions as a source for many of the potentials. Visual-evoked potentials in the cerebrum, moreover, are similar in form and duration to the large spontaneous waves. These slow waves are correlated after hatching with sleeping behavior, as in mammals, so that a chiefly forebrain origin may be suspected (*e.g.* Akert, 1965; Villablanca, 1965). The persistence of this electrical rhythm in the isolated forebrain of the chick (Spooner, 1964) confirms the existence of an intrinsic system for determining the temporal pattern in which the cerebral neurons are driven. A noteworthy aspect of the integrated forebrain system is the wide range of variation which is permitted in the amplitude, duration and distribution of successive cerebral slow waves. The analogous rhythm in the adult cat can be maintained indefinitely by an isolated cerebral cortex, whereas the isolated thalamus displays a quite different pattern (Kellaway *et al.*, 1966) and the slow waves disappear from subcortical structures following decortication (Jouvet, 1965). The intermittent activity which has been reported in most studies of isolated cortex, and which can be produced experimentally by hypoxic conditions (Kellaway *et al.*, 1966), might indicate an endogenous fluctuation of neuronal excitability. Intermittent output from the isolated hindbrain of anuran embryos can be made continuous by overstimulating the preparation, whereafter intermittency reappears as the activity pattern slowly returns to its previous level (Corner, 1964a).

After the cerebral slow potentials in the chick embryo have become essentially continuous and are almost of the mature amplitude, brief episodes of flattening of the electrical record (presumably desynchronization of neuronal potentials) begin to occur. Such stretches appear in a highly irregular manner during periods lasting several minutes, alternating with several minutes of relatively uninterrupted slow wave activity. Desynchronization of the electrical record then increases in prominence until the entire 'active phase' of each cycle is almost completely devoid of large waves while flat stretches occur frequently even during the 'inactive' phases. The facts that the embryonic behavior pattern does not change concomitantly, and that a similar cyclic variation characterizes 'activated' (*i.e.* desynchronized) sleep activity in the post-hatching chick, suggest that the system responsible for this phase of sleep has started to function several days prior to hatching. If its physiological basis is the same as in mammals, the activation pattern of the cerebrum originates in a small portion of the hindbrain reticular formation, normally independent of afferent impulses although proprioceptive stimulation can trigger it (Jouvet, 1965). As in mammalian development, activated sleep then becomes progressively less prominent as the animal matures still further (Jouvet, 1965). This decline begins in the chick on the last day of incubation and is practically completed by the time of hatching. The earlier appearance of the slow wave sleep rhythm has otherwise been reported only in the rhesus monkey (Meier and Berger, 1965). The processes by which the cerebral activity becomes largely desynchronized within such a short period of embryonic development and soon afterwards equally rapidly attains the mature sleep pattern, in which synchronized waves occupy more than 99% of the recording time, are completely unknown. The faster waves continue throughout all physiological stages without visible changes in amplitude or frequency.

The optic tectum begins late in the embryonic development of the chick to generate variable, spontaneous bursts of high amplitude fast potentials which sometimes also follow light-evoked responses. It is not known where this activity originates nor how the pattern of firing is regulated but it appears to be independent of functional patterns in the cerebral hemisphere. The bursts develop slowly through the first week after hatching until they become practically continuous. There is a reduction in amplitude during the waking state.

Somatic motility in the chick embryo can be regarded as the direct expression of activity patterns in motoneuron populations, in turn reflecting patterns originating in neuronal circuits and in sensory receptors. Isolation experiments (Alconero, 1965) have shown that, as in anurans (Corner, 1964a, b; Corner and Crain, 1965), all of the earliest motility originates in the central nervous system. Quantitative studies with deafferented chick embryos (Hamburger *et al.*, 1966) indicate that, at least into the final week of incubation, most or all of the somatic movements continue to originate centrally, despite the existence of functional reflex connections during most of this period. The rhythmic character of the short bursts which characterize motility thereafter (Corner *et al.*, 1966; and this volume) suggests that behavior continues to reflect a centrally-determined pattern until a short time after hatching. The possibility remains, of course, that afferent input during this latter period influences the rhythm in a quantitative way or affects the co-ordination of the motor discharges. Very similar bursts characterize early anuran behavior, however, and have been demonstrated to occur to the normal extent in the absence of sensory nerve fibers (Corner, 1964). In both of these classes of vertebrates the neural activity responsible for motility is generated both in the brainstem and in the spinal cord, with a decreasing cephalo-caudal gradient (*cf.* Hamburger, 1963; Corner, 1964b; also see Crain and Peterson, 1964; Corner and Crain, 1965; Crain, 1966). Even from the earliest stages of somatic motility, however, the degree of integration of the central nervous system is such as to permit propagation of excitation throughout all levels.

The earliest motor activity in vertebrate embryos consists of single twitches, and only gradually do bursts of repetitive twitching appear (see part II of this series, this volume; also Alconero, 1965; Corner, 1964). If the example of deafferented anuran embryos also applies to birds, this development must be attributed solely to loops within the central nervous system. Since a brief tactile stimulus typically evokes bursts of equivalent duration, endogenous motility possibly results from the triggering of a reverberatory neural circuit by a brief train of central pulses at varying intervals. The phases of relative activity and inactivity would then result from a cyclic fluctuation in the excitability of the motor circuit and/or in the quantitative parameters of the triggering pulses. The former possibility is implied by observations that the reflex thresholds fluctuate in a closely parallel manner and that a higher proportion of localized movements occurs whenever the overall activity level is reduced. Some of the motor neurons can evidently be fired by excitation which is too weak to spread throughout the central neuronal circuits. The reduction and greater localization of neuro-motor activity under conditions such as hypoxia and hypothermia likewise indicates a weakening of central synaptic interactions, whereas the later period of convulsive twitching during anoxia would be accounted for by actual depolarization of the nerve cells. A similar sequence is seen in mammalian cerebral structures where the electroencephalogram disappears several minutes before any signs of membrane depolarization can be observed (De Valois and Schadé, 1965).

The most striking development in the behavior of chick embryos, following the sudden drop in motor activity level around stage *42*, is the appearance of highly stereotyped bursts of movement. These are originally relatively long and variable but gradually become more consistent and shorter in mean duration. A similar process has been noted in anuran embryos (Corner, 1964) and seems to indicate the gradual addition of inhibitory elements to the reverberatory neuro-motor circuit. The reflex excitability is known to be reduced for several seconds following each burst, resulting in fewer responses and a higher proportion which remain localized. The finding of individuals at all stages in which the mean burst duration fluctuates slowly suggests that also this feedback mechanism has a cyclic character. Most of the individual differences recorded at each stage fall within the observed range of fluctuation, so that individuality would normally consist more of quantitative variations in rhythmicity than of distinct steady states. In the late embryo, most of the periods with much motility contain bursts with a mean duration of *ca.* 2 sec. The periods in which the mean value falls to around 1 sec would then be accounted for by increased strength of inhibitory feedback; the alternate periods in which the bursts are more variable and some last longer than 3 sec, approximating the pattern seen most often in many younger embryos, would resu't from a swing in the opposite direction. Study of stereotyped spontaneous motility in post-hatching chicks reveals that the system determining the burst duration undergoes little or no further quantitative development.

A slight decrease in variability and in mean length of the intervals between spontaneous motor bursts occurs in the chick embryo during the same period as the described change in burst duration. The similar trend which has been reported even in isolated portions of the basal hindbrain of anuran embryos (Corner, 1964a) implies that a purely local mechanism is responsible. The interval distribution at all stages can fluctuate over successive periods of strong motor activity, but this does not coincide with the cycle regulating the duration of the bursts. If this rhythmic type of behavior is made to again manifest itself after hatching, the intervals are considerably longer on the whole than in the late embryo. At about two days prior to hatching in the chick, without any change in the rhythm or duration, somatic motility acquires a co-ordinated character which must reflect the almost simultaneous differentiation of new excitatory and inhibitory pathways impinging upon the motoneuron pool. The ability of the isolated spinal cord or of the limb segments alone to exhibit typical locomotor co-ordination (*cf.* Denny-Brown, 1960) implies that intra- and intersegmental spinal mechanisms are sufficient to account for this change in behavior. The persistence in lower vertebrates of characteristic motor sequences following even total deafferentation of the trunk and/or limbs (*e.g.* Weiss, 1941; Yntema, 1943; Gray, 1950) suggests furthermore that the new pattern of efferent discharge is determined solely by the central organization rather than by patterned afferent impulses. Adequately intense pulse stimuli or weaker, repetitive stimuli from visual, auditory or tactile receptors trigger a visibly identical movement pattern in the chick embryo.

In the foregoing paragraphs, a rough picture has been sketched of the embryonic central nervous system as consisting of several sources of rhythmic excitation, each with its specific temporal pattern and pathways of distribution. Some of the generators may be distinct but intimately related, such as the systems which control synchroniza-

References p. 248–250

tion and desynchronization of cerebral activity. Others may be points within a single integrated system, such as the brainstem-cord motor region, all of which produce almost the same effect. The persistence of the normal interval distribution, and of the duration and character of the motility bursts for a time after the disappearance of electrical activity from the cerebrum, cerebellum and optic lobes confirms the impression that embryonic behavior in the chick is regulated essentially independently of the major brain structures necessary for adaptive behavior after hatching. Sensory input, furthermore, evokes vigorous movements without any obvious changes in the EEG's recorded from the hemisphere and optic tectum. The long, variable periods of quiescence which characterize the behavior throughout most of the final week of incubation could, however, conceivably be caused by inhibition originating from higher centers.

For mammalian embryonic development no studies have yet been made on spontaneous motor patterns and their neurological basis. The picture is the same as that given here for the chick, however, in regard to the following general features (*cf.* Carmichael, 1954): (a) spontaneous motility begins about the same time as the first tactile reflexes, or at most a few days earlier or later (according to the species); (b) it continues through most or all of gestation (reduction of the activity level towards term is more profound than in the chick); (c) total-body movements can be evoked from the time of earliest tactile sensitivity; (d) local reflexes too can be demonstrated at all stages, using minimal adequate stimulus intensities. These facts are incompatible with assertions in the literature about a universal principle of behavior development, a point made long ago by Kuo (1939) and more recently by Barron (1950), by Carmichael (1954) and by Hamburger (1963). Somatic motility patterns cannot be built up by the gradual integration of local reflexes, for instance, if total movements are already possible in the earliest stages and if sensory input is not required for local and generalized movements. The same considerations apply to the assertion that spontaneous, local reflex and generalized reflex motility appear as successive phases of development (Volokhov, 1961; Sedláček *et al.*, 1961), rather than being different modes which exist together at all stages. 'Individuation' from an originally total-motor pattern, on the other hand, can be said to occur only in that local reflexes become progressively easier to elicit. The situation existing at the onset of motility undoubtedly reflects the relative timing among groups of motoneurons and interneurons in the formation of functional connections. There is neither theoretical nor empirical reason at present for supposing that these processes must follow a particular schedule, but rather that they vary considerably according in part to the adaptive requirements of different species (also Anokhin, 1964). The neurological basis is complex and is in no sense to be understood as chiefly the addition of progressively more cephalad-located circuits (*e.g.* Volokhov, 1961; Sedláček *et al.*, 1961).

The first signs of sensory-evoked arousal in the cerebrum occur only after the chick has been out of the shell for some time. This implies a gradual excitation of the reticular-activating-system under the influence of increased sensory input. The source is likely to be proprioceptive since the same development occurs even when all other sources of stimulation have remained constant. Stretches of activation soon appear even without specific added stimulation and then persist longer and longer, accompanied by increasing postural tonus and by inhibition of the motility bursts. The complex effect of this alerting ('waking') system is later also seen clearly when stimulation produces inhibition of ongoing movements together with augmented postural tonus and reflex excitability. The cerebral activity always becomes simultaneously more completely desynchronized (disappearance of the low amplitude slow waves). The inhibitory influence upon certain lower motor centers is also seen in the absence of spontaneous struggling behavior and in its immediate cessation upon termination of strong sensory stimulation, in contrast to the prolonged activity which is triggered in the embryo. Simultaneous excitatory influences upon motor networks are revealed by the almost continuous walking, peeping and searching which characterize much of waking behavior, and by the intermittent occurrence of numerous types of movements which are never seen *in ovo*. A fluctuating level of small slow waves in the cerebrum accompanies this motor activity, and both are inhibited when the reticular activation is increased still further during attentive behavior. Mixed facilitatory and inhibitory motor efforts exerted by the reticular-activating-system have also been reported from mammalian physiological studies (*e.g.* Dell, 1963).

Transition to the sleeping state is characterized by gradual reappearance of high amplitude slow waves, reduced postural tone and lessened sensory reactivity. Since this constitutes a return to the embryonic condition, where motor activity is not dependent upon cerebral function, the simplest explanation for the role of the slow-wave system is that it inhibits the reticular and other systems which govern waking behavior. Even the inhibition which the latter exert upon the rhythmic embryonic mode of motility is lifted if sleep is deep enough. The sleep and waking systems are thus functionally linked by reciprocal inhibition so that they alternate between two steady states (also Akert, 1965). Each state shows fluctuating slow wave activity with a variable mean level, but always high amplitude in the former case and low amplitude in the latter. The transition from one state to the other often occurs in several steps and is determined in part by an internal cycle which is known to be sensitive to certain environmental parameters. Appropriate stimulation can produce a transient shift towards the opposite state, and if adequately intense will trigger the switch from one to the other. The threshold for these effects fluctuates considerably however, and complex homeostatic mechanisms have been implicated in the regulation of the reticular excitation level (Dell, 1963). The cycle is also a function of age, being initially relatively short with a high proportion of time spent in sleep. The physiological basis for the rhythm of interaction between arousal and sleep systems and for the quantitative changes in it during maturation is not understood.

B. MOLECULAR FOUNDATIONS OF NEURONAL CHARACTERISTICS

The incomplete maturity of the morphological network might partly explain the severely limited functional repertoire observed before the 17th day *in vivo* in the chick. As observed in Golgi-Cox and Bodian-stained preparations, the receptive surface of neurons in the superficial layers of the hemisphere and optic tectum still increases to a considerable extent during the last four days *in ovo* and the first two weeks post-

References p. 248–250

hatching. As the neurons develop mainly dendritic and axonal branchings during this period, the proportion of cell surface to cell volume will rise rapidly and most of the energy expended will go into building up the fine-structural and chemical architecture of the neuronal units.

In considering molecular parameters during maturation, two factors are of prime interest with respect to neuronal function, *viz.* ionic pumps which maintain concentration gradients across the cell membranes and energy requirements for these processes. The membrane properties of probably every type of cell in most animals depend upon the reaction of a single molecule, adenosine triphosphate (ATP). A sodium-potassium activated ATP-ase, first detected by Skou (*cf.* 1965, for review) in peripheral nerves, appears to constitute the enzymatic basis for active transport across cell membranes. This enzyme is present in all excitable tissues in high concentration in the cell membranes. A particularly high ATP-ase activity has been found in the cerebral cortex of mammals and, since this enzyme is glucoside-sensitive, the injection of ouabain causes severe neurological disturbances (Bignami *et al.*, 1966).

Samson *et al.* (1964) investigated the sodium-potassium ATP-ase activity during postnatal development of the rat brain and showed a rapid increase in the period between the 10th and 21th day. This marked increase in enzymatic activity coincides with significant changes in the development of a number of electrical parameters of the cerebral cortex. The same type of observation was made by Bignami and coworkers (1966), who observed a very rapid increase of this enzyme after 19 days of incubation in the chick. At hatching, the enzymatic activity per unit of weight reached about 80% of the adult value.

In none of the reported results have qualitative changes in the enzymatic activity been reported. It is therefore tempting to correlate the rapid increase in sodium-potassium ATP-ase with the increase in total area of excitable membrane per unit weight of cerebral tissue. During the above-mentioned periods of development in rat and chick brain, the number of neurons per unit volume of cerebral tissue decreases but the proportional volume of dendrites and axons increases considerably. A neuron apparently needs a certain receptive surface area and a minimum number both of excitatory and of inhibitory synaptic contacts before the mechanism for generating action potentials starts to operate continuously. Once this mechanism is established with a minimal amount of synaptic input, the further outgrowth of the synaptic surface area likely contributes only quantitatively to the pulse-generating properties of the neuron. Since the number of synapses increases proportionally to the receptive surface area, the connections with other neurons will increase in a logarithmic way, thus rapidly enhancing the integrative capacities of the neuron. The experimental data to date do not indicate any qualitative changes in the electrical parameters of developing neurons. If the membrane properties during successive stages were investigated quantitatively it would be possible to know the overall pattern of translation of input into output activity, which is a major basis for the changing functional patterns during maturation of the nervous system.

Concerning the energy requirements for establishing and maintaining membrane mechanisms, the mitochondria are the most likely organelles to consider in the neuronal cytoplasm. In addition to being involved in other functions such as providing energy for the overall structural integrity of the neuron, mitochondria play a key role as sources of power for the membrane pump mechanisms. Since the membrane area increases rapidly within a relative short period, the energy cost to maintain concentration gradients across the membranes will rise correspondingly in the same developmental stage. It has been shown for the rat that the average number of mitochondria per cell increases fivefold during the critical development period (Samson *et al.*, 1963). The greater power requirements of adult neurons are apparently met by an increase in the number of mitochondria per cell. Careful examination of electron micrographs shows that during development of the nervous system in the chick only the number per neuron and not the size of the mitochondria changes (Wechsler, this volume). This suggests that each mitochondrion has a unit capacity and that the potential for energy metabolism is thus precisely proportional to mitochondrial numbers. Since it has been reported that the oxygen consumption per gram of neuronal tissue rises during development, the inference can be made that the neuronal power requirement (*i.e.* energy per unit time) increases with maturation of the neuron. Corresponding to this increased power requirement there occurs a purely quantitative increase of the power-producing units, *viz.* the mitochondria. Although still speculative, the above-mentioned considerations indicate that the increases in functional capacity of the neuron are of a quantal nature.

C. EXTRINSIC FACTORS IN NEUROGENESIS

A rough mapping of the embryonic central nervous system was attempted in part A in terms of the origin and spread of functional activity. The overall pattern at each stage of development must be determined by the input-output relationships of the various neuronal units and by their mutual interconnections, about which not very much information is available. These properties, in turn, are an expression of the molecular organization and energy requirements of the functional units, *i.e.* nerve cells, aspects of which were treated in part B. The biochemical organization will itself be a complex function of the total spectrum of energy which impinges upon each cell. Since the formal relationship between such 'extrinsic' environmental factors and the 'intrinsic' factors which constitute the cell itself is often misunderstood, an attempt will be made at this point to clarify certain basic concepts. While doing so, available evidence concerning some of the factors which could play a role in neurogenesis will be discussed.

It was explicitly formulated by Wilhelm Roux in the introduction to the first volume of his *Archives für Entwicklungsmechanik* that future experimental embryology would consist largely of analyzing the extrinsic and intrinsic factors in development. The relationship between heredity and environment ('nature/nurture') in animal behavior development is, for instance, an application of this program to psychology. Confusion has arisen, however, because of the frequent tendency to seek answers to problems posed in these terms by *deciding between* them as if they were alternatives. Thus, it has been asked whether a given action pattern is 'innate' or 'acquired' ('instinctive *vs.* learned', *etc.*), or a combination of these, with the result that unrealistic extreme

References p. 248–250

viewpoints and not always fruitful controversies have arisen (for recent reviews and attempts at synthesis, see Konishi, 1966; Schneirla, 1966). In fact, however, *all* of the behavior of a system reflects its intrinsic processes, while these will all in some way be functions of the extrinsic forces operating upon the system. 'Internal factors', instead of being a distinct set of operators, become therefore simply the causal link between environmental parameters and the system's effector actions. The behavior is able to be described empirically solely in terms of present and past contingencies or 'experiences' (*e.g.* Skinner, 1966), while the inner workings of the system provide the 'explanation' for these empirical relationships.

In the case of the development of a neuron, the task at the cellular level becomes one of specifying the way in which its changing form and response-modes depend upon the entire range of impinging environmental influences (or upon aspects of special importance if the rest can be held reasonably constant). The factors known to be able to influence directly the maturation of nerve cells can be grouped broadly into the following, inter-dependent categories:

(1) *physico-chemical* factors such as temperature, pH, osmotic pressure;
(2) *metabolic* factors such as nutrients, oxygen, vitamins;
(3) *hormonal* factors such as 'Nerve Growth Factor' (*cf.* Levi-Montalcini, 1964) and thyroid hormone (Eayrs, 1964);
(4) *trans-synaptic* and other intra-neural factors (including glial), probably involving both trophic influences (*e.g.* Gutmann, 1964; Hughes, 1965; Hamburger, 1966) and functional activation.

The possible developmental role of neural function deserves some additional comment. With the demonstration of wide-spread endogenous, *i.e.* not sensory-evoked activity within the embryonic central nervous system (*cf.* Crain, 1966), the mere elimination of sensory input or the absence of motor output is no indication that neurons are not stimulating one another. Although the possibility has been pointed out, for instance, that the high level of excitation existing during the 'activated' phase of sleep may be important for normal neurogenesis (Roffwarg *et al.*, 1966), no information is presently available with which to answer this question.

Functional neural activity evoked by the stimulation of sensory receptors is of particular interest with respect to neurogenesis. The possibility has been sketched in detail (*cf.* Gottlieb, 1966) that embryonic behavior development is an expression of neural organization changing under the influence of afferent impulses, including 'self-stimulation'. The point has also been made that the formation of *co-ordinated*, adaptive patterns of motor activity may depend upon an adequate level of sensory input at or after the time of birth or hatching (*e.g.* Fox, 1966). Sensory input has been largely eliminated during development in amphibians by means of extensive extirpation of the sensory nerves (*e.g.* Yntema, 1943; Detwiler, 1947) or rearing in an anesthetic medium (Matthew and Detwiler, 1926; Carmichael, 1936). The normal limb and trunk locomotion pattern appeared in both cases, so long of course as motor nerve function had not been interfered with. Typical walking movements also appear in limbs which have been innervated after being either reoriented in maladaptive positions or completely deafferented (*cf.* Weiss, 1955). Developmental changes occur, furthermore, in the duration and in the rhythmicity of the swimming bursts generated by isolated hindbrain or cord fragments, whether or not any functional sensory nerve fibers are present (Corner, 1964). Sensory stimulation has also been excluded as a factor determining the specificity of retino-tectal functional connections, since rotating the retina or otherwise altering its normal orientation, even at pre-functional stages, results in a corresponding dislocation of the visual reflex actions and electrophysiological projections (*e.g.* Stone, 1960; Gaze *et al.*, 1965).

Early deafferentation of the chick embryo has had no noticeable effect upon the character of its motility nor upon the quantitative features of rhythmicity until early in the last week of incubation (Hamburger *et al.*, 1966). At that point, trans-neuronal degeneration of motor neurons (also see Yntema, 1943; Hughes, 1965) made it impossible to use motility any further as an indicator of the underlying neural activity patterns. The well co-ordinated locomotor or struggling pattern appears more than a day prior to hatching (Corner *et al.*, 1966; and this volume), and the example of the amphibian studies cited above suggests that sensory input need not be involved in this central re-organization. Additional deafferentation studies are in progress concerning the role, if any, of sensory stimulation in the maturation of this and other motor action circuits in the chick. Sensory-directed functional maturation has been demonstrated in the embryonic nervous system in the form of classical conditioning (Sedláček, 1966). The capacity to form such connections, rather than being a general property of nervous tissue, depends upon higher centers which in the chick begin to function only towards the end of incubation. A slight acceleration has been reported in the development of light-evoked brain potentials in the duckling as a result of prolonged stimulation by high-frequency flashes (Paulson, 1965).

While the capability of the embryonic nervous system to modify its organization in response to sensory stimulation, and the extent to which this normally occurs are not well known, there is no doubt about the dependence of much of *post*-natal neurogenesis upon the amount and distribution of afferent nerve impulses. Reducing sensory-evoked neuronal activity during particular periods of development, for instance, can lead to the regression of some already established functional connections as well as to impairment in the formation of new ones (for reviews see Riesen, 1961; Melzack, 1965; Sperry, 1965). In these cases it may be concluded that biochemical processes underlying the morphological or functional characteristics of the nerve cells are in some way sensitive to their level of activity, and that this level is under normal conditions largely determined by appropriate sensory stimulation. The developmental response itself will most likely be qualitatively the same as in neurons whose maturation normally is largely independent of such input, *viz.*, (1) migration and/or sending out processes along preferential sub-microscopic pathways, terminating with varying degrees of selectivity upon other cells (*cf.* Levi-Montalcini, 1964; Sperry, 1965), and (2) membranes becoming electrically polarized and responsive to specific transmitter agents. If the basis for mutual affinities lies in matching surface proteins, the patterns of RNA synthesis in neuroblasts will play a crucial role in the establishment of the organization of the nervous system (Bodian, 1965; also see Roberts, 1966a). RNA synthesis has indeed been shown in some neurons to be sensitive to the degree of

References p. 248–250

excitation, while the involvement of RNA and protein synthesis in learning and memory is a possibility which is currently of great interest (*cf.* Roberts, 1966a, b).

It will be clear that wherever neurogenesis depends upon the specific pattern rather than simply upon the intensity of the afferent input, changes in motor output can be expected which are recognizable as 'learned' behavior. It must be recalled, however, that the *character* of such a developmental response will still be a 'hereditary' property, presumably selected for via the adaptive actions which it has mediated during evolution.

REFERENCES

AKERT, K., (1965); The anatomical substrate of sleep. *Sleep Mechanisms. Progress in Brain Research, Vol.* **18**. Amsterdam, Elsevier (pp. 9–19).

ALCONERO, B. B., (1965); The nature of the earliest spontaneous activity of the chick embryo. *J. Embryol. exptl. Morph.*, **13**, 255–266.

ANDERSEN, P., (1966); Rhythmic 10/sec activity in the thalamus. *The Thalamus.* D. P. Purpura and M. Yahr, Editors. New York, Columbia Univ. Press (pp. 143–152).

ANOKHIN, P. K., (1964); Systemogenesis as a general regulator of brain development. *The Developing Brain. Progress in Brain Research, Vol.* **9**. Amsterdam, Elsevier (pp. 54–86).

BARRON, D. H., (1950); Genetic neurology and the behavior problem. *Genetic Neurology.* P. Weiss, Editor. Univ. Chigaco Press (pp. 223–231).

BERNHARD, C. G., KAISER, I. H., AND KOLMODIN, G. M., (1959); On the development of cortical activity in fetal sheep. *Acta Physiol. scand.*, **47**, 333–349.

BIGNAMI, A., PALLADINI, G., AND VENTURINI, G., (1966); Effect of cardiazol on sodium-potassium-activated adenosine triphosphatase in the rat brain *in vivo*. *Brain Res.*, **1**, 413–414.

BIGNAMI, A., PALLADINI, G., AND VENTURINI, G., (1966); Sodium-potassium adenosine triphosphatase in the developing chick brain. *Brain Res.*, **3**, 207–209.

BODIAN, D., (1965); A suggestive relationship of nerve cell RNA with specific synaptic sites. *Proc. Natl. Acad. Sci., (Wash.)*, **53**, 418–425.

BUREŠ, J., FIFKOVÁ, E., AND MAREŠ, P., (1964); Spreading depression and maturation of some forebrain structures in rats. *Neurological and Electroencephalographic Correlative Studies in Infancy.* P. Kellaway and I. Peterson, Editors. New York, Grune and Stratton (pp. 27–36).

CARMICHAEL, L., (1936); A re-evaluation of the concepts of maturation and learning as applied to the early development of behavior. *Psychol. Rev.*, **43**, 450–470.

CARMICHAEL, L., (1954); The onset and early development of behavior. *Manual of Child Psychology*, 2nd ed. L. Carmichael, Editor. New York, Wiley and Sons (pp. 60–185).

CORNER, M., (1964a); Localization of capacities for functional development in the neural plate of *Xenopus laevis*. *J. comp. Neurol.*, **123**, 243–256.

CORNER, M., (1964b); Rhythmicity in the early swimming of anuran larvae. *J. Embryol. exptl. Morphol.*, **12**, 665–671.

CORNER, M., AND CRAIN, S. M., (1965); Spontaneous contractions and bioelectric activity after differentiation in culture of presumptive neuromuscular tissues of the early frog embryo. *Experientia*, **21**, 422–424.

CORNER, M. A., PETERS, J. J., AND RUTGERS VAN DER LOEFF, P., (1966); Electrical activity patterns in the cerebral hemisphere of the chick during maturation, correlated with behavior in a test situation. *Brain Res.*, **2**, 274–292.

CRAIN, S. M., (1964); Development of bioelectric activity during growth of neonatal mouse cerebral cortex in tissue culture. *Neurological and Electroencephalographic Correlative Studies in Infancy.* P. Kellaway and I. Peterson, Editors. New York, Grune and Stratton (pp. 12–26).

CRAIN, S. M., (1966); Development of 'organotypic' bioelectric activities in central nervous tissues during maturation in culture. *Internat. Rev. Neurobiol.*, **9**, 1–43.

CRAIN, S. M., AND PETERSON, E. R., (1964); Complex bioelectric activity in organized tissue cultures of spinal cord (human, rat, and chick). *J. cell. comp. Physiol.*, **64**, 1–14.

CUNNINGHAM, A. W. B., (1962); Qualitative behavior of spontaneous potentials from explants of 15 day chick embryo telencephalon *in vitro*. *J. genl. Physiol.*, **45**, 1065–1076.

DELL, P., (1963); Reticular homeostasis and critical reactivity. *Brain Mechanisms. Progress in Brain Research, Vol.* **1**. Amsterdam, Elsevier (pp. 82–103).
DENNY-BROWN, D., (1960); Motor mechanisms — *Introduction*: The general principles of motor integration. *Handbook of Physiology, Section 1: Neurophysiology*, Vol. 2. J. Field and H. W. Magoun, Editors. Washington, D. C., American Physiological Society (pp. 781–796).
DETWILER, S. R., (1947); Further observations on the function and posture of limbs following the removal of the trunk neural crest in *Amblystoma. J. exptl. Zool.*, **106**, 299–312.
DE VALOIS, J. C., AND SCHADÉ, J. P., (1965); Conductivity changes in cerebral cortex and hippocampus during asphyxia under hyperbaric pressure. *Arch. internat. Physiol. Biochim.*, **73**, 569–579.
EAYRS, J. T., (1964); Role of thyroid hormone in the differentiation of the nervous system. *Proc. 2nd Internat. Congr. Endocrin.*, No. 83, International Congress Series. Amsterdam, Excerpta Medica (pp. 779–784).
ECCLES, J. C., (1964); The Physiology of Synapses. Springer, Berlin.
FOX, M. W., (1966); Neuro-behavioral ontogeny. A synthesis of ethological and neurophysiological concepts. *Brain Res.*, **2**, 3–20.
GARMA, L., AND VERLEY, R., (1965); Générateurs corticaux étudiés par électrodes implantées chez le lapin nouveau-né. *J. Physiol.*, **57**, 811–818.
GAZE, R. M., JACOBSON, M., AND SZÉKÉLY, G., (1965); On the formation of connexions by compound eyes in *Xenopus. J. Physiol. (London)*, **176**, 409–417.
GOTTLIEB, G., (1966); Conceptions of prenatal behavior. *Development and Evolution of Behavior*, Vol. 1. L. R. Lehrman, D. S. Lehrman, J. S. Rosenblatt and E. Tobach, Editors. W. H. Freeman, New York (in press).
GRAY, J., (1950); The role of peripheral sense organs during locomotion in the vertebrates. *Symp. Soc. exptl. Biol.*, **4**, 112–126.
GUTMANN, E., (1964); Neurotrophic relations in the regeneration process. *Mechanisms of Neural Regeneration. Progress in Brain Research, Vol.* **13**, Amsterdam, Elsevier (pp. 72–112).
HAMBURGER, V., (1963); Some aspects of the embryology of behavior. *Quart. Rev. Biol.*, **38**, 342–365.
HAMBURGER, V., WENGER, E., AND OPPENHEIM, R., (1966); Motility in the chick embryo in the absence of sensory input. *J. exptl. Zool.*, **162**, 133–160.
HUGHES, A., (1965); Some effects of de-afferentation on the developing amphibian nervous system. *J. Embryol. exptl. Morphol.*, **14**, 75–87.
HUTTENLOCHER, P. R., (1966); Development of neuronal activity in neocortex of the kitten. *Nature*, **211**, 91–92.
JONES, A., AND LEVI-MONTALCINI, R., (1958); Patterns of differentiation of the nerve centers and fiber tracts in the avian cerebral hemispheres. *Arch. ital. Biol.*, **96**, 231–284.
JOUVET, M., (1965); Paradoxical sleep — a study of its nature and mechanisms. *Progress in Brain Research, Vol.* **18**, *Sleep Mechanisms*. Amsterdam, Elsevier (pp. 20–62).
KELLAWAY, P., GOL, A., AND PROLER, M., (1966); Electrical activity of the isolated cerebral hemisphere and isolated thalamus. *Exptl. Neurol.*, **14**, 281–304.
KONISHI, M., (1966); The attributes of instinct. *Behaviour*, **27**, 316–328.
KUO, Z. Y., (1939); Total pattern or local reflexes? *Psychol. Rev.*, **46**, 93–122.
LEVI-MONTALCINI, R., (1964); Events in the developing nervous system. *Growth and Maturation of the Brain. Progress in Brain Research, Vol.* **4**. Amsterdam, Elsevier (pp. 1–26).
MATTHEW, S. A., AND DETWILER, S. R., (1926); The reaction of *Amblystoma* embryos following prolonged treatment with chloretone. *J. exptl. Zool.*, **45**, 279–292
MEIER, G. W., AND BERGER, R. J., (1965); Development of sleep and wakefulness in the infant rhesus monkey. *Exptl. Neurol.*, **12**, 257–277.
MELZACK, R., (1965); Effects of early experience on behavior: experimental and conceptual considerations. *Psychopathology of Perception*, chap. 12. P. H. Hoch and J. Zubin, Editors. New York, Grune and Stratton (pp. 271–299).
O'LEARY, J. L., AND GOLDRING, S., (1964); D-C potentials of the brain. *Physiol. Rev.*, **44**, 91–125.
PAULSON, G. W., (1965); Maturation of evoked responses in the duckling. *Exptl. Neurol.*, **11**, 324–333.
PURPURA, D. P., SHOFER, R. J., AND SCARFF, T., (1965); Properties of synaptic activities and spike potentials of neurons in immature neocortex. *J. Neurophysiol.*, **28**, 925–942.
PURPURA, D. P., FRIGYESI, T. L., MCMURTY, J. G., AND SCARFF, T., (1966); Synaptic mechanisms in thalamic regulation of cerebellocortical projection activity. *The Thalamus*. D. P. Purpura and M. Yahr, Editors. New York, Columbia Univ. Press (pp. 153–172).
RIESEN, A. H., (1961); Stimulation as a requirement for growth and function in behavioral develop-

ment. *Functions of Varied Experience*. D. W. Fiske and S. R. Maddi, Editors. Dorsey Press, Homewood, Illinois (pp. 57–80).

Roberts, E., (1966a); The synapse as a biochemical self-organizing micro-cybernetic unit. *Brain Res.*, **1**, 117–166.

Roberts, E., (1966b); Models for correlative thinking about brain, behavior and biochemistry. *Brain Res.*, **2**, 109–144.

Roffwarg, H. P., Muzio, J. N., and Dement, W. C., (1966); Ontogenetic development of the human sleep-dream cycle. *Science*, **152**, 604–619.

Samson, F. E., Balfour, W. M., and Jacobs, R. J., (1963); Mitochondrial changes in developing rat brain. *Amer. J. Physiol.*, **199**, 693–696.

Samson, F. E., Dick, H. C., and Balfour, W. M., (1964); Na-K-stimulated ATP-ase in brain during neonatal maturation. *Life Sci.*, **3**, 511–515.

Schadé, J. P., (1960); Origin of the spontaneous electrical activity of the cerebral cortex. *Recent Advances in Biological Psychiatry*, chap. 2. J. Wortis, Editor. New York, Grune and Stratton (p. 23–42).

Schneirla, T. C., (1966); Behavioral development and comparative psychology. *Quart. Rev. Biol.*, **41**, 283–302.

Sedláček, J., (1966); Some problems of elaboration of a temporary connection in the prenatal period. *Brain Reflexes. Progress in Brain Research, Vol.* **22**. Amsterdam, Elsevier (in press).

Sedláček, J., Svehlova, M., Sedláčkova, M., Marsala, J., and Kapras, J., (1961); New results in the ontogenesis of reflex activity. *Functional and Metabolic Development of the Central Nervous System*. P. Sobotka, Editor. *Plžen. lek. Sbor.*, Suppl. 3 (pp. 167–175).

Skinner, B. F., (1966); The phylogeny and ontogeny of behavior. *Science*, **152**, 1205–1212.

Skou, J. C., (1965); Enzymatic basis for active transport of Na^{+} and K^{+} across cell membranes. *Physiol. Rev.*, **45**, 596–617.

Sperry, R. W., (1965); Embryogenesis of behavioral nerve nets. *Organogenesis*, chap. 6. R. L. de Haan and H. Ursprung, Editors. Holt, Rhinehart and Winston, New York (pp. 161–186).

Spooner, C. E., (1964); Observations on the use of the chick in the pharmacological investigation of the central nervous system. *Ph. D. dissertation, Univ. of California, Los Angeles*. Univ. Microfilms, Ann Arbor (222 pp.).

Stone, L. S., (1960); Polarization of the retina and development of vision. *J. exptl. Zool.*, **145**, 85–96.

Villablanca, J., (1965); The electrocorticogram in the chronic *cerveau isolé* cat. *Electroenceph. clin. Neurophysiol.*, **19**, 576–586.

Volokhov, A., (1961); On the significance of various levels of the central nervous system in the formation and development of motor reaction in embryogenesis. *Functional and Metabolic Development of the Central Nervous System*. P. Sobotka, Editor. *Plzen. lek. Sbor.*, Suppl. 3 (pp. 141–147).

Weiss, P., (1941); Does sensory control play a constructive role in the development of motor coordination? *Schweiz. med. Wochenschr.*, **71**, 591–595.

Weiss, P., (1955); Special vertebrate organogenesis: Nervous system (neurogenesis). *Analysis of Development*, Sect. 7, chap. 1. B. H. Willier, P. A. Weiss and V. Hamburger, Editors. Saunders, Philadelphia (pp. 346–401).

Yntema, C. L., (1943); Deficient efferent innervation of the extremities following removal of the neural crest in *Amblystoma*. *J. exptl. Zool.*, **94**, 319–349.

Author Index *

* Italics indicate the pages on which the paper of the author in these proceedings is printed.

Subject Index